barebones

THE PRICE OF SUCCESS IN AMERICAN MEDICINE

barebones

A SURGEON'S TALE

AUGUSTO SARMIENTO, M.D.
with the assistance of Mark Dorfman

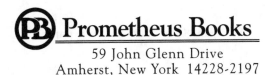

Prometheus Books
59 John Glenn Drive
Amherst, New York 14228-2197

Published 2003 by Prometheus Books

Inquiries should be addressed to
Prometheus Books
59 John Glenn Drive
Amherst, New York 14228–2197

716–691–0133 (x207). FAX: 716–564–2711.
WWW.PROMETHEUSBOOKS.COM

07 06 05 04 03   5 4 3 2 1

Library of Congress Cataloging-in-Publication Data

Sarmiento, Augusto, 1927–
    Bare bones : a surgeon's tale : the price of success in American medicine
    / Augusto Sarmiento.
        p. cm.
    Includes bibliographical references.
    ISBN 1–59102–049–2 (cloth : alk. paper)
    1. Sarmiento, Augusto, 1927– 2. Surgeons—Biography. 3. Orthopedists
—Biography. 4. Hispanic Americans in medicine. I. Title
    [DNLM: 1. Physicians—United States—Personal Narratives. 2. Hispanic
Americans—United States—Personal Naratives. 3. Orthopedics—United
States—Personal Narratives. WZ 100 S2463 2003]

R154.S253A3 2003
617'.092—dc21   2003041396
[B]

Printed in Canada on acid-free paper

To the many people who, in a
variety of ways, have made my life
a happy and productive one.

contents

preface

You fathers and you mothers fond, also,
If you have children, be it one or two,
Yours is the burden of their wise guidance
The while they are within your governance.

—Geoffrey Chaucer

"I can't do otherwise"

—Martin Luther

I almost gave up medicine on several occasions while I was still a student in Colombia. I later stood, near tears, in the U.S. Consulate in Bogota while an official explained that I did not qualify for a visa. Later, as my internship in a Passaic, New Jersey, hospital was coming to its end, I applied to every orthopaedic residency program in the United States, but came within days of having to return to Bogota. It seems strange now, but much later, I was to stand at the podium in the Convention Center in Anaheim, California, and receive the medallion marking my election as the next president of the American Academy of Orthopaedic Surgeons.

Along the way, in a small way, I helped bring total hip replacement surgery to the United States. My research has generated new concepts in and, I hope, an improved understanding of the way fractures heal. It has also changed the way that many fractures are treated. I chaired two medical school departments of orthopaedics—one at the University of Miami, the other at the University of Southern California. I also served as chief of orthopaedics at Jackson Memorial Hospital in Miami and Los Angeles County–University of Southern California Hospital. During my years in Miami and California, my colleagues and I transformed these orthopaedics residency programs into what are considered two of the best in the nation. We reached that goal at the cost of constant battles for survival with colleagues who resented our "intrusion" into their territory, as well as powerful hospital trustees and academic administrators.

9

After my California roller coaster ride as chief of orthopaedics, I sat in the empty operating theater of a luxurious new hospital in Scotland, waiting for patients from around the world, who never came. Upon my return to the United States, I experienced the life of working as an employee of a for-profit hospital and felt in a very personal way the trials and frustrations of the not-so-brave new world of American medicine.

I have witnessed the changes in American medicine from the days before Medicare—a time when poor patients were often treated by unsupervised interns and residents. I believe the era in which practitioners, in general, make the needs of their patients their first priority is at an end. And I watch in helpless frustration as unrestrained greed and the business interests of the health care industry overpower the philosophy, values, and ethics of medicine.

My family paid a heavy price for my career. I never gave them the time that should have been their birthright. I remember sitting at a table in a restaurant on the Via Venetto in Rome. I had brought my almost-grown children along on this trip, and was telling them a story about my youth in Bucaramanga, Colombia, before I came to the United States. They seemed surprisingly interested in my story.

Then my daughter, who was seventeen years old, interrupted: "You know, Dad, taking us on this trip is the best thing you've ever done."

"Why is that? What's so special about it?"

"This is the first chance that we've had to get to know you."

Janette, here is the rest of the story that I started so long ago, in Rome.

On that warm evening in the Eternal City I was displaying to my children my pride in the profession I had chosen and the excitement it had brought to me over the years. Little did I know then that within a short time I would begin to criticize medicine for the declining vigilance of its tenets and would be passionately expressing bitterness over the lax standards that it was tacitly accepting.

Such a transformation did not take place overnight. The metamorphosis evolved over many years of study and careful observations of events unfolding in front of me; events that many others would account as the normal evolution of society.

I have deliberately written this book in the form of an autobiography. The reason for following such a format was my belief that in such a manner I could better understand myself and be better understood by others. I have attempted to draw extrapolations of life events, which in different ways I thought had influenced my later attitudes about the critique of my profession, and in the development of my eventual philosophy of life in general. As Thucydides did in his writing of the Peloponnesian War, I felt the need to offer explanations of the events to better justify my comments. Like Dante Alighieri in the narrative of his *Divine Comedy*, in which Virgil and Beatrice serve as guides for the travel through Hell, Purgatory, and Paradise, I wished to guide readers in a way that would make easier their understanding of my actions.

I assume that some readers will be less interested in many of the events, but I hope that many will find interest in the continuously changing cultural perspective. Despite my success in becoming part of the U.S. medical establishment, I never tried to transform myself to a native-born American. My values and perspective continue to reflect my Spanish heritage and my Colombian birth. I sometimes suspect that my tendency to tilt at windmills also reflects my Spanish ancestry. Surely, it is no coincidence that my favorite possession is a remarkable bronze bust of Don Quixote facing his own madness. I bought it many years ago in Madrid. My wife, Barbara, hates it.

Throughout my career, I have remained aware of my status not as a foreigner but as an outsider. I have learned that my European-style education set me apart from most of my colleagues who graduated from U.S. medical schools. I have gradually realized that my values, standards, aspirations, and expectations differ from those of most native-born Americans. If that perspective somewhat isolated me from my colleagues, it also enabled me to see things a little differently than most. I hope you enjoy this narrative and its slightly out-of-kilter view of modern orthopaedics, academia, and the U.S. medical establishment.

In Geoffrey Chaucer's *Canterbury Tales*, a group of fourteenth-century pilgrims on their way from London to Canterbury Cathedral tell each other stories to help pass the time. The group includes a knight and a parson as well as a miller, a surgeon, and various other representatives of medieval English society. The tales and the encompassing narrative reveal a great deal about the travelers, their values, their principles, and their culture. With apologies to Chaucer, here is my own Surgeon's Tale.

Augusto Sarmiento, M.D.
Coral Gables, Florida

chapter 1.
roots

"Life's but a walking shadow, a poor player
That struts and frets his hour upon the stage
And then is heard no more. It is a tale
Told by an idiot, full of sound and fury,
Signifying nothing."

—William Shakespeare
Macbeth, Act V, Scene V

The corrosive anger is gone now, but I will never forget the devastating shock that shattered my certainties on that long-ago morning. I had learned that a small hospital in upstate New York was looking for a chief of orthopaedics. I decided to ask my department head at the University of Miami for his advice. He took me aside and said, "Gus, you are very smart and very talented. I think that you are smart enough to understand that with your name, your accent, and your background, you have no future in American medicine."

For many years, the scars of that moment brought frustration and resentment to my life. My memories of the incident may well have spurred my ambitions; the leaden bitterness endured despite many sweet professional successes. It lurked inside me for more than three decades. Then, unexpectedly, the lead transmuted into gold and filled me with the pungent sweetness of irony fulfilled. That paramount moment came on March 8, 1991, when I assumed the presidency of the American Academy of Orthopaedic Surgeons.

Most of the people assembled in the hall for my investiture did not know that medicine was not my lifelong ambition. As a child, I had always planned to become a lawyer. As a young man, I had seriously contemplated dropping out of medical school; actually I came close to doing so on several occasions. Many attendees knew that I had begun voicing growing doubts about current trends in the education, ethics, and values of my profession and my colleagues. That stand had already earned the enmity of an unknown number of influential leaders of the national and international orthopaedic community. Yet there I stood, despite improbabilities of every kind, about to assume the leadership of the academy.

My speech that morning covered many issues of interest to the profession, including concerns such as recertification, the need for greater interest in basic research, and the increasing fragmentation of our discipline and its erosion from without. I devoted most of my time, however, to a discussion of broader issues, which I considered of greater importance. I warned my colleagues that the public increasingly perceived us as insensitive and as lacking compassion and that we were rapidly losing their respect. "They accuse us of prescribing unnecessary tests and treatments, of performing too much surgery, and of charging too much for our services simply for greater revenues for ourselves. In short, they accuse us of greed and view us as materialistic and insensitive business people who have an unquenchable thirst for money."

This was not the message that my colleagues wanted to hear. It is, however, a message and a concern that increasingly occupies my attention. I believe that some business and entrepreneurial activity must remain an important part of the practice of medicine, but I sincerely believe that medicine must recapture its sense of mission and professionalism and restore the priority of healing and, more significantly, of caring.

Perhaps making such issues the centerpiece of my inauguration was not the most politically expedient thing to do. But then, my life has not been an easy one. Even as the convention guests honored me with their warm applause, my mind flew back over many years. In the few moments that passed as I stood before my peers, I remembered a lifetime of triumphs, disappointments, and fears.

For more than thirty years, I had fought for acceptance of my research into the treatment of fractures. Now my theories, once thought outlandish, had become widely accepted. I remembered my academic career and the countless frustrations as I fought to build two of the United States' leading departments of orthopaedics—one at the University of Miami, the other at the University of Southern California—two universities where my Hispanic heritage could prove less of a disadvantage than at other ivy-shrouded citadels.

Even as I stood before the academy's fifteen hundred guests and accepted the symbols of my new office from my predecessor, I wished that the honor had been given to me more than a decade earlier. I knew that many of my less friendly colleagues had fought hard not just to delay but to prevent this moment. Those thoughts made my ultimate triumph all the sweeter.

According to conventional wisdom, my career was totally impossible. By rights, I should never have been able to overcome the prejudices and traditional practices that have long dominated professional medicine in the United States. I have had few friends and never learned to attract the help of mentors. I have never accepted or fully understood the need to prioritize "prudence" or "expedience." Had such been my character, I would probably have remained in Bucaramanga or Bogota. In Colombia, at least, I knew the language and could have drawn strength from my family's deep roots.

Throughout my life, it seems, I have always done everything the hard way. At every crossroads, I have always chosen the most difficult path—not necessarily the best way, rarely the most profitable way, sometimes the most interesting way, but always the most demanding way. I present this aspect of my life only as a fact—a quirk of personality that I did not always recognize. Certainly, I do not offer it as wisdom or as advice to readers seeking guidance in this narrative.

My path has been as unusual as my background. The U.S. medical establishment takes great pride in its own institutions. Only recently has it been forced to look beyond its increasingly archaic citadels. I have long felt that my career as a physician, educator, researcher, and administrator was defined to a great extent by my birth in Colombia, my slight Spanish accent (which intensifies in direct proportion to excitement), and my education at a foreign medical school.

Colombia is a remarkable and beautiful country with proud traditions and a rich heritage. Two oceans shaped the national history, the Caribbean Sea to the north and the Pacific Ocean to the west. Both coasts host ancient cities with beautifully sculpted, welcoming harbors. Colombia should be known and loved for the richness of its soil and its remarkable landscape, dominated by three mountain ranges and a remarkable network of rivers. It is a modern tragedy that this lovely nation has become known primarily for corruption, banditry, and the export of narcotic drugs.

Colombia has a reputation as a violent land. It may well be that violence, like the mountainous landscape, is a defining facet of the national heritage. Many of Colombia's native tribes were fiercely barbarous. The sixteenth-century arrival of the Spanish conquistadors only focused and precipitated that endemic culture of violence.

It has become fashionable, especially in the United States, to revise the work of historians who taught of the heroism of the conquistadors. To some extent, such revision has been useful. The introduction of the Catholic religion and Spanish culture to Latin America was accomplished at great cost. No one, however, should ever challenge the courage, heroic spirit, and adventurous nature of men like Hernan Cortez, Francisco Pizarro, and Sebastian de Belalcazar. The largest native tribe in Colombia, the Chipcha, did not offer much resistance to the conquistadors. But other native peoples, especially along the Andean plateau, fought fiercely and exacted a high price from the Spaniards, who invaded on three fronts. According to the contemporary accounts of Bernal Diaz del Castillo, some of the indigenous defenders ate their prisoners on the battlefield.

The conquistadors founded Santa Marta, the first city in Colombia, in 1525, almost a century before the British had begun to build permanent settlements in North America. Pedro de Heredia, an aristocrat from Madrid, laid the first stones of Cartagena in 1533. Gonzalo Jimenes de Quesada, a lawyer by profession and the descendant of Spanish nobility, conquered a Chipcha stronghold and began the building of Bogota, the modern capital of Colombia, in 1537. His success marked the completion of the Spanish conquest of Colombia.

I trace my roots to sixteenth-century Spain. One of my aunts (a gracious and proud lady who sometimes may be carried away by her enthusiasm) insisted that she had identified a connection to the migration of many Spaniards to England, following the 1501 marriage of Catherine of Aragon (daughter of Ferdinand of Aragon and Isabella of Castile) to Prince Arthur of Wales. Catherine, you may recall, later married Arthur's brother, who ascended the British throne as Henry VIII. Their subsequent divorce strained English/Spanish relations and forever fractured the hegemony of the Catholic Church. My aunt claimed that Meruel, the last name of my maternal ancestors, was the Spanish version of Merrill. When a Merrill, from Kent, England, married a Spanish woman and moved to northern Spain, the spelling of the name changed forever.

My earliest definitively documented direct ancestor in the Americas, Francisco Rosillo y Meruel, the Marques (Marquis) del Garrote y Fuerte, was born in Spain in 1714. He was an *hidalgo* and a captain in the Spanish infantry. One of his sons, Andres Maria Rosillo y Meruel, served as president of the Universidad del Rosario (Bogota), one of the oldest universities in the Western Hemisphere. Andres later became a member of the revolutionary movement that won Colombia's independence from Spain. He was in prison in Bogota on the day the Charter of Independence was signed. His younger brother, Miguel, my direct ancestor was, however, one of the rebels whose name is affixed to the historic document.

More recent members of my family also led distinguished lives and influenced the history of the land where I was born. My father and grandfather both served in the State of Santander legislature and its the Supreme Court. At the time of my father's death at the age of forty-nine, he was state director of the Conservative Party. Well after I left Colombia, one of my uncles was elevated to the position of archbishop in the Catholic province of Pamplona, in Colombia.

The separation between the U.S. medical establishment and me was brought on, in large part, by my foreign name and accent and helped to produce in me a valuable objectivity. In part, because the power elite originally denied me a place "in the box," I responded by thinking and acting "outside the box." That vantage point led me to ask new questions and develop new theories. It helped me to play a part in reshaping orthopaedic thinking and practice, and in the creation of contemporary orthopaedics.

Those accomplishments empowered my rise to a position of international influence with the world of orthopaedic surgery. I have chaired the department of orthopaedics and rehabilitation at the University of Miami, and the department of orthopaedics at the University of Southern California. I have served as president of the Hip Society and the Association for the Rational Treatment of Fractures and the American Academy of Orthopaedic Surgeons—the largest and most prestigious orthopaedic organization in the world.

Yet even as I occupied these powerful positions within the health care community, I have always been more critical of my chosen profession than many of my colleagues. I have freely expressed concerns about impending crises of values and ethics in medicine and have raised questions regarding the wisdom of accepting a system that makes medicine a for-profit business. Like Greek mythology's Cassandra, whose predictions were doomed by the gods always to be ignored, I spoke of coming threats that have been realized in health care "reforms" of the 1990s.

These days, I continue to serve as a guest speaker at conventions and universities around the world. I persist in warning colleagues of the increasing threats produced by the changing relationship between U.S. society and its health care industry. My warnings seem to be ignored or disparaged by many in my audience, as depicted by the fact that rather than improving with the passing of time, the situation has worsened.

Many times, I have felt that it would have been better—and certainly much easier—had I expressed my ideas in different ways. Acquaintances have sometimes said to me that I would have been able to accomplish much more if I had ever learned to temper my remarks. I do not agree. Political finesse may have helped me to make more friends, but I do not believe that I would have been more productive or happier. In fact, I have come to believe that I have enjoyed the life-long series of battles as much as I have relished my many victories.

From the perspective of my "senior citizenship," those victories did not come without great cost. Over the years, I was not as close to my wife, Barbara, and our children as they (and now I) wish. My daughter, Janette, is a practicing attorney. My older son, Gus Jr., works in information technology at the University of Southern California. My younger son, Gregory, is a member of the orthotic and prosthetic profession. But while I happily share the pleasure of the accomplishments of my children, I cannot take credit for them.

As I said earlier, my daughter told me while we were sharing a rare family moment at a restaurant in La Via Venetto in Rome that she was only then getting to know me. She was seventeen years old. At the time I realized that I had become one of those people whom Nietzsche describes as "loving work more than it deserves." I also feared that it was too late to change.

Or maybe not. This book is one more chance for my family to get to know me. It explores my efforts to provide a context for my professional life, my experiences at the nexus of orthopaedic medicine, and my struggles with the medical-industrial complex. It presents my often heterodox views of the United States' changing health care and social environment, my scattered successes, and my many frustrations and failures.

It must also be the account of a life that has taken me down many unexpected pathways. I have a difficult time explaining why I became a medical doctor. Throughout my youth, I never gave a thought to spending my life caring for sick people. I had known, virtually since birth, that law school would inevitably follow college. My path had already been charted by my father and his father. No one had ever tried to change my mind about that dream. No other path appealed. No other profession even lay within the realm of contemplation.

Then, when I was thirteen years old, the entire world as I knew it collapsed.

chapter 2.
a troubled adolescence

"People do not lack strength—they lack will."

—Victor Hugo

My earliest years were dominated by my close relationship with my father and grandfather. Only much later in life did I come to fully appreciate the remarkable qualities of my mother. While my father was alive, my family lived in a nice, comfortable house. We did not own it. It was rented from a distant relative. But that is the kind of thing that children do not think about. I knew only that we had a comfortable place to live, that we often entertained guests, and that we were treated with respect by the community. Later I would learn that my father never made enough money to buy a house, and that we lived well only because we spent every penny he earned. His earnings must have been reasonable, however, since he was a successful attorney who served in the state of Santander's legislature and in the State's Supreme Court of Justice.

My paternal grandfather also served in the Santander state legislature, as a congressman in the National Assembly, and a judge in the Santander State Supreme Court. He was even, briefly, secretary of state for Santander, and, later, an alternate in the Supreme Court of Justice for Colombia.

My grandfather lived five years after the death of his son, my father. So, it was the "old man," *El Viejo*, who sustained my intellectual curiosity during those critical years of disruption and disillusion. My grandfather fascinated me with stories about local and national politics—a rough and tumble business filled with vibrant and active personalities.

He loved to tell the story of a debate between two of his colleagues, Congressman Montana, nicknamed *"El Gato"* (the cat), because of his questionable ethics, and the other, a congressman named Rincon (which translates, "the corner"). During the debate, Congressman Rincon took the floor to smear his adversary by commenting that "my opponent apparently has forgotten why it is that he is called 'the cat.'" With that, *El Gato* took the floor. "I would like to thank Congressman Rincon for giving me the opportunity to set the record straight. The real reason for my nickname has nothing to do with my ethics or personal life. I am called 'the cat' because I defecate in 'the corner' (*el rincon*)."

My grandfather would tell this story repeatedly, always enjoying it immensely, filling the room with his laughter at the forty-year-old memory. The actual events of that debate took place almost a century ago, yet the memory of it survives to this day.

Of his fourteen children, only twelve reached adulthood. They formed a sophisticated, cultured family. The six girls were musically talented. I vividly recall the days when the family would get together to celebrate special occasions. Some of them played the piano, others the violin, while others sang. There were wonderful memories of a childhood so rich in artistic and intellectual experiences.

Because of my family's interest in music, my sister (one year older) and I were registered to take piano lessons. From the very outset she demonstrated amazing talent. I did not. Soon I became extremely jealous of her, so much so that I could no longer tolerate the situation. I stopped attending classes, much to the displeasure of my parents and relatives.

Though I was only a ten-year-old child, I think my jealousy turned into hatred of her. Two years later, at the age of thirteen, she died from a complicated case of appendicitis. During the next fifteen years I experienced a nightly recurrent nightmare in which my sister and I stood at the top of a hill, in front of a precipice. Suddenly I pushed her over the cliff. I saw her body fly until it finally hit the ground. Then I woke up and jumped out of bed while my heart pounded fast. I had killed her. For fifteen consecutive years I killed her every night. For a long time I thought I would have to live with that terrible nightmare every single night of my life. Suddenly, the nightmare stopped.

My paternal great-grandfather was not a lawyer. Instead, it is to him that I can trace my family connections not only with the practice of medicine but even with my own specialty. My great-grandfather operated the only drugstore in his own native city of Convencion, in the neighboring state of Norte de Santander. We have no records of his attending medical school, yet we know that he also served his community as a physician.

One night, when he was 101 years of age, he was summoned to attend at a birth. As he returned home, he slipped, fell, and broke his hip. Unable to move, he spent the rest of the night lying on the ground. He developed pneumonia and died a few days later. How ironic that his descendant would become an expert in the field of hip replacement surgery!

From both my father and grandfather, I learned that politics can be a noble profession. I suspect to this day that the ancient Greeks (in contrast to the even older Hindu civilization) were correct in proclaiming that to be true, in spite of the corruption that seems so frequently to infest the profession. Now that my daughter has returned to the traditional family business and become an attorney, I delight in seeing her stubbornly insisting on being an ethical practitioner. In her decency and pride I see my father's greatest values reborn. I can only hope that I had some role in transmitting them to her.

A MAJOR LOSS

My father died suddenly, when I was just thirteen years old. While the medical records are incomplete, family memories suggest that he suffered either a heart attack or a stroke. My own diagnosis, based on his symptoms and the events described by family members, suggests that he suffered a ruptured aortic aneurysm.

At the time, I was nearing the end of my elementary education. (In the United States, I would have been finishing ninth grade.) We discovered that he had made no financial provision for his family if he were to die. On the day that my father died, my mother learned that all the money she had in her possession was 200 pesos, and that the rent on the house we lived in would be due in a few days. One of her brothers owned a small coffee plantation; he invited us to come live with him. Other family members also offered to open their homes to our newly destitute family. Relatives and friends also collected a small fund—several thousand pesos—to help with the immediate crisis.

My mother chose to use this money to open a small grocery store in a poor neighborhood of our hometown, Bucaramanga, the capital city of the state of Santander. The store included a small living quarters with two bedrooms. There was just me and my brother Hector to care for. (Our two sisters, Lucila and Esther, had preceded my father in death. Lucila, the family's first-born child, had died in infancy. My sister Esther, a victim of appendicitis, had died at the age of thirteen just three years before my father.) My mother was forty-three when she bravely took her two sons on this quest for independence. The three of us shared a bedroom. We used the second bedroom as storage for the grocery store, my father's books, my mother's sewing machine, and a few other household possessions. We proudly called the room "the library."

On my thirteenth birthday, my father had instructed me to stop by his office on my way home from school. We left his office together and walked a few blocks to a local bookstore. There, I found that he had purchased a complete set of the works of Jules Verne. When we returned home, I found that my bed had been moved to another room, and that I would, from then on, be sleeping in the company of my father's books. What a remarkable birthday gift!

Just a few months later, my father was dead, and I never really had much of a chance to learn who he really was. Was he the "attorney's attorney" described in his many glowing obituaries? Why had he not been interested in amassing wealth, or in wielding political power? Why had he chosen to live a simple, almost spartan life? While I would enjoy many conversations with my grandfather, I would never learn the answers to these basic questions. I still think about him quite often. I still wonder about the values that lay so deeply imbedded in his complex soul.

Forty years later, during one of my occasional visits to my native town, I commented to a cousin of mine how unfortunate it was that I never had a chance to meet any of my father's colleagues. I would have had the opportunity to learn about the type of person he really was. She responded that just a few blocks from her house lived an attorney named Domingo Arenas, younger than my father, but a contemporary of his.

We immediately walked to his house. Sitting behind his desk in a poorly lit room was this old man in his mid-nineties, wearing a Lenin-like cap, poring over some document. His daughter interrupted his work to introduce the son of Ernesto Sarmiento. He raised his head, looked at me with intense curiosity, and attempted to get up. I urged him to remain seated and proceeded to apologize for the interruption.

His first words were "What a coincidence," and handed me the paper he was studying. It was a handwritten document. I immediately recognized my father's handwriting. He explained to me that my father, in the 1920s, was the judge who oversaw the purchase of a certain property by the local nuns. Fifty years later the city was planning to construct a street where the nuns' property was located. The nuns were trying to fight the issue. The old man sitting at the desk had been the original young attorney who represented the convent; this is how he found himself working as a consultant in the case.

For some fifteen minutes he chatted about my father and grandfather. Prompted by me to summarize what kind of person my father was, he remarked that what distinguished him the most was his "impeccable integrity." He was the attorney to whom other attorneys went whenever they had personal problems. Then he shared a few trivial episodes in the life of the city in those early days.

I was amazed at the lucid mind that this man had retained at his age. When I indicated to him that I did not want to trouble him any longer, he stood up. Then I realized that though the ravishes of old age had left his mind almost intact, his body was frail. I assume he must have died not many years or months later. Nonetheless he provided me an unforgettable experience.

MY MOTHER'S SACRIFICE

The years following my father's death were incredibly difficult. My mother began work in the grocery store at 5:00 in the morning and finished at 11:00 at night. The store was open seven days a week. She left it only to attend mass. We sold bread, sweets, a few vegetables, firewood, and cigarettes. During the holiday season, business was at its best, and we might earn as much as 10 pesos per day. As soon as my brother and I came home from school, we would relieve my mother behind the counter. Later, she would relieve us, when it was time for us to do homework and seek respite in "the library."

Living under these new conditions was particularly traumatic for me. I now recognize that it must have also been difficult on my brother. At the time, I preferred to assume that my brother was too young to care about the change. I also felt that my mother had chosen this new path herself, and I held her responsible for the environment in which we now lived.

I know that I was so embarrassed by our living conditions in the poor neighborhood that during those five years I never invited a single friend to my house. I did not want them to know where I lived, although I realized that they must have known of our financial distress.

Once, a classmate offered to walk with me to the house to pick up a book he wanted to borrow. To keep him from coming and seeing my mother in the store, I pretended that I had to return to school to retrieve something that I had forgotten. Eventually, my former friends came to accept the isolation that I had imposed on myself.

At Christmas time, our relatives always gathered to celebrate with feasting, dancing, and fireworks. The family parties would last through the night. Every Christmas, I would fantasize that I was still part of that life. The next day, however, and the rest of my school holidays, I spent helping my mother at the store.

I grew up bitter and increasingly angry at a world that I had not made and did not like. We could not belong to the country club. Before long, even the occasional invitations from former friends stopped coming. Gradually, we stopped attending birthday celebrations and other fiestas. I took to keeping a list of every unpleasant occurrence in a little black book that I always carried with me. I wanted revenge, like Electra and Orestes in the Greek plays, for every slight—some real, most imagined. I looked forward to the day when I could show them the book, make them remember, and prove to them that their offenses had not "broken my back." I looked forward to forcing them to recognize my success, to realize that I had succeeded despite their offenses.

I no longer have the book. I know now that keeping it was incredibly childish and a frightful waste of time, effort, and energy. Yet, although I know that I destroyed the book, I cannot remember any details about my decision to do so, or about its actual destruction. I am proud that I eventually recognized the futility of keeping the book and the real danger of the emotions behind the practice. As Mahatma Gandhi wrote, "An eye for an eye and the whole world will go blind."

Yet, I know that I was not alone in my discontent. I inherited my distorted and pathological inability to forgive directly from my mother's side of our distinguished family. Feuds dating back years before my birth kept the Rosillos divided from each other. I grew up never having spoken with my mother's older brother. Only when I was nearing completion of my medical school years was I able to bridge that gulf and bring my mother and her brother back together.

MY HOMETOWN

My memories of Bucaramanga are neither warmer nor fonder than my memories of those difficult years. Bucaramanga is not particularly well known outside of Colombia. The city occupies a plateau nearly a thousand meters above sea level. It is not particularly remarkable for its scenery, history, or architecture. It has never attracted large-scale tourism. Today, the city hosts a population of about three quarters of a million within a metropolitan area of over one million.

Bucaramanga attracted substantial numbers of immigrants from Britain in the early part of the nineteenth century, and a large wave of German immigrants toward the end of the century. Possibly because of this strong Germanic influence, Bucaramanga has always been in the technological forefront. It was the first city in Colombia to have electricity and natural gas. It also built the country's first commercial airport. If this all sounds rather cold, perhaps that is due to the unpleasant nature of my memories, or to the distance and isolation from Bucaramanga that I now feel. My only ties to Bucaramanga are the ties to family members who still live there. Even those ties largely ended with the death of my mother.

My mother outlived my father by sixty years. She died as she approached her ninety-ninth birthday. Until nearly the last three months of her life, she retained her full intellectual capabilities. Sadly, she remained alert enough to be vitally aware of her own final deterioration. I spent many pleasant hours over the years talking with her. I always stopped by during my frequent visits to South America, and made it a point to visit her at least twice a year. We discussed everything: abstract intellectual concerns, national politics, my own life and career, local gossip, and the most minute family matters.

For her entire life, she remained a devout Catholic. I grew accustomed to her fanatical views, although I never shared them or became fully comfortable with them. But that is only fair. I know that my eventual marriage to a Protestant woman caused my mother more distress than her orthodoxy caused me.

I always listened to my mother with respect. As she grew older, she began to mellow. Her views became more tolerant in religious matters. The change always amazed me, especially because I had fully expected her childhood views to harden, rather than soften, with the passing years. Once, when I came home to visit, I was asked by relatives to use my influence with her to convince her that she needed to eat better and to walk more. As instructed, I told her, "Mother, you should eat more. It is good for you."

"Good for what?" she asked.

"Well, it is good," was all that I could say. When I attempted to emphasize the need for her to walk more and to exercise more, she offered the same defense: "What for?"

"Son, it appears that I may be unfortunate enough to live one hundred years. I never wanted to live so long, but apparently, God has other plans. I no longer want to eat better or to walk much. I don't feel like doing those things any more. I have walked for more than ninety-seven years, and I think that I have walked enough."

Such was her simple way of stating a coherent philosophy that she had followed all of her life. For me, her simple statement holds as much power and depth as Samuel Beckett's *Waiting for Godot*, or James Joyce's *Ulysses*. I have learned to understand and respect her viewpoint. She was right, of course. She *had* walked enough.

She did not say very much about my father. On one occasion she wrote a short poem in which she discussed the very short time they were together, before fate took his life. She lamented that he was gone before she even got to know him.

More than once she said to me that every night she prayed to God that she be allowed to die in her sleep. "I want to die like a bird, in private, with no witnesses." She asked me if I had ever given thought as to the way that animals die. "Even on the farm, where birds and other animals die by the thousands, you never see many of the dead. Very few, as a matter of fact. They like to die in private, even though all other things that they do are done in the open, like having sex."

When my brother, Hector, told me of her final decline, I traveled back to Bucaramanga to be with her again. I wanted to see her one more time while she was able to recognize me and to have one last conversation. Her final slide toward oblivion, however, proved too rapid. By the time I reached her home, she had lapsed into silence and almost constant sleep. During her waking moments, the only sounds she made were her gasping for breath and from the accumulated fluids in her lungs.

I do not think that she suffered much during her final days. My brother and I did the suffering for her. To watch her nearly lifeless body hanging on, failing slowly, dying by inches, tore my heart. I held her hands. Toward the end, her blue veins showed clearly through her thinned out skin, as her heart struggled to regain her life's blood. As she neared death, her pale blue eyes, the remarkable eyes of the Rosillo family, lost their ability to focus and faded to expressionless emptiness.

Pressing professional obligations forced my return to the United States before my mother actually died. I made it clear to my brother that I would not return for her funeral. I wanted to leave, never to come back, with the memory of those painful last hours with her. On the way to the airport the next morning I stopped by her house to look at her one last time. I wish I had not done it. I kissed her forehead, but she never knew it.

My mother died two weeks later. My brother told me that her last hours were tranquil. I hope that he spoke truthfully. I was alone in the house in Miami when he called to tell me of her passing. No one was there to share my grief, but also, no one was there to witness my agony.

More than five years have passed since her death. Memories of my mother still haunt me daily. I am struggling to write, surrounded by the desperate loneliness and irrepressible sadness that remain.

chapter 3.
shattered dreams

"The only way to have a friend is to be one."
—Ralph Waldo Emerson

When my father died, my firm anticipation of a university education and a future of law and politics died with him. So did my emotional security, my confidence in the rightness of the world order, and my sense of self.

A local pharmacist offered me a position as his assistant. I was briefly tempted to accept. Although it would also have meant the end of my formal education, it would also have rescued me from the grocery store. Continuing my formal education appeared to be beyond my grasp in any case.

Happily, the Jesuits who ran the local school where my brother and I were enrolled offered to allow us to continue attending the school for the remainder of our studies—through the U.S. equivalent of college—without cost to my family. At the time I had no great appreciation of the importance of their generous offer. Only in retrospect did I recognize that only their intervention made my future possible.

Throughout my life, I have thought about that remarkable crossroads in my life. It has made me recognize the casual way in which we often make, without any attempt at systematic, rational, appropriate thought, the most important decisions. We often spend days or weeks agonizing over choices, which at the time seem to be vital, yet soon show themselves to be totally insignificant. But more often than not, we make decisions and set off down new roads, taking steps that will become crucial to our futures, without hesitation, recognition, or any sense of proper appreciation.

In fact, it has taken me many years to appreciate the importance to my life of that small order of Jesuits. They not only provided a good academic foundation but also instilled in me, in my brother, and many of our classmates the social, cultural, and ethical values we were to carry throughout life.

Secondary education in South America follows the European rather than the North American model. College is completed in six rather than four years. Medical school also requires six years to complete. Europeans and South Americans pay more attention to the liberal arts. Their studies are much broader than the curricula of U.S. pre-med and medical students. Europeans do not ignore the liberal arts. They study history, philosophy, and literature, preparing to take their place as leaders of their communities as well as medical professionals.

North Americans spend less time in school but more time studying the physical sciences. They delve deeply into these required subjects. Consequently, their scientific background is much more intense, but they largely ignore such topics as religion, philosophy, and political science. As a result, they tend to view all problems in narrower, more technical ways. A humanistic psychologist once wrote, "When the only tool that you have is a hammer, all problems tend to look like nails."

I have often discussed these differences with my children, all of whom were born and educated in the United States. I have always sought to stimulate them to broaden their own education through their own reading. My success in this endeavor has been limited. While they have all extended their horizons beyond those defined by their various professions, none of them share the love of learning that, it seems, has always been such a central part of my life.

I must admit, however, that my full appreciation of the value of broad studies came only with increasing maturity. In my youth, I was, at best, a mediocre college student. The intense pleasure that I had always taken from learning disappeared almost entirely after my father's death. I began first to dislike mathematics. That difficulty would continue throughout my life.

Only now that I am no longer responsible for multimillion-dollar budgets as I was during my tenure as professor and head of orthopaedics at the University of Southern California, I admit that I have always hated to work with numbers. Throughout my career as an academic and as the administrator of a professional society, I totally despised every aspect of financial administration.

When I completed my term as chairman of the finance committee of the American Academy of Orthopaedic Surgeons, I told the board of directors of a dream that I had on the previous night. I told them that I had dreamt that I had died and appeared before St. Peter. He had looked at my record on Earth and concluded that punishment was due. He proceeded to appoint me chairman of Heaven's Finance Committee.

Ever since my adolescence, I have also hated to memorize dates (which made the formal study of history something of a challenge). Yet, I believe I was blessed from an early age with an uncanny sense for knowing what is and what is not important, and an ability to anticipate the essential core of any issue or topic. I was always fascinated with the "big picture" and always able to concentrate on aspects that I believed to be important. Often, what I viewed as important had been long ignored by some of my colleagues. Often I would find myself ignoring things that others thought to be important. That attitude may have been unhealthy in school, but it has proven to be invaluable throughout real life.

Still, I might well have left my future career on the classroom floor had it not been for a classmate of mine, Reynaldo Rodriguez, who had lived next door to my family during our more financially comfortable days. Reynaldo proved to be a remarkable individual—one of the few friends from my youth who remained a friend during my years of poverty. He was not only a true and devoted friend, he was also extremely bright.

Reynaldo allowed me to copy, with great frequency, the homework assignments that he had invariably completed, as ordered, the night before. (While I am being so open about this, I should also admit that my behavior on examinations may not have been the most appropriate, either. I occasionally sought the help of "crib notes" concealed on my clothing.) In the fashion of today, I should probably dismiss any lingering concern for this behavior as the result of "misguided youth." In fact, the memories of this behavior have haunted me ever since. I can only hope that this public confession will help me to exorcise this particular demon.

Certainly, my friend Reynaldo never expressed any concern over my inappropriate behavior, though I am sure that he found it distasteful. Sadly, later in life, others would abuse his trusting nature even more than I had done. He became an extremely successful engineer, but proved too trusting a businessman. Embezzlement by his partners left him bankrupt. At the same time, his older brother managed to lose most of the family's inherited wealth. Reynaldo therefore spent many years working in Saudi Arabia for an American firm. Despite poor health he worked in the hot Arabian Desert until he finally retired at the age of seventy-three.

When I was leaving Colombia for the United States in 1952, Reynaldo purchased my small collection of books. Among them were the biographies of Napoleon and Goethe by Emil Ludwig, and Stefan Zweig's *Stellar Moments in the History of the World*. He also purchased my small stamp collection, a product of our shared interests. In this way, Reynaldo endowed me with money that would prove crucial during my first days in the United States.

I lost touch with Reynaldo when I came to the United States, but we reunited briefly when he came to my office in Los Angeles. He apologized that he did not have an appointment, and hesitantly gave his name to my secretary. Filled with excitement, I immediately went to meet him. There, instead of the energetic friend of my youth, stood a hesitant, white-haired old man. He timidly extended his hand as if greeting a stranger. Only when I embraced him with all of the warmth of a countryman and fifty years of friendship did he relax.

He had come because his oldest son, a youngster in his mid twenties, had just been diagnosed with cancer of the pelvic bone. The cancer was inoperable, Reynaldo had been told. How sad it is that only the desperation of a frightened father had driven him to seek me out. Fortunately, this part of the story had a happy ending. With a few tests, my colleagues were able to rule out cancer. They diagnosed an infection, which responded quickly to surgery and antibiotics. Reynaldo's son recovered completely, and my friend soon returned to the deserts of Saudi Arabia.

Reynaldo and I shared many memories while his son was undergoing treatment. We spent many happy hours revisiting Bucaramanga in our minds. We also revisited our shared reading from the library that he had purchased. We talked about Dostoyevsky and Tolstoy, about Napoleon's Waterloo, and about Sutter and the California Gold Rush. We also talked about postage stamps. He still had the stamps that he had purchased from me so many years before, on the eve of my departure for the United States. He had continued to collect stamps, and took great pleasure in his extensive collection.

Reynaldo and I met once more, quite by accident, on the streets of Bucaramanga. Our mothers had been close friends as children, and now both lay ill. Both of us had come home to visit. Together, we walked the streets of the town and re-created the trip from our respective homes to our school. Together, we discovered that the dirt streets and the cobblestones were all gone. Together, we found that while our college was still at the same location, it had been totally remodeled.

Despite all of that discouragement, we managed to revisit the past. We found the rooms to which we had once been assigned and joyously recollected the names of various teachers. We recalled the many student pranks that we had played, and laughed at the joyous memories. We sought out old college publications and found photographs taken in those years from long ago. In Reynaldo's company, the memories of my youth became much more enjoyable. I found that I could take great pleasure from my memories of those days in Bucaramanga. When I think about those days while I am alone, my memories are much more troubled, much angrier, and much sadder. But then Reynaldo was my only true friend.

On the way home, we looked for the houses where we had spent our early childhood, only to find that they had given way to development. While the gracious homes of the wealthy had fallen victim to modernization, the little house where my family had moved after my father's death still survived. The store appeared to me to be unchanged from the way it had been some fifty years earlier. The counter, the shelves, the doors were the same. Only the person behind the counter was different.

I wanted very much to look again at the two rooms where my family had spent those years, so long ago. With Reynaldo at my side, I think that such a visit may well have helped me come to terms with those difficult and frightening years. But the woman behind the counter refused to allow me to visit our old house. I do not think that she believed that I had once lived and worked there.

That night, it rained heavily in Bucaramanga. The torrential tropic rain brought intense memories of rain on the tile roof of my childhood and the tin roof of my adolescence. That night, it seemed as if the rain were a Mozart piano sonata, full of passion, playfulness, and tenderness.

"There was a roaring in the winds all night," wrote Wordsworth. "The rain came heavily and fell in floods." That night, however, the sounds of the rain were muffled by the sealed glass windows of the air-conditioned hotel. The next morning, I sought to find a vantage point from which to view the well-remembered rain-soaked Spanish tiles of Bucaramanga. Even from the hilltops, however, the tiled roofs no longer dominated the landscape. Tall buildings had replaced the colonial houses. They took with them the most beautiful part of those long ago years. Beauty is fragile. Ugliness endures.

SEEKING A TRUCE

During that sentimental visit to my hometown, Reynaldo and I walked by the home where my Uncle Miguel, my mother's older brother had lived. I recalled that my mother had told me several times that Miguel had played an important part in raising her. They were extremely close. Yet, my mother's wedding became the source of a family schism that divided my family from my brother and his family for many years. My Uncle Miguel was out of town when the family was making wedding plans. In his absence, the family decided that Miguel's girlfriend was not socially "suitable." In an effort to discourage the relationship, they refused to invite her to the wedding. Miguel became furious when he returned to town and discovered what the family had done. He walked out of the house, out of their lives, and married the woman he loved. For many years, Miguel, his wife, and his children refused to speak to any member of his family.

I grew up without ever having spoken to my Uncle Miguel, although his family lived just a few streets away and his two children were of the same ages as my sister and me. I knew who he was, however, and that I was not to speak with him or have anything to do with him. Frequently, I would watch him walk past our house without ever turning his head or greeting any of us.

His daughter was a lovely girl. She was tall and had a graceful walk. She had golden blond hair and had inherited the blue eyes of the Rosillos—beautiful blue eyes that fate had denied to both my brother and me. For many years, I wanted to talk to my uncle and my cousins, but I never did. I never knew how to bridge the split.

Years later, I came home during a break from my medical school training. Again, I saw Uncle Miguel walking past our house. This time, he noticed me and looked at me, briefly, with curiosity. The next day, I knocked at the door of his home.

"I am Augusto Sarmiento," I said. "I am the son of your sister Teresa and I would like to talk to you."

He froze in the doorway. Then he asked me to come inside. I trembled with nervousness as I greeted him and his wife. "I do not understand why, after so many years, you cannot forgive things that at one time must have been painful to you. But after all, you, and my mother, and me, and your children, we all have the same blood. You are my uncle. Your children are my cousins.

"I want you and my mother to forgive each other and become the brother and sister you once were. I want your children to be my cousins."

He paused and did not reply. I was sure that I had failed and that the family feud would continue.

"Uncle," I said, "I will be back again to beg you to meet with your sister again. Neither one of you are young any more. Let us not postpone that meeting very long."

Remarkably, he put his arm around my shoulder. "I am so glad that you came to see us. Tell Teresa that we had this talk and that I am looking forward to seeing her again."

I saw him a few more times after that. I became a good friend of his children. My mother and he were reunited. When I saw them together, I experienced special warmth. I had done something worthwhile! To this day, I think that it may have been one of the best things I did in my life.

chapter 4.
uncertainties

"The mass of men lead lives of quiet desperation."
—Henry David Thoreau

Anger and resentment remained constant companions during my younger days. No doubt, my perceived social deprivation in relationships with girls dramatically accentuated all of the resentment that accompanied our family's loss of wealth and social position.

As I grew into a smoldering adolescent, it seemed that an adoring female companion constantly accompanied every other male in my world. I believed every word of their constant tales of conquest and advance to adulthood. I alone did not have a girlfriend. Worse, I was convinced that I simply could not afford to have one, and certainly not a girlfriend of an appropriate social class. Where would I go with her? We no longer belonged to the social club. I had no allowance.

Yet I had been brought up to believe that my family, though of no financial means, was part of the upper class, and therefore my friends and relationships had to be held within those circles. The idea of establishing amorous relationships with a girl from a lower stratum of society was therefore out of the question. What a senseless and stupid thing to teach to children. It took me a few years and some better appreciation of such practices to realize that my native country in the middle of the twentieth century was still stuck in the traditions that Jane Austen had so vividly described in her classic book *Pride and Prejudice*.

Adolescence is hell on earth, everywhere on earth. But Latino culture has found a remarkable number of ways to take this dreadful time of life and make it a hundred times worse. Since medieval times, we have built twin, parallel cults of machismo (which requires the conquest of every female in sight) and virginity. To this mix, we have added the idiocy of class consciousness, the passion of the tropical climate, the influence of the Catholic Church, and the intensely violent influences of the native cultures. Only the United States, where sexuality is defined by the constantly changing whims and fads of popular media, rather than by any constant culture, has made more of a mess of things.

Upon leaving school late one afternoon, I passed a group of girls who were leaving their classes and heading for home. A sixteen-year-old girl caught my attention. She was pretty and flirtatious and wore her hair combed into a ponytail. (Today, fifty-five years later, I can still see the proud and inviting way that her ponytail responded to every movement of her head.)

I began to look for her whenever I left school, and she soon realized that I was waiting, every day, for her class to be released. I'm sure that my adolescent stare left little doubt as to my interest. (Today, I would probably be cited for stalking.)

I was seventeen years old and had no idea of how to approach her. I also had neither father nor older brother to ask for guidance. One afternoon, it began to rain as I waited for her to walk by. The hard driving tropical rain made it impossible to do anything other than to seek shelter. Remarkably, the girl and two of her friends sought shelter under the very canopy where I was waiting.

With the rain drumming onto the stretched fabric of the awning, we began to talk. I learned that her name was Gloria and that she lived just a few blocks up the street (as if I had not followed her home and did not already know exactly where she lived). Despite my fervent prayers, the rain began to let up, and Gloria insisted on running home. I followed, and was with her as the rain returned, drenching both of us, completely soaking our clothing, soaking us to the skin. We were enjoying the warm rain and laughing together as we reached the corner where we said good-bye.

My family soon learned about my "girlfriend." They also quickly discovered that Gloria was the illegitimate daughter of a local taxicab driver. They did not approve, but I was totally infatuated—filled with a potent concoction of puppy love and adolescent lust—and willing to risk all consequences.

My mother pretended not to know anything about it. She remained silent, and let other relatives make their feelings known. Few of them missed an opportunity to express their disapproval and offer stern cautionary advice.

Then, one afternoon as the school term neared an end, Gloria asked me to come into her house to meet her mother. Gloria and I sat on adjacent chairs while her mother sat in the next room, with a full view of us. Gloria turned on a radio, and the music of a bolero, a popular slow dance, filled the room. Gloria's mother watched our every movement as we danced together and held hands for the first time.

I wish that I could tell you that love conquers all and that our passion overcame my family's objections. I will never even know if that could have happened, because that afternoon, I did not pass the test. I can only surmise that Gloria's mother did not approve of her daughter's relationship with me. I know only that she was forbidden to meet me. I never even had a chance to ask the reason for those instructions. I never had a chance to argue my case. If I were more inclined to consider myself a passive victim of life, I could probably blame Gloria's mother for all the poor decisions I may have made in the last fifty-five years.

In truth, I never really tried to find out what had happened. I was deeply hurt by the experience, which I still think about whenever I see people running in the rain. When I see that, especially when I see a young couple running without thought of taking shelter, I remember the torrential rain that afternoon in Bucaramanga and the soft, romantic melody of the bolero a few weeks later.

I saw Gloria again several years after we parted as I was about to graduate from medical school and was already planning my move to the United States. We ran into each other in Bogota, where she was visiting some relatives. She had lost the soft curves of her youthful figure. She looked emaciated. The bouncing ponytail was gone. Her hair hung straight down to her shoulders. She moved more slowly and seemed exhausted.

We had lunch together that day. She told me that she had been sick with tuberculosis. The doctors told her that she was cured, but she still had not really regained her energy or her full health. We parted after lunch. I never saw her again. So ended the one and only great romance of my adolescence.

I suspect that much of my later ambition was rooted in the disappointments of those early years in Bucaramanga. I have often wondered if my drive and intense motivation came from the bitterness of those high school and college years. Yet those years were not entirely bitter, and my anger was often softened by intellectual discoveries.

While my Jesuit teachers may well have approved of my nonexistent social life, they would have been horrified had they known more of the avenues my mind was starting to explore. I am certain that in those days, I read more of the writings of the agnostics and the atheists than of the classics of Christianity. For every day that I spent in the company of Augustine, Aquinas, Suarez, and Pascal, I spent a week rejoicing in the iconoclastic philosophy of Epicurus, Lucretius, Hume, Rousseau, and Voltaire, and the forbidden fruits of Marx, Nietzsche, Gide, and Schopenhauer.

AN UNFORGETTABLE MAN

Jose, one of my father's younger brothers, was the primary source of much of my youthful intellectual radicalism. He was probably the smartest of the six brothers and, at first, the one who seemed destined for the brightest future. He left Bucaramanga for medical school in Bogota during the early 1930s, in the midst of the worldwide Great Depression. It was a time when the philosophy of Karl Marx was winning converts throughout the old world and the new. In Latin America, radicalism was central to student life—much as beer and football are in the United States.

My uncle's involvement with radical politics led to many adventures with his classmates. One such episode, almost literally borrowed from Joyce's *Ulysses*, led to his expulsion from medical school. For the rest of his life, he claimed that the punishment was "unjust."

That episode became a crossroads in his life. Within a short time, he left the church and made himself a social hermit. He became mesmerized by Simone de Beauvoir, Sartre, and Camus, and became a total atheistic existentialist. He remained intellectually fascinated by the devout Christianity of Kirkegaard, but would never again be tempted by the faith of his fathers.

Jose stimulated me to read the European classics and talked often of the need to make my education as eclectic as possible. Though consumed by his interest in international politics, he remained an avid reader of classical literature. It was he who first introduced me to Dostoyevsky, Hugo, Dickens, Chekhov, Stendahl, and Joyce. After a few drinks, his romanticism would surface. He would begin to recite Spanish translations of Byron, Keats, Goethe, Wilde, Poe, and Valerie. His enthusiasm grew several levels as he discussed the short and restless rebellious life of the intellectually revolutionary Keats. He was, however, at his best reciting Latin American poems composed by Guillermo Valencia, Pablo Neruda, Juana de Ibarboru, and Porfirio Barba-Jacob.

On one occasion, he lent me the original typewritten manuscript of his own translation of Binet Sangle's *La Folie de Jesus*. I was spending a few days of vacation with my father's family, and tried to hide the work from his sisters. They found it, however, and took the book to the Jesuits at our local college—the same college that had sheltered and educated all the male members of my family, including my brother and me.

The Jesuits refused to return the manuscript. Jose had no other copy. He forgave me and his sisters, but not the church. I, too, found it impossible to accept their actions. Their theft of my uncle's manuscript severely weakened my faith in the teachers who had so much to do with the shaping of my character.

My uncle Jose left Bucaramanga shortly after the Jesuits stole his manuscript. He moved to a small town on the Pacific coast. I never knew what he did there. He later killed himself. He left no note. I suspect that he had concluded that without faith and without a belief in an afterlife, his life had no meaning. What a shame. He had so much to offer.

POLITICAL RESTLESSNESS

My own intellectual radicalism took a more productive route for a while, and detoured to take me down one of the strangest byways of my life. Together with several of my college classmates, I became involved in the education of adult laborers from the suburbs of Bucaramanga. The owners of an empty building, a former movie theater, let us use it to hold reading, writing, and basic arithmetic classes for these uneducated peasants. Of course, they did not have to pay us any tuition, but in return for our help in teaching them basic skills, they had to listen to our ideas on religion, history, and politics.

At first, our social radicalism came wrapped in political conservatism. We feared the growth of communism. My fellow students and I sought reform, but we feared revolution. It seems so odd now, but it seemed so clear at the time.

Then things became much less clear. Today, it is easy to look back and see the internal conflicts and logical inconsistencies of our youthful political excesses. I can see that in the early 1940s we were caught up more in the excitement and drama of the moment than in commitment to any clear political philosophy.

Colombia had enjoyed more than forty years of political stability. Two generations of my own family had played an active role in the democratic government. Yet somehow, my fellow students and I became convinced that the government in power would not be able to make the needed reforms. Yet, we feared the growing power of the communists more than we resented our own weak leaders. Gradually we made the transition from moderate political conservatives to right-wing revolutionaries.

Or perhaps the change was not so gradual after all. One moment, it seems, we sought only to protect our government from threats of the left. In what I can now only recall as the next instant, we found ourselves allied with the militaristic radicals. I suspect that we had allowed ourselves to be seduced by a particularly talented group of leaders and organizers. Yet, no single particularly inspirational leader stands out in my memories of this remarkable episode.

It may have simply been the infectious excitement, the romance, and the drama. Civil war had swept through our beloved Spain just a few years earlier. Now it was our turn to deal with similar questions. I wish that I could tell you that we followed the courageous lead of the Spanish loyalists, but we did not. Instead, we followed the leadership of our own, home-grown fascists. Twice weekly, we met with political instructors who taught us the proper way to view current events at home and abroad. We read Mussolini's proclamations, Hitler's *Mein Kampf,* and the writings of Primo de Rivera whose thoughts had shaped the Spanish Civil War.

Our teachers were sincere revolutionaries following a messianic calling. In my youthful passion for action, I thought that I was bringing my ancestor Andres Rosillo y Meruel back to life. Andres had played a vital, revolutionary role in the history of Colombia. He had helped, from the high position as president of the prestigious Universidad del Rosario, in Bogota, to free our country from the Spanish oppressors. Now, I honestly believed, it was my responsibility on behalf of the family to again carry the torch and lead my beloved Colombia to freedom. May Andres forgive me!

During the week, we went to school. On the weekends, we made bombs. Our officers locked us in a small room on the outskirts of town where we filled aluminum cans with dynamite, pellets, and rocks of various sizes. A few times, we walked to the mountains to test our homemade products. The results proved quite satisfactory. We believed that we were preparing for glory. We anxiously awaited our orders to take to the streets and inspire the poor, downtrodden peasants to follow our example.

We believed that our "troops" would be the working people who attended our evening classes on reading, writing, and the Hegelian dialectic. We were confident that when the great day came, they, like us, would be ready to battle in support of a cause that none of us understood.

My only salvation lies in the fact that the call to arms never came. Something must have happened at a high level, and the planned coup took its place on the cutting room floor. We were devastated, of course. Today, I can only be thankful that my misguided, confused, abused, and absurd passion never resulted in anyone's death.

World War II ended all thoughts of domestic revolution, if not of domestic discontent. Colombia had declared its support for the Allies, though it was no secret that most Colombians held the Germans in greater esteem. Bucaramanga, especially, was home to a large number of German immigrants. Memories of U.S. imperialism and exploitation of the "Banana Republics" made friendship between the United States and Colombia somewhat less than firm.

In Colombia, we had another grievance. We had sought, with the aid of the French, to build a canal through Panama in the mid-1800s. In 1903 the imperialist President Roosevelt masterminded Panama's break from Colombia, and in that manner made it possible for the United States to successfully accomplish the gigantic task that Colombia had been unable to perform. So, while we admired the power, technology, and accomplishments of the United States, we did not love the giant to our north.

During the war, Radio Berlin broadcast the news in Spanish every evening at 7:00. The broadcast began with a series of loud gunshots— one shot for every allied ship that the Germans had sunk. The Allies showed neither the concern nor the creativity of their enemies, and ignored us entirely. In fact, the war held little meaning for us. Some families in Bucaramanga, including my own, had relatives who had married German emigrants. They and their immediate families were kept under surveillance. The German families had lands and possessions expropriated. When the war ended, the United States (and its corporate companion, the United Fruit Company) resumed its unquestioned suzerainty over Colombia and the rest of Latin America.

I still remember how much my countrymen and I resented this assumed power of the United States. Almost half a century later, I would find myself guilty of the same kind of arrogance. In 1994, I became part of group led by the Harvard University Foundation, which sought to establish a medical center in Glasgow, Scotland. The clinic was designed to meet the needs of wealthy patients from throughout the world. We firmly believed that everyone thought that U.S. medicine and medical technology were the best in the world. The faith of the investors (and their lavish promises) led us to anticipate extraordinary success for our state-of-the-art, U.S. medical outpost abroad.

In 1994, I packed my life and, in the company of several other distinguished physicians, moved to Glasgow. I would have done better had I then remembered my own feelings, and the feelings of my neighbors, during and after World War II. But then, as the German philosopher Hegel wrote, "The only thing that we learn from history is that no one remembers the lessons of history." In any case, the events surrounding Health Care International belong at the end of my story, and we are still just at the beginning. But then perhaps the beginning makes sense only when examined in the light of the conclusion.

chapter 5.
facing reality

"The problem of living is learning the problem of how to die"
—Socrates

"The eternal silence of the infinite spaces frightens me."
—Blaise Pascal

I have been a practicing physician for more than forty years. I have been a teacher, headed two of the most prestigious departments of orthopaedics in the United States, and served as the president of several medical professional associations. I have lectured in more than three dozen countries and published more than 170 articles in refereed medical journals. I have replaced the hips of more than 4,000 patients and consulted at the bedsides of thousands more. In all those years and different medical contexts, I never once thought about what it must be like to be a patient.

In the summer of 1997, I was told that I had cancer of the prostate. The oncologists offered a guardedly optimistic prognosis. They told me that cancer had advanced sufficiently to require aggressive treatment. They did not believe it would prove fatal. They had every reason to anticipate a favorable outcome, but they could not offer any guarantee of a cure.

For the first time in my life I found myself asking questions about health instead of answering them. I was not the doctor, but the patient. I found the unanticipated role reversal to be an emotionally devastating but intellectually exhilarating experience. I felt helpless and powerless, in ways that I found embarrassing to the point of awkwardness. I learned more about illness during the following few weeks than I had learned in all my years of medical school. Only now do I know about what it means to go through the denial state of a potentially fatal disease and to feel the pangs of frustration and desperation. As a physician, I had always known about denial. I had also believed it to be a highly exaggerated phenomenon. And only now do I fully understand and appreciate the all-encompassing nature of the fear of imminent death.

Laypeople frequently joke about the way in which we doctors come to think of ourselves as gods. I understand now that the real joke is on us. We truly come to believe in our own ability to deal routinely with life and death, to alleviate pain, to improve the quality of life. Only when faced with the inevitability of a patient's imminent death do we confess, with all due modesty, to our own limits. It never occurs to us that our own eventual deaths are just as inevitable.

I now understand the limits of my own mortality in a way I had never suspected. Those feelings and experiences, however, have not devastated me. Rather, I have found them to be reassuring, humbling, and liberating.

Just a few days prior to learning about my cancer, a young man came to my office. He believed that he had injured his knee during a sporting activity. He had already consulted a sports medicine specialist, a modern-day medicine man who had taken him to surgery for an arthroscopic procedure on the knee. He was among the thousands of people who fall victim of a wonderful procedure that is being abused to an obscene degree. Arthroscopy is often recommended at the sight of any history of even mild trauma to the knee joint and without waiting for spontaneous improvement to take place.

The procedure had proven negative, however, so the sports medicine man had performed the latest ritual—a long period of physical therapy. At the conclusion of several weeks of intense treatments and even more intense exercise, the young man found his condition unchanged. His gait was still abnormal. He could not swing his foot normally and was now experiencing substantial back pain. So, the physical therapist referred him to a foot specialist.

The foot doctor did exactly what many foot doctors around the world always do: he prescribed special supports and indicated that if they proved ineffective, surgery might be required. Unfortunately (but not surprisingly), the corrective device did nothing but make matters worse.

By this time, his back was troubling him a great deal and long walks had become impossible. He was now in the hands of a back specialist who ordered a multitude of tests including X rays, MRIs, and CAT scans, and more physical therapy. He also ordered a specially designed back brace. The man's gait continued to deteriorate, his knee was still sore, his foot continued to ache, and his back pain was becoming disabling.

After all of those consultations, he was sent to me, the hip specialist. With all of the physicians he had consulted, I was the first to examine his hip. Within minutes, I realized that his primary pathology was in the hip. In the original sporting event, he had torn the labrum, a major ligamentous structure in his hip. The problems with his foot, knee, and back had all stemmed from that original injury.

My own specialty, and the only surgical procedure that I personally perform, is total hip replacement. In this case, it was clear to me that hip replacement was not the appropriate treatment. Instead, I recommended arthroscopic reconstruction of the ligament. The young man had that procedure performed by one of my colleagues, and was soon back to normal.

We physicians have narrowed down the scope of our expertise so dramatically that we have lost much of our ability to diagnose the illnesses afflicting our patients. All too frequently, we miss the most obvious pathology if it does not fall within our territory.

The attitudes and expectations of our young physicians-in-training are only accelerating this trend. A few years ago, I was giving a lecture on the healing process in fractures. In the midst of the lecture, I noticed that one resident's attention was directed toward his newspaper. At the end of the session, I approached him and questioned his actions.

He looked at me with total self-assurance. "I really do not care how fractures heal, Dr. Sarmiento. I simply want to know how to fix them." He was expressing comfort with the fact that in some segments of the discipline the orthopaedist was becoming less a physician and more a cosmetic surgeon of the skeleton.

At first, I thought the young resident was an aberration and that others reasoned differently. After probing further into the matter, I concluded that he was, in effect, speaking on behalf of many of his contemporaries and expressing, quite accurately, the ethos of the times. After all, his education had taken place in an environment that emphasized technique over the biological sciences. The lectures he listened to were, for the most part, related to the technical aspects of treatment modalities. "What operation does this fracture need?" was the question the sight of an X ray depicting a fracture instinctively provoked. It had replaced the traditional "What is best for this patient." He had never learned to appreciate the need to understand the healing process.

Overspecialization and excessive faith in medical technology are presenting a viscous, two-edged threat to the medical profession. If we allow it to progress, it may well reduce the art of medicine to the level of computer technicians. This realization—that our physicians may have become overspecialized and that our U.S. medical education has become too technological—is hardly startling to the professional medical community. We recognize the problem, however, as a theoretical and philosophical professional issue. Only when my cancer transformed me from physician to patient did I recognize the extent of the crisis or its terrible impact.

Upon learning of my own cancer, and in full-blown denial, I cast a wide net searching for other, more optimistic opinions. As a result, many medical professionals and other (some self-appointed) authorities were quick to contribute their opinions. I read every conceivable article dealing with the subject; I spoke to friends and colleagues who had gone through the same experiences; I found myself listening to all kinds of horror stories; I was entertained with endless accounts of splendid outcomes. In short, I received so much advice that within two weeks, I had acquired a massive data overload that crashed into complete confusion. Without exception, the experts who I consulted had little understanding or concern with the way in which my cancer was consuming my entire life. They cared only about the way in which it was destroying cells in my prostate gland.

The urologist who first identified my cancer recommended surgery. I had a great deal of respect for his opinion. He was an intern when I first came to the University of Miami. We have known each other casually for almost thirty years. He probably expected me to simply take his advice and to begin treatment.

But I have long recognized that in many fields of medicine, especially my own specialty of orthopaedics, surgery is widely recommended, even when it is not necessarily the best treatment for a specific case. I was very aware of the complications that can follow surgical treatment. I also question most surgeons' lack of involvement with their patients. They come in to treat a specific condition. Many have little knowledge or concern with the person they are treating, but only with the part of the person that is not hidden by the surgical drapes. I have been philosophically opposed to this kind of medicine for many years. I found myself remarkably reluctant to seek surgical treatment.

So, I traveled across the country seeking opinions from the leading gurus of prostate cancer. As I anticipated, the surgeons recommended surgery and the radiation therapists recommended radiation therapy. I realized that alternative medicine practitioners would recommend their approach, and that snake oil salesmen, should I encounter any, would tell me that my only salvation lay with their particular potion.

Then one surgeon, an expert who is internationally recognized as among the best in his specialty, proved to be more candid than most. Shielded by a rather aloof and somewhat arrogant attitude, he nonetheless reached out with a refreshing approach. "Your cancer is in its early stage of malignancy," he said. "It is likely to be curable by whatever method you choose."

I pressed him for a more precise answer. "What would you do if your were in my position?" I asked.

His answer surprised me: "I would go for radiation."

I followed his advice (and my own original inclination). Soon, I found myself going through the treatment protocol, keenly aware of the many uncertainties and likely complications. Later I was told (by someone who may just have been jealous of the surgeon's success rate), that the surgeon had recommended radiation therapy only to protect his own reputation; that he operated only in cases where the good prognosis was exceptionally high. His accuser claimed that it was his skill in selecting cases, rather than his skill with the scalpel, that had produced his extraordinary success rate.

For a few moments, I thought that perhaps this critic was right. Then I rejected his mean-spirited and probably scurrilous argument. Now, I must recognize that a patient has no way to be sure about such things. Overspecialization, excessive reliance on technology, arrogance, and greed have exacted a price. We professional men and women of medicine can no longer assume that we have the full faith and respect of our patients. We have taught our patients to recognize our weaknesses.

When I informed my urologist that I had decided against surgery, he seemed pleased. He told me that he, too, under my circumstances, would probably have made the same judgment. He helped me coordinate the entire treatment program and has acted throughout as a totally professional, caring, sincere, and dedicated physician.

He and others have assured me that the survival rate with radiation therapy can be higher than fifteen years. If that proves true in my case, I will be more than content. I have had a good life. My death would come at the right time. I do not wish to live to be ninety-nine, as my mother did. I have learned to accept not only the theoretical limits of mortality but also the fact that I, too, am mortal. I just try to remember the old saying "I am not afraid of dying; I simply do not want to be there when it happens."

I went to my library seeking advice and read once again books that describe the ultimate event in different but unforgettable terms. None of them totally satisfied me. Albert Camus in *The Myth of Sisyphus* and *The Stranger* addresses the inevitability of death in his inimitable existentialist and rather morbid way. The reading of his works did nothing but aggravate my confusion. Arthur Miller's *The Death of a Salesman* depressed me further. The resignation of the seventeen-year-old boy in the face of impending death, as described by his father John Gunther in *Death Be Not Proud*, was not something I could picture myself capable of displaying. Ajax and Mark Antony chose suicide, a very distant and unlikely option. Only Leo Tolstoy's masterpiece *The Death of Ivan Ilyitch*, with its realist details, came close to assuaging my dilemma. The existentional dissection of the novel by Martin Heidegger made it even more palatable. Though written over one hundred years ago, the words of Ilyitch, "for Christ sake let me die in peace" resonate in contemporary ears with clear meaning.

My mother used to tell me that the best way to get ready to die is to read a bit of Thomas à Kempis's *Imitation of Christ* every day. I gave that book to her on her fiftieth birthday. I returned it to my library when she died half a century later. It may well come in handy one day, but I have not yet begun to read it.

I then planned to resume my tennis game. When I was a child, the game was played at the country club. Many of the other children my age took lessons, but my family could not afford them. I first took tennis lessons the year that I celebrated my fiftieth birthday. I enjoyed the game, but tennis elbow ended my interest, or so I thought.

Shortly after I returned from the ill-fated Health Care International venture in Glasgow, Scotland, in 1995, I took up tennis again. I took lessons two or three evenings a week, from a man forty-five years my junior. I enjoyed the game immensely, but never played against other opponents in spite of my teacher's urgings. I hate to lose, and refused to play with others until I could play a competitive match.

The cancer brought my tennis career to another hiatus. I anticipated substantial debilitation from the therapy. Surprisingly, the treatment did not totally drain my energy, although I went through both the external beam radiation and the subsequent implanting of radioactive "seeds." The external beam consists of the traditional radiation technique, where a relatively large area of the abdomen is exposed to radiation. Small radioactive needles are then manually inserted into the prostate in an attempt to further expose the cancerous cells to the radiation effects.

I refused to allow the treatment to incapacitate me. Instead, I remembered the observations that had originally led me to advocate major changes in the treatment of fractures. When I was first trained in orthopaedics, we learned to treat a fracture by immobilizing it and by immobilizing the joint above and below the fracture. In the case of the tibia, the large bone below the knee, this heavy, rigid cast was kept in place for approximately sixteen weeks. While it allowed the fracture to heal, it caused substantial deterioration of the affected muscles and joints, and created the need for physical therapy after the cast was removed.

As I was undergoing treatment, I found myself frequently thinking about my life and my career, and about my philosophy of healing. "Physician, heal thyself: then wilt thou also heal thy patient," wrote Friedrich Nietzsche in *Thus Spake Zarathustra*. I remembered that I had insisted throughout my career on the importance of the healing process, and the relative subordination of the technology of treatment. I decided to take my own advice.

I came home every evening and swam one hundred laps. Every weekend, I walked a minimum of fifteen miles. My PSA, the blood test that helps diagnose and monitor the progress of prostate cancer, suggested that the cancer was under control. Good news, but I will continue to take it cautiously. And I will continue to maintain the highest possible level of activity. I am having my tennis racket restrung.

During my first visit with the radiation oncologist I inquired about his experience with prostate cancer and asked him about his own personal results. In a convincing way, he told me of his high incidence of cures and the small number of complications associated with radiation treatment. I assumed that he had his position well documented, and looked forward to participating in the follow-up studies necessary to appropriately document clinical results. (As a hip surgeon, I continue to stay in touch with every patient I have treated. I seek annual X rays and have records that go back more than thirty years.) As I write this, many months have passed since my radiation treatment. To this day, the radiation oncologist has neither called nor written. He has not sent a personal note inquiring about my health. He has not requested follow-up data.

To my chagrin, I have learned that most therapeutic facilities do not maintain long follow-up data concerning their patients. They refer to the experience of other institutions and other physicians. They assume that their own experience will be similar to the published results of work done by others. That is scientifically and morally indefensible.

I have done well, so far. I do not question the competency of my radiation oncologist. But I think that I would have preferred treatment by a physician who had carefully and honestly recorded his own results.

As I look back at those troublesome days and ponder on the factors that made me reach a reasonably calm attitude about my illness, I think that my wife's example is probably the most important. Barbara has had four bouts with cancer—the kind of experience that can break the spirit of even the strongest people. Throughout the course of repeated surgeries, radiotherapy, and chemotherapy she has remained unflappable. Though I am sure that in some hours of solitude she must have despaired and quietly cried, never once has she shown any signs of desperation. She seems to have accepted her fate as being beyond her control. Perhaps the example was set for her by her stepfather, who, totally blind and deaf, continued to look at his life as a blessing to be enjoyed to the fullest.

I have maintained an active lifestyle and continue conducting surgery. Happily, the radiation treatment does not seem to have had much of a long-term effect on my energy level, except that sometimes, these days, I feel the need for a late afternoon nap.

In retrospect, perhaps that would not have been such a bad idea much earlier in my life. In my native Colombia, as throughout the Hispanic world, the afternoon siesta was a regular practice. My father came home for lunch every day. Afterwards, he took a twenty-five-minute siesta. He always woke up on time, without the aid of an alarm clock. Now that I am past the age of seventy, I have found this traditional practice to be remarkably refreshing and rejuvenating. It seems to make it easier for me to work late into the evening, into the hours of solitude when I can listen to my music, read my books, and sift the trivialities from the enduring truths.

chapter 6.
choosing a medical career

"Those who live are the ones who struggle."

—Victor Hugo

My days in the early 1940s, attending San Pedro Clarer College in Bucaramango, Colombia, were marked by indecision and frustration. Questions, doubts, and other considerations of my future and lifelong calling dominated my thoughts.

My conscience spoke clearly on the subject. It frequently reminded me that it was unfair to continue to ignore my family responsibilities. It said that an additional six years of professional schooling would force my mother to continue to support the family. In the end, however, my mother prevailed. Only at her insistence— and with the continued help of the Jesuits (albeit indirectly)—did I begin to contemplate a professional career.

This time, it was my father's younger brother, Raphael, who upon my graduation from college came to the rescue. He provided me with an allowance—24 pesos (about $12) per month. This was not much money, even back then, but it was sufficient for me to pay 10 pesos for rent and 10 pesos per month for meals in a student dining area.

To this day, I do not know the basis on which I decided I should pursue a medical career. I like to believe I thought I would make a wonderful doctor and somehow feared that the law was not my calling. I can assure you that there were many occasions during the years that followed when I would be convinced that medicine had been a poor choice.

I was not the only beneficiary of my uncle's kindness, generosity, and faith. His great wisdom and strong personality attracted attention throughout the Catholic hierarchy in Colombia, and my uncle was later made bishop in the city where his father had been born one hundred years earlier. Subsequently, he won promotion to archbishop of

Pamplona, Colombia, the city that his maternal ancestors, the Peraltas, had helped to found when they first arrived from Pamplona, Spain.

He died in 2002. He called me to tell me that he felt that in spite of apparent good health, he had the feeling that something serious was unfolding inside of him and that his remaining days in this world were rapidly coming to an end. I traveled to Bogota for one last conversation with him. He did not look good. He had lost weight and fatigued easily. His mind, however, was clear. We talked for nearly an hour about life and death. With sincerity, I suspect, he claimed to be ready to die and held no doubt that a better life was awaiting him. He was probably recalling that several times in the past I had asked him if he really believed in the afterlife. I returned to the States the next day filled with grief and the uncomfortable feeling that Hobbes was correct when he said, "Life is solitary, poor, nasty, brutish and short."

My first few months in medical school at the National University of Colombia were enchanted. I found anatomy fascinating. I also thoroughly enjoyed the rigorous studies and the intellectual ferment in noisy public coffeehouses where tables lining the walls were reserved for medical students. We often brought dried human bones to those coffeehouses, where much of our study took place.

The coffeehouses served both coffee and alcoholic beverages. Sometimes, the noise of fights between drunken customers was all that kept us awake after the coffee lost its ability to hold Morphia at bay. Today, I wonder how we managed to concentrate on our books and our work. Several years later, I returned to Bogota and sought out the café where my friends and I had studied dried bones at the tables lining the walls. The café and the tables were still there, but the students had moved on. I suppose it had never been a particularly important or appealing tradition, but I mourned its passing.

My fascination with medicine and medical study waned early in my career. I found the increasing intensity of required science classes especially troubling. I yearned for more focus on the humanities. I sought continued discussions with friends about philosophy, history, politics, music, art and literature. They sought discussions with me about chemistry and pharmacology.

I was also increasingly concerned that difficulties with my eyes might prevent me from achieving success in medicine. When I was twelve, our entire grade in school was taken to the local doctor for a complete physical examination. When my turn came for the eye test, I had a rude surprise. While my right eye was able to read the entire chart with no difficulty, my unaided left eye was unable to read even the top line.

Since I had never had trouble with my sight, I first thought that I had contracted some kind of a condition and was suddenly going blind. My parents shared my concern, and quickly took me to an eye specialist. Incredibly, he told us that my left eye must have been almost blind from birth. My "ambliopia," he said, might improve somewhat with time. It was too bad, he said, that we had not discovered the condition earlier. Had we done so, we might well have been able to force the "lazy eye" to develop better.

Strangely, however, I never suffered any problems from this condition. While the vision in my left eye did gradually improve, it has never been able to see details sufficient, for example, to recognize a face. Yet, the condition never prevented my participation in sports or other activities with other kids. In fact, I was better than most at target practice, and quite talented with the slingshot.

As a medical student, I feared that my ambliopia might create difficulties performing surgery. One day, during a physiology class, I was required to sit on a low stool. With my eyes at the same level as the tabletop, I held two strings attached to vertical wooden sticks that moved over parallel tracks. My assigned task: move the sticks back and forth until they stood exactly opposite one another. The task clearly was designed as a test of depth perception. Despite my childhood skill with the slingshot, I failed the test miserably.

Today I look back in horror on this episode. By rights, I should never have been allowed to continue and to go into surgery. Yet, despite my inability to bring those two sticks into the proper position, my ambliopia has never been a problem. I can still thread a needle as quickly as anyone with perfect vision; I can look into the depth of the canal of a long bone; I carry out any surgical detail. So despite this physiological handicap, I became a successful surgeon.

CRISIS OF FAITH

In fact, far greater obstacles than ambliopia lay before me. First among them, both in time and in the difficulty it presented, was my own increasing dissatisfaction with medicine. I resented the need to work at many menial jobs to support myself. I found myself increasingly frustrated by the absolutism of my science classes. Worse, I began to doubt myself and increasingly to question my religious faith.

While I had never been numbered among the most faithful of religious devotees, the faith of my family and my long association with the Jesuits had created a strong foundation. While I may have questioned the actions of individual priests, I had never challenged the doctrine, rituals, and teachings of the church. Now I found myself questioning values, beliefs, and commitments that had always been beyond doubt. I found myself enveloped in an emotional crisis, living the experience that St. Augustine describes so brilliantly in the *Confessions*. I began to feel somewhat embarrassed by what appeared to be myths and superstitions that belittled the dignity and rational foundations of my religion.

Perhaps the hours in the coffeehouses were taking their toll. The atheistic Marxism and the existentialism of Sartre and Camus had reached great popularity, and I had read them with enthusiasm. Sartre himself visited Bogota, and I attended one of his lectures. Sadly, my skill with the French language proved inadequate. Yet, I emerged from the hall with a sense that I totally understood him and agreed with every word. The occasion only aggravated my own crisis.

I began to neglect my medical studies and delved into classical Catholicism. I read Saint Paul and Thomas Aquinas, then Blaise Pascal and Francisco Suárez. I read the Protestant Søren Kierkegaard with enthusiasm. Their ideas seemed staid and outdated. Kierkegaard, especially, seemed to defuse the brilliance of existentialism and return to repetition of ideas that I had heard week after week for my entire life. I turned to Thomas à Kempis's *Imitation of Christ*. I found great solace in this simplest of all religious treatises. It helped me contain the crisis and retain some control over my life, but it did little to resolve the swirling questions. I suspect I must have accepted Pascal's wager that there is nothing to lose by "believing."

I shared my thoughts with my most admired classmate, a man whom I had come to regard as the smartest and most promising among us. He and I had shared a cadaver when we started anatomy dissection. Working at such close quarters had formed a bond of mutual respect. I sought his council to total expectation that he would defuse my doubts and return me to the calm, dispassionate, professional pursuit of knowledge.

Instead, he told me that he would be leaving medical school at the end of the term. He was planning to join the order of Benedictine monks. He told me that he had gone through the same crisis that I was experiencing. As his doubts had grown, a close friend had advised him to seek help from the Benedictines. He urged me to meet with the brothers and to learn from them.

I was reluctant, at first, to meet with the monks. Then I found myself troubled by my own hesitation to seek knowledge and understanding, whatever the source. Soon I acquiesced. The Benedictines assigned a particularly bright and overpoweringly logical brother to speak with me. After several sessions with him, I began to think that, like my classmate, perhaps I should also abandon medicine and take to the robes and the cloister. I knew beyond doubt that my personality would fit easily within the embrace of the monastic life.

I recognized, however, that I could not leave my mother totally dependent on relatives after she had sacrificed herself so long to finance the education of my brother and me. My brother, an architecture student, was talking about leaving for Europe to finish his studies. He was also contemplating the possibility of practicing architecture abroad. He would only be able to follow his calling with some financial contribution from me.

I attended the impressive medieval ritual by which my friend left the world and entered the Benedictine cloister, but I stayed behind. I hoped that he found the answers and the peace of mind that he sought behind those walls, but I have never regretted my own decision to remain in the secular life. Recently, I learned that he eventually left the Benedictines, returned to medicine, and became a successful physician.

I continued to question my calling as a physician and law school continued to tempt me. Eventually, the thought of starting that long (and expensive) path made a career change seem out of the question. So, I continued to study medicine and to advance toward my career as a doctor.

PLAYING DOCTOR

At the end of my fourth year in medical school in 1949, I spent one and a half months providing medical care to the residents of a small town about four hours from my home. My Uncle Raphael had asked his superiors to allow him to serve as a parish priest. They had assigned him to this small, poor community, which lacked most of the civilities that people usually take for granted. The community's only doctor had not had a vacation in more than twenty years. My uncle asked me to join him there, to provide his flock with some basic medical care while the local physician had a break.

I was not at all prepared to take care of sick people. My knowledge of medicine was minimal; my class work in medical school had been confined largely to basic sciences. I had had only one year of clinical work. Happily, the residents of the town survived through the interlude, even if their visiting "physician" barely made it.

One evening, my presence was requested at the home of the mayor. His wife was delivering a child. I had never helped in the delivery of a baby. In fact, I had minimized my exposure to obstetrics as much as possible. I had even gone so far as trade tours of duty so that other classmates would deliver all the babies assigned to me. I took the obstetric examinations, consisting of both written and oral questions, without difficulty. Happily, they had never insisted on a hands-on demonstration.

This time, it was another story. They mayor's wife was quite insistent that I provide more than verbal assistance. Fortunately, the local midwife was already on site. She quickly assessed the situation. She graciously assumed responsibility while allowing me to pretend to be in control. Happily, the delivery was uncomplicated. I caught the baby, handed it to the midwife, and said, "Please, take over. I believe that you can finish."

She took over and I watched her work, well aware that the next time around, I might have to do it all myself. The next day, I discovered that the entire town knew that "Dr. Sarmiento successfully delivered the mayor's fifth son."

I wish that I could tell you that I found such experiences exhilarating and that they became the foundation of my desire to help patients and care for their needs. In fact, the experience only increased my self-doubts and intensified my concerns. I continued to question my suitability for a medical career, and my desire to practice medicine.

Toward the end of my fifth year of medical school, with only one year of study remaining, I simply could take it no longer. Although law school was no longer possible, I could not continue to study medicine. I told my friends. They told me that I was being stupid, but that they respected my choice because they knew how long I had agonized over it.

Then I had to tell my family. My mother, especially, had spent all those years waiting for the completion of my medical studies. Now I had to tell her that I was starting over, with no real idea of where I was headed. It would be difficult, but I knew that nothing could stop me.

I sought the advice of a cousin by marriage whom I had long admired. He was a successful man of business, who had been a good friend of my father. I told him that I was "considering" quitting medicine, but he could tell that I had already made up my mind. He assured me that he could help me find a job. He told me about a tin mine that was opening, about 150 miles from home, and asked if I would be interested in supervising the employees. I found the idea quite appealing. I could live far from the city, in solitude, and enjoy reading the many books that my medical studies had kept me from.

Armed with the security of his job offer, I approached my mother. She heard me out with a somber expression. She said that she had expected me to make such a choice for some time. She added that she was prepared to help me in any way she could. I told her that I planned to become a tin mine operator, and would not need her help. She nodded as if she were accepting the idea as a completed concept. To me, it seemed that my decision to quit had become a "done deed." As Sartre might have said, "*Les jeux sont faites*." All bets are down.

Then she asked if I had given any serious thought to the idea of finishing medical school before quitting my chosen profession. She added that if she were in my position, she would do just that. "You never know. Some day you might feel differently. Having a medical license might come in handy." She shrugged her shoulders as if the burden of such choices were too much for her, and went back to her housework.

To this day, I do not know exactly what happened next. I hope that I was not overpowered by the simple logic of her argument. I hope that I had, in fact, previously considered her suggestion. I hope that guilt, or belated wisdom, or recognition of the enduring power of past promises swayed the day. I know only that I could not disappoint her. In retrospect, she proved to me that day that she was a great deal smarter than I had given her credit for being. I hope only that my wife and I have been able to guide our children with such gentility, grace, courage, and wisdom.

LAW AND ORDER

So I returned to Bogota and to medical school. There would, however, be at least one substantial change. Instead of working at any of the menial jobs that had helped finance my first five years, I was determined to find a new way to complement my medical work. I would no longer work through the night as a clerk in the post office. I would no longer spend hour after hour, taking the mail out of huge bins and sorting it into little pigeonholes lining a giant wall. I would find something more meaningful and more exciting. I became a detective in the secret police.

I suppose that I should have known better. In my own defense, I can only remind my readers that these were the days before *Miami Vice* or even now-ancient television shows like *Dragnet* or *The F.B.I.* I had no idea, no Hollywood image, and no concept of what lay before me. I knew only that it offered an increase in salary and a way out of the post office with its mail-sorting operation.

There was no "secret police school" or special training. I was given a gun, a badge, and commanding officers. I volunteered to work nights. The duties were light enough that continuing medical school presented no problems. For a while, we had almost nothing to do. We just sat around, waiting for "the call."

Then the liberal candidate for the presidency of Colombia was assassinated. Riots broke out in Bogota and most other cities. The masses took to the streets and began looting businesses. The government declared a state of emergency. My group of secret police went out on patrol. Without any noticeable contribution from me, we restored the rule of law. The country went back to relative tranquility.

Yet, something intangible had changed. For more than forty years, Colombia had enjoyed peaceful democratic stability. Now, a new era had dawned; a new era of political instability had begun; the *violencia* that has crippled Colombia ever since had made its debut.

The political and social *violencia* has since given way to the problems of drug production and export. This hellish combination has virtually destroyed my native land. Colombia is a nation rich in resources. It is a land capable of supporting its people and providing all with a comfortable, healthy lifestyle. Yet, Colombia and her people will remain confined to hell until the consuming countries find a way to stop their demand for drugs. Until that happens, neither political, nor religious, nor military institutions will be able to save my native land and restore its people's birthright of domestic tranquility.

The new era brought new duties to the secret police. One night, my superiors ordered me to arrest a well-known and distinguished journalist of Bogota. I knew the respect that surrounded this man, but no one told me what charges had been lodged against him. At twenty-one, I was the youngest man on my team. The others wanted me to "learn the ropes," so they made me the arresting officer. I displayed my badge and told him that I had instructions to take him to police headquarters. He asked me to sit down and wait while he got dressed and prepared to go with me. He asked my name. I told him. He asked why such a young man was not in school. I told him that I was a medical student, working nights. He asked how I was doing in school.

It was terribly disheartening and embarrassing. Fifty years later I met a young Colombian student in Miami. When he gave me his name, I suddenly realized that the distinguished journalist I had been ordered to arrest in Bogota had his same last name. Soon we came to the conclusion that it was a direct ancestor of his who I had led to the police station in my younger days. He was a Caballero Calderon, a member of one of the most distinguished families in Bogota.

Other experiences were more troubling in other ways. One night, at about 2:00 in the morning, a large contingent of both uniformed and secret police descended on one of the poorest neighborhoods in town. We banged on doors, broke them in, and intimated the residents. We were looking for weapons, we said. We never found any.

I did, however, see how the poorest people in Bogota were living. The houses were meager in every way, with almost no furniture. Adults and children slept together on bare dirt floors. Stolen electrical equipment and appliances were everywhere, but none were in use since the houses had no electricity. Until that moment, I had no idea how much misery lay in the hidden underbelly of our capital city. I began to understand their still unvoiced discontent. I understood the reality of the social injustice described by the likes of Dickens, Balzac, Zola, Flaubert, Tolstoy, and Dostoyevsky, which until that moment had been little more than a political concept badly described by Marx and other left-leaning theoreticians. That experience exacerbated my already strong disgust with social injustice—a feeling that maturity has not assuaged. That feeling explains my admiration for the likes of Mahatma Gandhi, Robert F. Kennedy, and Martin Luther King Jr.

During the Christmas holidays in 1950, the police transferred me to the eastern coast of Colombia. In Cartagena, the beautifully preserved colonial city, I first saw the ocean. You who have traveled throughout your lives and enjoyed the benefits of movies and television have no idea of the shock of that first sight of the topaz waters of the Caribbean Sea. In the evenings, I sat by the water and rejoiced in the sounds and timeless parade of the waves. I walked the soft, seductive length of the sandy beach under the azure dome of the tropical sky. I had never even imagined it. I wept for my father, who in the forty-nine years that he had lived, had never stood on the edge of the world, had never seen or smelled the sea. That first day I fell in love with the ocean with the passion that Ishmael must have felt when chasing the white whale described in Herman Melville's *Moby Dick*, the most classic of American novels.

My duties as a detective consisted primarily of spying on small merchants and checking the accuracy of the scales at the open markets of Cartagena. Once I participated in a sting involving smuggled guns. I later found that the chief of detectives subsequently sold the guns, which we had seized, to other merchants of death. The same man once asked if I would be interested in going to Panama by boat and bringing back some "merchandise that can not be brought in by air." I declined the invitation. Those who accepted the invitation later told me that it had proved "profitable and rewarding."

I resigned from the force shortly after my return to Bogota. In some ways, my year with the secret police had proven more educational than my last year in medical school. But it seemed wise to return to a more physiological focus on the nature of man.

My next job brought me closer to the path that would eventually lead to my future. I went to work in the office of an orthopaedist, a government employee who held office hours from 3:00 to 9:00 every evening. It proved to be the best-paying and the most rewarding job that I held during my six years of medical school. Like the police force, it proved to be educational in unexpected ways. The orthopaedist was a kind man. It was from him, not from medical school or from colleagues, that I learned, above all, how to treat patients with respect and empathy. It proved to be a lesson that has lasted my whole life.

chapter 7.
a rude awakening

"The teacher affects eternally; he can never tell where his influence stops."
—Henry Adams

In the end, my mother won the battle and lost the war. I agreed to return to my studies, to complete my sixth and last year, and to obtain my license to practice medicine. It was clear that she was right. She had said, "You never can tell what the future holds, and a license to practice medicine might come in handy."

And so in 1951 I emerged from my crisis of faith and resumed my destined path. Then my life took a strange twist that the Fates had hidden from both my mother and me. Before long, I would turn from the well-traveled highway to follow a previously unnoticed, less traveled side road. I would obtain my medical license and begin my lifelong career in medicine. That career, however, would take place thousands of miles away from Bucaramanga.

My brief stay in the small community where my Uncle Raphael had served as parish priest had taught me all that I wanted to know about rural medicine. Instead of taking the year of "rural medicine" licensure requirement, I applied for an internship at the Central Military Hospital in Bogota. At the time, the hospital was considered one of the best training programs in Colombia because it had well-trained full-time staff and resources superior to many other hospitals where medical training was provided. I was somewhat surprised and extremely pleased to learn of my acceptance.

In medical school, I had greatly enjoyed my rotation in psychiatry. I found both the theory and the practice to be pleasing and rewarding. On those occasions when I contemplated specialization (rather than simply abandonment of medicine), I thought most frequently about specializing in psychiatry.

At the Central Military Hospital, my first rotation brought me to orthopaedics. For the first time, I thoroughly enjoyed being a doctor. I reveled in the glamour of surgery and found myself enchanted by the concrete, early results that can usually be obtained from the treatment of bone and joint disorders. This rotation in orthopaedics became the turning point of my life.

GUILLERMO VARGAS: THE MOST INFLUENTIAL MENTOR

The credit (or blame) goes to a brilliant teacher and gifted surgeon named Bill Vargas. Dr. Vargas was a human dynamo, full of energy and overflowing with excitement. A young orthopaedist, he had just a few months earlier returned to Colombia from Boston, where he had spent several years learning from some of the world's leading orthopaedists.

It seemed that Dr. Vargas imagined that within a short time he could change Colombian medical tradition and raise its standards to those he had found in the United States. He peppered every conversation with references to Boston, Harvard University, Children's Hospital, and Dr. William T. Green, a professor at Harvard and chief of orthopedics at Children's Hospital. He continuously spoke of the rigorous training, the brilliance of the teachers, and the excitement of the lifestyle.

Vargas came from a wealthy Bogota family. I recognized his brilliance and his ambition, though I questioned his discipline. I found his enthusiasm and excitement about the medical life in Boston to be contagious. I never let myself recognize the difference between the rigors he described and the undisciplined style he pursued.

We found him a magnetic personality. Often, after working late into the evening, he would invite us to dinner at some restaurant in the heart of the city. When I accompanied him, it meant that it would take me more than an hour to return to the hospital by bus, since the hospital was located in the outskirts of Bogota, and the buses ran infrequently. Despite the inconvenience, I never declined his invitations, and to my knowledge, none of the other interns did either.

The Central Military Hospital was extremely busy. Military hospitals throughout Colombia referred their more difficult cases, and we witnessed an enormous amount of clinical material. The orthopaedic service was particularly active. Colombian troops fought in Korea, along side North Americans, under the United Nations flag. Many Colombians were seriously wounded. All soldiers with peripheral nerve injuries were sent to Central Military. Bill Vargas was particularly interested in those injuries, and conducted much of the surgery on them. I followed his work closely. Eventually, I wrote and defended my doctoral graduation thesis on the subject of nerve injuries.

Once a week, he held rounds with the medical and nursing staff. During rounds, one intern would present every one of the approximately one hundred orthopaedic in-patients. This was Dr. Vargas's opportunity to show us the Boston way to conduct medical rounds and to teach orthopaedics.

In accordance with the protocols he had learned in Boston, he demanded that all patients admitted to the orthopaedic service, regardless of their medical condition, undergo a complete physical examination, including a complete description of the function of all central and peripheral nerves. He required all of us to fill out forms copied from those used for the purpose in Boston. We began to dread the phrase "in Boston."

I was told that cheating would be a grave mistake. The credibility of any report is destroyed by the inclusion of false information. If caught reporting fake data, we were warned, Dr. Vargas would fire you on the spot. No lesson learned before or since has stayed with me more deeply. To this day, I regard research data as sacrosanct. To me, there is no greater sin than falsifying, fabricating, or "messaging" research data. It infuriates me to discover misrepresentation or deliberate distortion of research. I credit Bill Vargas with teaching me this lesson in ways that have stayed with me. I only wish that all others in my profession had learned to value research data so highly.

At Central Military Hospital, the Vargas system of rounds required every one the three interns to know something about each patient. The resident had to know it all. Vargas would arbitrarily assign one of the interns to preside over rounds without previous notice.

One day I was chosen to lead. I presented the patients. He asked me questions. It soon became obvious that I had not prepared myself appropriately. I had not met his standards or his expectations. He made it clear that this would never do "in Boston." Obviously, it would never do in Bogota, either, as long as Bill Vargas was in charge.

He embarrassed me in front of the entire entourage. I could have quit on the spot. Instead, I swore I would never let it happen again.

Until that moment, I had been a poor student, studying just enough to pass tests, but never to be as good or better than anyone else. This episode changed that forever. The next time he asked me a question, I had the answer. I began to enjoy "being good." He noticed the change and began to pay attention to me. I enjoyed the attention. I felt that he was proud of what he had done. I wanted to carry it even further, and sought out his direction. He even gave me a list of articles to read.

Gradually it became clear to me that while Vargas was somewhat undisciplined, he demanded absolute professionalism from those around him. He required that everyone on his service be on-call seven days a week.

Having a "second job" was absolutely forbidden. I knew the rules when I was assigned to his service, but thought I could break them without being caught. So, I had continued the last job I had held while in medical school, working for the public health service orthopaedist in the late afternoons and evenings. After all, I rationalized, I had been able to continue working while a medical student. And my hospital salary was not sufficient for me to continue to assist my brother's subsistence while he attended architecture school.

The public health service orthopaedist excused me whenever I was late, because he knew of my responsibilities at the hospital. He was also aware of Vargas's idiosyncrasy and of his erratic schedule.

Vargas usually left the hospital for his office in town around one o'clock in the afternoon. I would then slip out of the hospital and report to my other job. One day he returned to the hospital unexpectedly. The next day, he asked me where I had been the previous afternoon. I told him the truth. He angrily reminded me that such a practice was forbidden. Without further discussion, he sent me to the office of the medical director for reassignment.

Ophthalmology was my next assignment. For the next few weeks I learned about the new specialty and began to get used to it. I was disappointed, however, because by that time I had developed an extraordinary liking for orthopaedics.

During the subsequent days, I avoided running into Vargas. One day, around noon, I was by myself having a cup of coffee in the doctors' lounge when he walked in. I quickly finished drinking the coffee and started to leave the room. He remarked that I did not have to leave simply because he had come in. I apologized. He told me to sit down. He asked about my new rotation and I responded that it was great. I had already tried telling this man the truth, and it had not worked out well. This time, I was not going to give him any satisfaction.

Unexpectedly, he asked why I had ignored the rules and held a second job. I decided to try the truth. "I need to have a second job in order to meet family responsibilities. I cannot satisfy those responsibilities with the salary I earn from the hospital."

"Why didn't you inform me of your circumstances?" he asked.

"Because you never asked me," I replied. "And you never gave me an opportunity to explain." The force and anger of my answer amazed me, even as I spoke. My bitterness and disappointment must have been evident to him. Clearly, he understood my love of orthopaedics, perhaps even better than I understood it myself.

"Would you like to come back to orthopaedics?" he asked.

I was back in orthopaedics the following day. Shortly afterwards, Vargas began to suggest that once I finished my tour of duty at the Military Hospital, I should go to the United States to pursue residency training. Boston was the place to go. Children's Hospital would be perfect for me. He would help me secure a position.

I had spent six years worrying about whether or not medical school was the best path for me to follow. I had agonized over my family obligations, my religion, and virtually every other aspect of my life. It took me only an instant to make the next decision. I would go to the United States and the sooner the better. I should have thought about things a little longer and more thoroughly. I would also have done well to remember the lack of self-discipline for which Bill Vargas was famous around the hospital.

The next day, I began to make plans for my trip to the United States. The airfare was about $110; those dollars were much harder to earn than they are today. My family did not have access to that kind of money. I had only one asset of great value—my father's library.

I loved those books. The deprivation of my childhood had not motivated me to sell them. I had chosen to work countless hours at dreadful jobs through medical school rather than sell those books. I thought about the ten-volume *History of the World* written by the Italian historian Cesar Cantu, published in Spanish in 1880. My grandfather had bought that beautiful set of books. He had presented them to my father when my father graduated from law school. I treasured those books.

The books were my introduction to history and led to my interest in the humanities. My father had encouraged us to read them. He had read many of them aloud to me. From them, I first learned of the English, American, and French Revolutions. Later, I spent many hours listening to the husband of my mother's sister reading those books. That was my introduction to Alexander the Great, Julius Caesar, and Mark Antony. Those books introduced me to Cicero and the lives of the Medici family, to Machiavelli, to Savonarolla.

Now, my only concern was, how quickly could I sell them. Would they finance the journey to Boston? Would they cover my expenses until I could start my residency at Children's Hospital? My other tasks would not be nearly as time consuming. I had to obtain the necessary papers, of course. That would be simple enough, since the American Embassy was located in Bogota. Then I needed only to purchase the tickets and tell my mother. Without further thought, I put my books up for sale and submitted my resignation.

The conversation with my mother went much more easily than I had anticipated. She received the news with enormous equanimity. In fact, she appeared happy that I was making a move to better myself, and that I had abandoned the idea of quitting medicine. She had only one question: How long would it be until I returned?

I assured her that I would be gone only two or three years. That would be sufficient time for me to obtain the necessary training in orthopaedics, especially since I already had completed more than a year of internship under Bill Vargas. At the time, I spoke the complete and absolute truth. I had every expectation of returning to Colombia, where I would practice orthopaedics, raise a family, and eventually die.

I never contemplated remaining in the United States. My brother, to the contrary, was planning to immigrate to Europe to pursue his graduate training in architecture. My mother was delighted that I would return within a few years. She feared that my brother would be gone forever. As things turned out, she would be wrong about both of us. My brother eventually returned home to live. I would return to Bucaramanga only as a visitor.

chapter 8.
on to the colossus of the north

"The world is a book, and those who do not travel, read only a page."
—Saint Augustine

My first disappointment came when I learned how little my books were worth on the open market. In fact, their sale financed little more than the cost of the ticket to the United States. And I realized the small sum because a considerate relative chose to purchase the entire collection. It seemed that all that learning and all the wonderful thoughts and experiences of Western civilization, gathered lovingly over three generations, counted for little on the open market. I should have taken it as an omen. Instead, I charged blindly ahead.

I approached the task of obtaining my United States visa with the same optimism. Again, at first it seemed that there would be little difficulty. Even the fact that I spoke no English presented little challenge. The kind and helpful employee at the consulate spoke fluent Spanish. He told me that he had been to Boston as a young man. He thought it a wonderful city. He assured me that I would enjoy living there and would find it to be an exciting place to work. My excitement and enthusiasm continued to rise. Where, exactly, would I be employed? he asked.

With great pride, I responded that I was going to be a resident in orthopaedics at the Children's Hospital, the best hospital in Boston and one of the most highly regarded hospitals in the United States. I told him that Dr. William T. Green, "a good friend" of my chief at the Military Hospital in Bogota, was head of the department. The official congratulated me, assured me that I would be on my way shortly, and asked to see my contract with the hospital in Boston.

Contract? Not only did I did not have a contract but it had never occurred to me that such a thing was necessary. In Colombia, such arrangements did not require contracts; they were arranged between men of honor. Dr. Vargas was a "friend" of Dr. Green. He had assured me that he would take care of everything. It had never occurred to me that there could be any problem or that formal arrangements were necessary. I assumed that the two great men had taken care of the details. All I needed to do was show up and go to work.

Highly embarrassed, I apologized to the consul who by that time had realized I was in trouble. I suspect that he wanted to help me. He asked what would happen to me if, for some reason, Dr. Green did not have a position to offer me. I replied that I would be surprised and disappointed, but that I could wait for a vacancy to open. I assured him that I could work somewhere else in the meantime.

He asked about my family's financial resources. When I admitted to him that my financial situation was not good at all, he stated that it was impossible for him to grant me a visa. Furthermore, I would need to secure a position in the United States before I could even reapply. I tried to soften his heart by saying that I was only twenty-five years old: I had a medical diploma in my pocket and the courage to put up with whatever inconveniences I might have to face. I added that I did not speak English, but I was certain that within a short time I would learn it. He rose and politely extended his hand to me.

Angry, frustrated, crushed, and desperately trying to hold back (or at least hide) my tears, I returned to the Military Hospital. There was nothing else to do. I would have to withdraw my resignation. The job, however, was no longer available.

Fortunately, I had developed a good relationship with the medical director. He told me that his youngest brother was a surgical resident at a hospital in New Jersey. He suggested that his brother might be able to help me out. He telephoned him immediately, and was told that there were several jobs available right away at the hospital. Saved!

My next interview with the American consul was brief and cordial. The embarrassment of the initial experience hung in the room. Still, he completed the paperwork and wished me well. In a few days, I would be on a plane, flying to a new life in the United States. I would not be going to Boston, but New Jersey sounded appealing.

American immigration historians have written poignant accounts of those who fled the deprivation of the Old World for the hope of starting life anew. They wrote of people who agonized over the decision to leave ancestral homes, and the difficulty of leaving families and friends behind. They wrote of the emotional and physical distress that dominated the immigrants' journey, and wrenching shock of arrival in the great port cities of the United States—Boston, New York, Philadelphia, and Charleston. I wish that I could confirm their account, or present something even nearly as dramatic.

Instead, I can only tell you that no decision I made ever seemed simpler or more obvious. Even the flight to the United States onboard an Avianca DC-4 airliner was relatively uneventful. The DC-4 was slow, extremely noisy, and vibrated constantly. I was cold going over the mountains as we left Bogota, and hot as we flew over the ocean. I remember the constant noise and the vibration. I later read in a book called *Fate Is the Hunter** that the DC-4 had a bad safety record, and that many crashes occurred during winter flights in Latin America. I am glad that I did not know that at the time.

During an stopover in Miami, a gentleman, probably in his sixties, boarded the plane and sat next to me. He was tall, blue-eyed, of light complexion, and addressed me in broken Spanish. I instantly decided that he was clearly a citizen of the United States, and assumed that he would be just the man to help me when we landed in New York. Surely, he would be able to assist me through customs and help me find the McAlpin Hotel.

An hour after we left Miami, I asked him if he would mind helping me when we arrived in the city. He smiled gently, and told me that he was not an American, would not be staying in New York, spoke little English, and his final destination was Europe. He did, however, prove to be an experienced traveler and helped me find my way to the proper lines when we went through immigration and customs. Much that followed would also turn out less successfully than I had so quickly assumed.

I arrived in New York on the afternoon of December 7, 1952. My trip into the city from the La Guardia Airport took forever. The taxi driver must have realized that he had a "greenhorn" onboard his cab—a visitor without a clue, who would be willing to pay whatever he was charged. I had left Colombia with 200 dollars in my pocket. By

---

*Ernest K. Gann, *Fate Is the Hunter* (New York: Simon and Schuster, 1986).

the time I reached the hotel, I had a lot less money. I probably should have taken a bus into the city, but I did not know that. I also did not know who to ask for help.

I was unable to sleep that night. The next morning, carrying around a big trunk with all of my possessions, I left the McAlpin Hotel and ventured into the streets of Manhattan. My destination: the West Side Bus Terminal. A uniformed policeman, who seemed to me to be much bigger than anyone I had ever before seen, pointed me in the direction of the Port Authority.

At the time, New York's Port Authority Bus Terminal was one of the world's greatest transportation centers. It was crowded with throngs of people going to and coming from everywhere in North America. I suspect that more American immigrants passed through the Port Authority Bus Terminal than ever stood on line in the Great Hall at Ellis Island. The sight and sounds were simply staggering. I thought that I had witnessed ethnic diversity in Colombia, but I had never seen anything like the crowds that jostled through the Port Authority Bus Terminal.

Remarkably, with only a little more help, I found the right train. I asked the person sitting next to me to let me know when we reached Passaic, New Jersey. I was not quite sure that the man had understood my request, but he shook my shoulder and pointed to the sign as we pulled into the Passaic train station.

Finding the hospital proved almost as easy. I approached people who looked like they were in positions of authority, and repeated the name of my destination. Almost everyone proved helpful, and soon I found the hospital. And at the hospital, I soon discovered, the most widely spoken language among the staff was Spanish, not English. Most of the interns and residents spoke Spanish. There were also several doctors from other nations.

From the front desk, I was taken to a room that I was to share with Dr. Kim, an intern from Korea. He had been in the United States only for a few months. Even to me, it was obvious that his English was poor, and my English was even worse than his. Neither of us could understand a word that the other said. I realized that while I had learned to read English by studying medical texts, I had never spoken the language, or even heard it spoken to any extent. Dr. Kim had more experience with the spoken language, but he knew less English medical terminology.

Unbelievably, the hospital had scheduled me to be on-call on the day that I arrived. When the phone rang for the first time, Dr. Kim picked it up and then passed on it to me. I held the receiver and listened to what might just as well have been Greek or Japanese. Embarrassed, I gave the receiver back to Dr. Kim. Displaying his unforgettable grin, he said slowly, "You are needed in the Emergency Room." I still did not understand. In the way that he could have learned only from other Americans, he repeated his message more loudly. "You are needed in the Emergency Room."

Finally, he held me by the hand, like a little child, and took me to the ER. There, lying on the table was a six-year-old girl, with long blonde hair, who had sustained a small laceration on her right temple. I greeted everyone in the room with a serious "good night." The instruments needed to stitch the laceration were already on the table.

Having already exceeded the limits of my English, and with no additional conversation possible, I proceeded to repair the cut on the pretty girl's face. The nurse dressed the wound. I followed the precedent I had just witnessed from Dr. Kim, bowed in the Oriental fashion, and left the room. I had survived my first experience. I was now an American doctor, and extremely pleased with myself.

The phone rang several more times that night and I went back and forth to the Emergency Room. The scenario would be repeated hundreds of times during the course of the next year. During the day, I was assigned to the various services on a rotating basis. There was no teaching, no conferences. There was a monthly morbidity-mortality conference, where deaths and major complications were discussed, which I surmised was only a formality. To make matters worse, while my English was beginning to improve, I was still not in a position to understand the rapid-fire give and take of the conferences, and missed much of what was being said.

I have vivid recollection of being on call one evening when I was summoned to "pronounce dead" a woman in her forties. She had succumbed to the ravages of breast cancer. After carefully rehearsing the appropriate words to use, I went to the waiting room to inform her husband of her death; he grabbed my shoulder and said, "Doctor, is there anything you can do?"

I understood his words and his anguish across the language and cultural gap. He raised a question that night that I have never been able to answer. How do you respond to such a plea? What do you say to such a painful and totally irrational cry? Oh, how I wished I had been able to speak his language, to talk to him and to try to console his grief. I could not do it, and simply remained silent, shook my head, and left the room.

Since that night, there have been thousands of occasions when I have heard people speak of the cold, aloof posture of many physicians, and especially surgeons. On occasion, I, too, have been known to criticize colleagues for a lack of personal concern. But I sometimes wonder how much of this seeming lack of compassion really stems from our own devastation. There is nothing we can do. There is nothing we can say. I have become proficient in the language of my adopted land, but that night, speaking to that woman's grief-stricken husband, none of my acquired linguistic skills would have helped. I still have not learned any words that would have eased his grief.

With the passage of time, however, I was rapidly acquiring other skills. I was also acquiring an understanding of the obligations one assumes when accepting employment at a hospital in the United States. So, it did not take long for me to realize that I would not be departing from Passaic and moving to Boston in the near future, as I had assumed. I had failed to read the contract with the hospital, which committed me to work there an entire year. In fact, for better or worse, I was stuck at Passaic General Hospital for the entire year.

Fortunately, the staff senior orthopaedist, Samuel Yachnin, soon recognized my passion for his specialty and invited me to scrub with him every time he did surgery. He also held a clinic for indigent patients that I could attend. My year in Passaic could have been a professional and emotional disaster. Instead, his kindness and professional skills made it a productive, exciting year, and I learned a great deal from him.

About two months after I arrived in Passaic, Dr. Yachnin invited me to go with him to the annual meeting of the American Academy of Orthopaedic Surgeons, which was taking place at the Waldorf Astoria Hotel in New York City. I accepted the invitation with alacrity, and for once, the event exceeded my expectations. For the first time, I realized how large the United States must be, and how many people practiced orthopaedic surgery. I attended sessions led by famous men whose clinical and research articles I had read. I did not understand the sessions, but that did not slow down my fascination with the event. Then, from a distance, I saw Dr. Green from Boston.

Since I assumed that I would be Dr. Green's resident in the near future, I was tempted to introduce myself. Dr. Yachnin said that he did not think that doing so would be a good idea. He told me that in the United States, doctors often behaved with a rigid view of social and professional protocol. He convinced me that approaching Dr. Green at the conference would be perceived as rude, clumsy, and overly ambitious. I did not fully understand what he was saying, but I allowed him to convince me, and I heeded his advice.

I have since, of course, come to understand the social and political hierarchy of American medicine. I now recognize the instinctive wisdom of Dr. Yachnin's advice that morning, so long ago in New York. But I have never fully accepted it. I can also say with total honesty and conviction, that I have never followed it. Throughout my career, I have tried to remain available and accessible to patients and colleagues alike. I have sought out the company of residents in training. I can only hope that no one has ever been told that it would not be a good idea to approach me.

As I discussed in previous pages, I had developed, during my medical school days, a strong dislike for obstetrics. I had managed to graduate without ever having delivered a single baby; other students assisted in the delivery when my turns came up. During my internship in New Jersey, I worked out a similar arrangement with other interns. It was the practice at the hospital to have one intern deliver the baby and for the other one to give the anaesthetic to the mother. My fellow interns agreed to deliver every time while I always handled the anaesthetic.

Surely, you know where this anecdote is headed, but you only think that you know the whole story. One Saturday afternoon, the inevitable happened. The other intern on call went across the street to get his hair cut after having assured me that there was no one in labor. A few minutes later the telephone rang. I heard a woman's voice say something that suggested that I was needed for a difficult or complicated delivery. My first reaction was to run to the barbershop and get the other intern off the chair. I quickly realized what would happen if any harm came to the baby or the mother because of the delay. On my way up to the Labor Room, I tried frantically to remember everything that I had observed, years before, in the small Colombian town with the mayor's wife.

When I arrived on the obstetric floor, I found the nurses sitting around a table having coffee. I told them about the call I had received. One of them suggested that perhaps it was the emergency room calling. I ran down to the ER and found out that no one there was in labor, either. I knew, however, that I had received an urgent call from someone in the hospital. I decided to call the telephone operator—to ask her where the call had come from.

When she heard my question she started laughing and suggested that I come to the switchboard. She said that she was having a hard time understanding me. When I reached the switchboard, the two operators were still laughing. They told me that there was no one delivering a baby. There was, however, a special delivery letter for me. They thought that the whole thing was extremely funny, and could not stop laughing. I laughed about the incident, too, but only years later.

Seven months after I began my internship in Passaic, I traveled to Boston to meet with Dr. Green at the Children's Hospital. I wanted to ask him for a residency position. His secretary informed me that he was not available that day but would be happy to give me an appointment for another day. When I told her that I would be leaving town that evening, she suggested that I wait. Perhaps Dr. Green would give me a few minutes of his time.

About an hour later, Dr. Green came into the office. He was courteous and asked why the meeting was urgent. I told him that I was a former intern of Dr. Vargas in Bogota. He expressed what appeared to be genuine interest in finding out about Dr. Vargas, but assured me that he had no position to offer me. That day, July 1, 1953, was the beginning of the new academic year. The new residents were already starting their tours of duty. My request was simply impossible.

I do not really remember how I reacted, but it must have been dramatic. Dr. Green asked me not to despair, telephoned the chief of orthopaedics at the Lahey Clinic in Boston, and set up an appointment for later that day. He also invited me to spend the next two hours following Dr. David Grice, his associate, who was making his daily rounds with the new and old residents. Finally, I had the opportunity to witness the academic process that Dr. Vargas had described so often. It was wonderful, and I ached to be part of the group making their rounds.

At the Lahey Clinic they took my name and told me they would consider me for a rotation the following July. Again, however, fate would intervene and send me down a different road. A year later, the Lahey Clinic tried to contact me to offer me the position. By the time I received their letter, however, I was already a resident in South Carolina.

I saw Dr. Green again several years later, when he came to Miami as a visiting professor. A few years after that, I was invited to be a visiting professor at Harvard, and was negotiating the possibility of joining the faculty at Massachusetts General Hospital. Dr. Green asked me to sit next to him during the presentation. I could not help but think of the day, years earlier, when I had sat in his office and begged him for a job.

chapter 9.
facing a daunting crisis

"Man is not made for defeat."

—Ernest Hemingway

My lack of success in securing a Boston residency left me disheartened and discouraged. Like Tantalus of Greek mythology, I had been allowed to almost touch the prize but not to hold it. I was also feeling alone, totally isolated from family and friends, and, for the first time in life, a little afraid. I returned to Passaic wondering what would happen if my student visa expired before I could secure a resident position. I wrote letters applying for residency to every single orthopaedic program in the country.

I was slowly learning that U.S. hospitals were not exactly anxious to hire foreign-born, foreign-educated medical students for their residency programs. I had learned to read English well enough to read medical journals and charts. I had not yet realized that my inability to converse comfortably in English had become a major handicap. Nor, despite many encounters with confusion that resulted from my lack of English-language fluency, had I come to accept that Spanish could no longer be my only language.

I was especially disappointed that I had not heard from the people at Leahy, and that the Hospital for Special Surgery in New York had not responded to the letter I had sent them shortly after my arrival in the States. In those days, the Hospital for Special Surgery was known as the Hospital for the Ruptured and Crippled. In my letter, I had indicated that I was seeking residency and that I had been an intern under Dr. Enrique Botero in Bogota. Dr. Botero had trained in orthopaedics at their hospital, and was highly regarded. I wrote a second letter repeating my inquiry.

In response to my second letter, they wrote to "remind" me that they had contacted me by phone several months earlier. They also reminded me that, during that call, I had scheduled an appointment with Dr. Thompson, head of the department. I had failed to appear for that interview, they wrote, and they no longer had any interest in my candidacy.

I was devastated, but I understood. Shortly after I began my internship in Passaic, I had received a call from somewhere in New York. I had not really understood what the lady on the telephone was saying; it could have had something to do with an appointment. I had not even been able to understand the name of the hospital, although she had repeated it several times. Finally, I had simply been too embarrassed to ask her to repeat it, or to seek help from someone else at my hospital in Passaic. It was the first, but not the last, time that my inability to understand English got me into trouble. It had proven to be a high price to pay for not having learned the language prior to my move to the United States.

The experience with the Hospital for Special Surgery convinced me that I had to begin to study English in earnest. The vast majority of the interns and residents in Passaic were Latin American with a sprinkling of Russians and Koreans. The official language of the house staff was, for all practical purposes, Spanish. Therefore, I had few opportunities to learn English. From that day on I banished my beloved classical music station, WQXR, from my radio. I tuned only to programs featuring conversations in English.

I started going to the movies—often watching the same show two or three times. I began reading English-language newspapers and magazines. I knew that if I continued to speak Spanish most of the time, I was never going to learn to speak acceptable English. I resolved to speak only English as much as possible.

My new plan was not well received by the other Spanish-speaking interns. They accused me of being aloof, a traitor, and ashamed of my background. Their feelings could not have been further from the truth. To the contrary, I have always taken great pride in my Hispanic heritage and my Latin American education. I still believe that Americans could learn much from Hispanic culture, if they were only willing to learn to appreciate it, rather than being so condescending toward it. American students need to study Cervantes instead of simply laughing at Don Quixote. They need to know more about Garcia Marquez and less about Seinfeld.

I told myself that the resentment of my colleagues and associates really did not matter. Within a few months I would be leaving Passaic and would probably never see them again. I also knew that my failure to learn English would severely limit my ability to learn, grow professionally, and practice orthopaedics. Those thoughts, however, only reminded me that the end of my contract was rapidly approaching. Unless I succeeded in finding a residency, my visa would also expire.

I was losing my ability to choose my own destiny. Unless options opened quickly, I would again be in a position where events would move me along a seemingly predestined path. I had to have a place to take my residency in orthopaedics, or I would have to return home to Colombia without full training in the medical specialty that I had come to love. I knew that unless I succeeded in finding a residency, I would probably end up abandoning medicine entirely, and seeking a new profession.

As the days passed, I continued to receive only negative responses to my letters. On some days, I received no response at all. It was already November of 1953. My visa expired the following month.

Then, remarkably, I received a letter from Dr. Yount, chief of orthopaedics at the University of Pittsburgh. Dr. Yount wrote that he had received my application and was interested in granting me an interview. He was going to be in New York at the Waldorf Astoria and wanted to set up an appointment for one evening the following week. I had never heard of the University of Pittsburgh. I had to consult a map to find the city. But I welcomed the opportunity to meet Dr. Yount with great relief and excitement.

It was the first time that I was to be interviewed in the United States. I was not prepared. I knew that I would be a disaster. I dreaded the meeting and, to this day, I am sure that I must have presented an appalling performance. At the end of the interview, however, Dr. Yount said that he had been impressed. He promised that he would write to me within a few days, with a definite answer. My spirits rose, and I returned to Passaic, sure that my visa was safe. Every day, I waited for Dr. Yount's letter to arrive. Several days—then a week—passed without word from Pittsburgh. It was already the middle of November. I had only three weeks left before my visa—and probably my career in medicine—expired.

Then a letter arrived from Columbia, South Carolina. It was an official letter offering employment as a resident at the Columbia Hospital of Richland County. I was not only immensely relieved but also quite delighted. I knew from my reading of the orthopaedic literature that Columbia was the city where Dr. Austin Moore practiced. I had been intrigued by his writings on hip fractures and his new artificial replacement for the hip joint. His work seemed incredibly fascinating. I looked forward to meeting him, and learning more about this remarkable procedure. One day, perhaps, I would be able to work with him.

I immediately began to make plans for my departure. As I prepared myself for the journey south, Dr. Yount's letter offering me a position at the University of Pittsburgh finally arrived.

Now, more than fifty years later, my ignorance and naïveté continue to amaze me. At the time, however, I saw no difference between the sophisticated academic program in Pennsylvania and the nonuniversity residency that I had been offered in Columbia, South Carolina. I still believed that Boston was the only *real* place to get an education. After that, I thought, all other programs were the same. Again, I made a critical, vitally important decision without giving it the research or attention that it deserved. I made no effort to research the programs. I did not attempt to seek advice. I simple decided to inform Dr. Yount of my acceptance of the job in South Carolina. I sometimes wonder how Dr. Yount reacted when he read of my decision!

Today, I look back on my first year in the United States, particularly at my New Jersey experience, with mixed emotions. That year, and the friendships that came with it, provided a good introduction to the North American way of life.

To a boy from a mid-size Latin American city, the glitter of nearby New York had irresistible charms. I discovered that New York's fast pace and cosmopolitan culture fit quite comfortably with my growing independence. I began to learn about the looser fabric of the family and the more casual attitude and practice of religious beliefs. New Jersey gave me the opportunity to start the long process of cultural assimilation, and for that I will always be grateful.

A GIRLFRIEND

During that year, I made several good friends who made my stay in Passaic more pleasant than it might have been. I will always remember Norma, a young woman of Italian descent and a newly graduated nurse. I arrived in Passaic in early December. Christmas came about two weeks later. I would have spent it alone in my room if Norma had not come to my rescue. She invited me to come to her house and to share the holiday with her family. That invitation saved me from a terrible first Christmas in the United States.

Norma and I eventually became very close. We traveled to New York City frequently after work hours, sometimes as often as twice a week. Norma was taking advanced courses at Columbia University, where she was working toward her master's degree. We fell in love and seriously discussed wedding plans. But they never materialized.

After I left New Jersey we saw each other a couple more times but the flame had been extinguished. Twenty years later I received a letter from her children. Norma had died. They had found some love letters from me while going through her papers, and thought that I would want to know of her death. I expressed my gratitude for their thoughtfulness, and shared a few memories of those days when we had both been young. Norma had taught me a great deal.

On the other hand, I am forced to remember with disappointment and some anger the lack of training and support that I received at Passaic General Hospital. As a medical internship, my year was nothing more than a farce. The other foreign-educated interns and I simply provided cheap labor. We never had an educational conference. We were never escorted on rounds. Our work was never reviewed. We did not receive rudimentary training, much less an advanced education. Only the friendship, support, and teaching of the staff orthopaedist, Dr. Samuel Yachnin, saved the year from being a complete waste of time professionally.

I now know that Passaic General Hospital was not alone in its abuse and exploitation of its interns. Nonuniversity-affiliated teaching hospitals often place young physicians in an environment where they only provide services. These services are basic to the practice of medicine. The interns need to acquire high-level skills in providing them. There is much more, however, to the practice of medicine. When basic services are performed daily and repeatedly, to the exclusion of more meaningful duties, they become offensive and demeaning to the fledgling doctors.

For my year in New Jersey, pronouncing people dead, breaking fecal impactions, and starting intravenous injections constituted the bulk of almost every night's work. Community hospitals like Passaic

General are now disappearing. Most have been replaced by for-profit corporations. Since the Unites States currently bars large immigration of most foreign-trained doctors, graduates of North American medical schools now fill many of the internships at these hospitals. Native-born North American medical students refuse to tolerate the kind of exploitation I experienced at Passaic. Consequently, the responsibilities that dominated my evenings on duty have now been assumed by nurses, physicians' assistants, and even people without medical degrees.

chapter 10.
southern exposure

"If a man begins with certainties he will end in doubts, but if he will be content with doubts, he will end in certainties."

—Francis Bacon

On December 1, 1953, overflowing with more enthusiasm than I had had since leaving Bogota, I boarded the train headed for Columbia, South Carolina. For the next few years, I would be working at the Columbia Hospital of Richland County. It was hard to believe that just two weeks had passed since I was in the depths of depression, convinced that my stay in the United States and my medical career were both nearing their ends. I was soon to discover that my new enthusiasm would be equally unsupported by coming events.

At the hospital in New Jersey, Spanish had been the unofficial language for the residents in training. When I arrived in Columbia, South Carolina, I had a rude shock. The language spoken at the hospital was, most assuredly, not the English that I was finally learning to speak and understand. In fact, learning to speak "Southern" English required almost as great an effort on my part as had learning to speak English in general.

Furthermore, for reasons that everyone involved seemed to understand and take for granted, "colored" and "white" patients occupied separate quarters. While I did not understand the system, neither did I question it. I accepted it as one more of the many strange customs that made up life in North America. I put it alongside the relative insignificance of family and the weak influence of religion.

For most people in the hospital I was the only South American they had ever seen. They had just as much trouble understanding my English as I had with theirs. Many of them could not understand me. A patient in the "colored hospital" referred to me as "the Chinese doctor." Taking a medical history, particularly from the poor and uneducated black patients, proved to be a major ordeal. In retrospect, I suspect that our language gap rendered many of my early histories incomplete or inaccurate.

In more recent years, I have given much thought to the problems experienced in large city hospital in the United States where the massive immigration of people from other nations means that patients and doctors frequently do not speak the same language. In the United States, I have learned that relatively few people in the medical professions have even rudimentary skills in any language other than English.

The Los Angeles County Hospital, the main teaching hospital for the University of Southern California (USC), where I was later to spend fifteen years, is a good (or horrifying) example. The majority of patients in the institution speak only Spanish. Most of the medical staff spoke only English. An intern or resident in training attempting to obtain the medical history of a patient's illness or injury would find the task virtually impossible. Inevitably, a great deal of important information—some if it, from time to time, a matter of life and death—was missed in the process.

I discussed this matter with the professor of psychiatry at the USC medical school. I asked him how his discipline was taught to medical students and residents in light of the fact that so many patients did not speak or understand English. Psychiatry requires a great deal of personal contact between doctor and patient. The discussion typically involves intimate matters and extraordinary, subtle shades of meaning and a relationship of close trust. How does a student achieve such a relationship with patients who literally do not speak the same language?

He answered that somehow, they managed to do the job through interpreters, who they typically found among other patients and nurses. What nonsense! What arrogance! I find it impossible to believe that patients could have any faith in confidentiality. Under those circumstances, no wise psychiatrist could place any faith in the strength of the doctor-patient relationship. Yet, the psychiatry profession has made no attempt to demand that practitioners become fluent in the languages of their patients. I am pleased that I can assure you that within a few months I had become somewhat comfortable with the southern dialects of English. I cannot, however, provide any such assurance concerning the ability of my patients to understand their doctor's English.

The chief of the orthopaedic program at the Columbia Hospital of Richland County, South Carolina, was Dr. William Boyd, a Southern gentleman of social distinction. He had been the first orthopaedist in South Carolina. He was a legendary figure in the community, though within a short time it became clear that the medical staff did not hold him in especially high regard.

He was no longer a young man and seemed to be more interested in medical politics than in medicine. I was the only resident in orthopaedics, although he had apparently sought to entice others to join the program. I eventually realized that Dr. Boyd's last-minute invitation had not been extended to me because he had suddenly recognized my "extraordinary" qualifications. Rather, he had turned to a Spanish-speaking South American, a graduate from a nonapproved medical school, only with reluctance. They needed a pair of hands, and they were willing to be stuck with me for a while. Nevertheless, to Dr. Boyd's great credit, he was extremely kind to me and sought to be as helpful as possible, under the circumstances.

Shortly after my arrival, I met the renowned Dr. Austin T. Moore, a tall, handsome gentleman of Scottish descent, endowed with a distinguished demeanor. I looked on him as a physician of heroic proportions. Beyond my wildest expectations, he treated me with respect. He became extremely important to me and to my career in orthopaedics.

He invited me to assist him, and I went to surgery with him as often as my other responsibilities allowed. He left printed orders in all his patients' charts, indicating that I should be asked to visit them. Soon, I concluded that there was no comparison between Dr. Moore and the other orthopaedists on the staff. The flamboyant, gracious, accomplished Dr. Moore simply towered over all others. His surgical skills were extraordinary.

Even from the perspective of my many years in the profession, I still regard Dr. Moore as an extraordinary individual. He had a restless and innovative mind that made him able to improvise when necessary. I also now recognize that he was a showman par excellence. He was able to make the most of every situation. Certainly, he was able to blind and create an almost mindless hero worship in a naive, impressionable young resident from Bucaramanga.

For three consecutive years, I saw every patient he admitted to the hospital. I scrubbed in with him in most of his surgeries. Eventually he displayed paternal feelings toward me and took seriously my education, growth, and future development. He and his wife welcomed me at their home. They even invited me to join them on rides through the magnificent countryside of South Carolina on sunny, clear days.

On one occasion, when Dr. Moore served as Charles Herndon's visiting professor at Case Western University in Cleveland, I traveled with him and assisted him in his surgical demonstrations. One another occasion, I accompanied Dr. Moore to New York and participated in his meetings with manufacturers of hip prostheses.

To prepare for the meeting with the engineers in New York, I accompanied him to the morgue at the hospital where we obtained human bones. Together, we filled the marrow of the bone with putty, split the bone, and removed the injected material. It was a crude way to do research when compared with modern methods, but it enabled him to further plan for his modified surgical implants. With a dull knife, we carved the desired shape of the implants.

Fifty years later, the hip prosthesis created by Dr. Moore remains in widespread use. It is still the benchmark by which all newer implants are judged. Countless new designs have been discredited and abandoned. Recollection of my small part in assisting Dr. Moore in creating his modified hip prosthesis still fills me with excitement and gratitude.

Before long, however, I was forced to pay a substantial price for my close association with Dr. Moore. I was extremely naive in those days, and slow to recognize that Dr. Moore was not liked by most of the orthopaedists on staff at the hospital. It may have been a mixture of envy and jealousy. It may have been a failure to understand the complexity of a man substantially ahead of his time. Most likely, it came from his innate pride and arrogance.

I lacked the political savvy to avoid being identified too closely with him, and I was soon perceived as not being interested in working with the other surgeons. I was bluntly reminded that Dr. Moore was not the chief of the program and that I had to assist all the other attending surgeons. I responded to the marching orders dutifully, but I was somewhat disappointed that I could not spend as much time with Dr. Moore as I had in the past. In a short time, however, I realized that there were many other good surgeons on the staff. I could also learn a great deal from them.

I made good friends with many Americans during my three years

(1953–1956) in South Carolina. I was a good student and read medical journals and textbooks with passion. In spite of all my medical work, I managed to find time to continue my reading, including both medical journals and many other subjects. I found, however, that I missed conversing with others about the humanities. None of my fellow residents were the least bit interested in anything outside of medicine, baseball, fishing, or football. As you my well imagine, none of those things interested me. I had played a game that we called *futball* in my youth, but it was nothing like the game played in the United States. I later learned that my *futball* was called "soccer" in the United States, but that almost no one played it. Ironically, I understand that in the last few years the Carolinas have become an important center of amateur and collegiate soccer. Today, in Colombia, a young doctor from Bucaramanga would probably be in high demand to coach a local team.

In the early 1950s, however, I suspect that the few Carolinians who thought about South Americans at all probably assumed that South America lacked any kind of serious civilization. Many, no doubt, visualized Colombia as the home of wild-eyed *bandidos* and natives running naked in the jungle. Several asked me if coming to America had been a great "cultural shock."

At first, I did not know how to respond because I was never "shocked " in the implied sense. New York had been a major change from Bogota. The winter climate in Passaic had been a shock, as well. But otherwise, Passaic, and Columbia, too, had much in common with Bucaramanga and Bogota. I responded that yes, I had been shocked but primarily "by the lack of culture among most of my peers in the United States." That lack of culture was evident in the 1950s. It is even more evident today. I never ceased to be amazed that so few physicians are able to appreciate the traditions of their own culture and know so little about other cultures with which they share the planet. They do not seem to appreciate the pleasures of intellectual conversation, but prefer to gossip about celebrities (including each other), television, movies, the stock market, golf, or football. They seem to regard the continued search for knowledge and inspiration as a dubious activity that is clearly inferior to hitting little balls into little holes, or watching grown men hit each other while fighting over a bigger ball.

In the United States, medicine seems to consume the minds of many of its practitioners and prevent them from indulging or developing a passion for serious subjects outside its purview. I know there are many in my profession who, like me, would prefer a night at the opera to a day at the football stadium, but there are not enough of us. Elsewhere in the world, the medical community plays a leading role in the intellectual lives of their communities. In the United States, many physicians seem to have delegated that responsibility to their wives, while they go golfing or fishing.

      🐿 🐿 🐿

I was still the only resident in the orthopaedics program when the Board of Orthopaedics announced that the residency program at the Columbia Hospital was to be reviewed for reaccredidation. I had no idea what such a review might involve. And as usual, I was not given any information regarding it. During my entire three years at Columbia Hospital in Richmond County, I had never attended a scheduled educational conference or lecture. The closest thing to didactic education had been the quarterly meeting of the Columbia Orthopaedic Society, held at the home of one of its members, where members of the group discussed "interesting cases" and had dinner and drinks.

On one occasion, I was told by Dr. James Green, one of the older orthopaedists in the group, to prepare a talk and to present it at the next meeting of the Columbia Orthopaedic Society. The assignment that he tossed off so casually would become an extremely painful ordeal with long-term consequences.

For several days, I spent every leisure moment working on my presentation and refining it. I was still terribly insecure about my skill with the English language and worked endlessly editing my comments. I had never before made such a presentation. I was so petrified at having to stand up and give a talk that I felt I needed to experience the soothing effects of alcohol. Before arriving at the home where the meeting was to take place, I stopped at a local bar where I had two strong drinks. The alcohol had the desired effect, and I felt myself relaxed enough to get through the trial that lay ahead. My presentation went well. My colleagues seemed pleased.

My concern over my imperfect English usage and heavy Spanish accent continued to overwhelm me. In 1963, I was called on to speak in front of a large audience at the Miami Beach meeting of the American Medical Association. On the day of the speech, I had lunch with Dr. Eugene Jewett, a distinguished orthopaedist from Orlando, Florida, who had been especially kind to me. The old anxieties began their familiar patterns, so I ordered a martini. Then I ordered a second, and a third. By the time I got up from the table I was more than relaxed. I do not know whether anyone noticed that I was drunk, or if they were just too polite to say anything.

It took several years for me to feel slightly more comfortable at the podium and to assuage the anxiety and embarrassment that my foreign accent provoked in me. Even up to this day, some fifty years after I first landed in the United States, I am sensitive about it. I still experience the "odd kind of trembling" that affected Cicero, "the founder of Roman eloquence" whenever he began to address a large audience.

I continue to make efforts to get rid of my accent, although I know that it will be with me for the rest of my life. I have concluded that, with few exceptions, it is impossible for anyone to speak without an accent and to totally think in an acquired language, if the new language was learned after the age of twenty. There are certain things that time seems unable to change. For example, I find that I still prefer to carry out mathematical calculations in Spanish. I can do it in English, but find it easier in my native tongue.

I continued to drink before any public comment of any kind. I found that I could not even stand up at a meeting to ask a question if I did not first take a drink. I realized that such a pattern could eventually become a problem, and so I stopped drinking. It was obvious that the "treatment" could become worse than the "disease."

Sudden breaks seem to be the only way I can stop a pattern. For example, after fifty years of consuming a minimum of ten cups of coffee a day, I stopped. I did not taper off. I just stopped, overnight. I simply decided that I did not really need all that coffee. I could work just as well without it. I did not touch a cup of coffee for nearly six years. Lately, however, I began to drink a couple cups of coffee every day.

I did the same thing with salt. For as long as I can remember, I had salted my food even before tasting it. I did it virtually unconsciously. One day, some twenty-five years ago, I decided to stop this bad habit. I have not picked up a salt shaker ever since. Sometimes I have chosen to alter a pattern of behavior just for the sake of self-discipline, just to test my ability to change. Once I prove my point, I go back to the behavior with renewed insight. I seem to enjoy the challenges.

MAKING A MORAL CHOICE

The reviewer from the Board of Orthopaedics arrived to evaluate the hospital's residency program. I had assumed that when the reviewer came to the hospital to inspect the program I would be taken aside and questioned about my medical knowledge. That did not turn out to be the case. Instead, Dr. Boyd informed me that the reviewer was a close personal friend of his and that all I needed to do was to be in the operating room performing surgery when Dr. Oscar Miller, from North Carolina, came to the hospital the following week.

Dr. Boyd had selected a patient for surgery before Dr. Miller's visit. He had also assigned an intern to help me. The patient was a black child of approximately ten years of age, afflicted with the sequella of poliomyelitis. One of his legs was partially paralyzed. Some of his muscles were completely functionless, but others were in good condition. The child walked with an obvious limp and was unable to tiptoe.

I prepared the child for surgery and discussed with Dr. Boyd the type of tendon transplant most appropriate for his condition. The night before surgery, I went back to the hospital ward to give last-minute instructions. I wanted to assure myself that everything was in order. I was stunned to see that the surgery schedule read differently than what Dr. Boyd and I had agreed previously. The operation indicated on the schedule was, in my opinion, inappropriate. I was certain that if I carried it out, the child's condition would be made worse.

Thinking that Dr. Boyd had inadvertently made a mistake, I tried to contact him at home. I could not reach him since he was out entertaining Dr. Miller. I decided to wait until the next morning to inform him of what I perceived to be an error.

The morning came and I succeeded in reaching Dr. Boyd at his home. I attempted to inform him of the mistake in the listing of the procedure. The conversation that ensued must have been memorable. I only wish that we could have had access to modern technology, and I could have recorded it.

Dr. Boyd was partially deaf, and probably feeling the after effect of the previous night's drinking with Dr. Miller. My own English was still far from perfect, and the more excited I became, the more I moved from English to Spanish. Eventually, Dr. Boyd understood that I was going to carry out a different operation from the one that appeared on the schedule. He began yelling at me over the telephone. He ordered me to do the transplant as he had written it. I was to proceed with the surgical procedure as indicated. I was an insubordinate, untrained, uncouth idiot.

Thinking that perhaps he had not yet understood me, I tried to tell him again that if I performed the indicated procedure, the child would suffer the consequences for the rest of his life. Dr. Boyd only yelled even louder: "God damn it, Sarmiento. You do what I am telling you to do or *you* will suffer the consequences for the rest of *your* life." The phone went dead.

I was scared and simply did not know what to do. The anesthesiologist was already concerned that Dr. Boyd might arrive at any moment. He knew that Dr. Boyd would be furious that surgery had not yet started. I tried to explain the consequences of proceeding with the wrong surgery. He reminded me that if I canceled the surgery, both he and I would be in serious trouble. He urged me to proceed.

I finally acquiesced, and he put the child to sleep. I watched the anesthesiologist do his work through the glass window that separated the operating room from the scrub room. My stomach tensed, poisoned by the aftertaste of orange juice and my half-eaten breakfast.

I knew that I was facing not some a silly, simple test of will of my own devising, but a serious personal test of the highest order. The stakes could not be higher. The health of a child; my career; my self-respect. This was an ultimate test of my humanism and my faith. My mind filled with the words and thoughts of the world's greatest ethicists and philosophers. St. Augustine told me that I had no choice; I could not accept that, but I knew that the choice facing me would shape everything to follow. Immanuel Kant's categorical imperative reminded me that only one of the alternatives facing me was the ethical choice; Hippocrates reminded me that, above all, I must do no harm.

Then, I knew that there was a simple decision to be made. Augustine was right after all. I had no choice. Regardless of the consequences, I could not go ahead with surgery. I told the anesthesiologist to awaken the child and return him to the ward.

The anesthesiologist pleaded with me again, and others joined in, warning me about the risk I was taking. "Do you have any idea what Dr. Boyd can do to you?" I left the operating room and waited for Dr. Boyd to call, but the call never came.

Late that afternoon, I was summoned to the office of Mr. Daniels, the hospital administrator. When I walked in, Dr. Boyd, with his hands in his coat pockets, was standing there, his face a portrait of anger itself. Mr. Daniels, like administrators everywhere, seemed to think I had gone out of my way to make problems for him. He said that he had never before found himself in such a difficult position. He handed me a sheet of paper, and asked me to read and sign it. It was a letter of resignation.

I looked at them both and told them I was not interested in resigning. The administrator said that if I did not sign, he would be forced to fire me from the residency program. I repeated that I was not interested in resigning, and acknowledged their authority. Mr. Daniels asked me again to resign. He said that if I forced him to fire me, it would be virtually impossible for me to find a residency position in any other hospital in the United States.

I told him that I knew that too, but at least my conscience would be clear for the rest of my days. "In that case," he said, "this meeting is over." I left the room. I felt the way Antigone, in Sophocles' masterpiece, must have felt when, aware of the likely dreadful consequences of her refusal to accept King Creon's orders, she dared challenge the powerful monarch.

The entire episode was a nightmare. I did not have a job and there was no way I could get another one. Who would hire a foreign trainee who had been fired for insubordination? I had no other option but to return home to South America.

The next day I went to see Dr. Moore at his office and apprised him of the situation. He was deeply disturbed. "Dr. Boyd would never listen to me. There is nothing I can do," he said. I had heard that before. I would hear it many times again from many different people through the years ahead. Dr. Moore asked about my plans. I told him that I would be returning to Bogota.

Dr. Moore then offered me temporary work in his office. He invited me to help him by working in the plaster room, until my departure from the country. I accepted his offer and went to work. There was nothing else for me to do. When I received my next and final paycheck, I would return to Colombia. I wrote to Dr. Vargas in Bogota to inform him of my premature and unexpected return, and to ask if I could join him in his office. He was out of town, taking a long vacation. I therefore did not receive a response. Nonetheless, I proceeded with my plans to return home.

Even as I was completing my last-minute preparations to leave, I received a message that Dr. Boyd wanted to see me in his office. When I entered, he did not respond to my greetings. He proceeded to scold me for having done so much harm to him by questioning and challenging his authority in the presence of Dr. Miller. Incredibly, he seemed to expect an apology. He pointed his index finger at me. He was willing to reinstate me, he said, if I promised "never to do anything like that again." I told him that I did not feel I had anything to apologize for. He did not respond. We both stood there in silence. Occasionally we would look at each other, then we would both look away. I looked up at the clock on his wall. The second hand crept around with agonizing slowness. More than a full minute passed in total silence. Then he looked up and said, "Go back to work right away."

About seven years after I left Columbia, South Carolina, I ran into Dr. Boyd at a meeting of the South Carolina Orthopaedic Society, where I had been invited to present scientific material. At that time, I was a junior member of the faculty at the University of Miami. That night, during a cocktail party, Dr. Boyd suddenly put his hand on my shoulder and held me in an intense, powerful grip. "This young man embarrassed me and challenged my authority some years ago," he said to a group of orthopaedists. "I was very angry and I tried to fire him. He was right, but I never admitted it." Then, he shook my hand, and introduced me to several of the people standing around. I thanked him for all he had done for me. Our feud was over.

chapter 11.
life as an orthopaedic resident

"The law of the desperate is wrong."

—Plato

During my three years of residency in South Carolina, I had not done much surgery, though I had seen a great deal performed by Dr. Austin Moore. In spite of the good relationship we had, Dr. Moore had never felt comfortable letting any resident do surgery. On the few occasions when he tried to serve as my assistant, he had taken over the surgical procedure within minutes.

Dr. Moore's associate, Dr. Barney Freeman, an excellent surgeon and a warm human being, did allow me to operate. Every Friday afternoon, Dr. Freeman and I would go to the State Hospital, at that time the largest psychiatric hospital in the South. At the State Hospital, we would perform as many as six surgical procedures. Primarily, we stabilized fractured hips. It was at the State Hospital, under the direction of Dr. Freeman, that I first learned to deal with the pathology of the hip. That interest would continue to fascinate me for the rest of my life.

So, although he had never seen me operate, Dr. Moore had good reason to know of my growing surgical skill. Those skills would stand him in good stead on one highly memorable occasion.

Following a national meeting in New Orleans, several orthopaedists stopped by to visit Dr. Moore. He invited them to observe him perform surgery. He did a few prosthetic hip replacements and a couple spinal fusions. On the last day of their visit, he was to demonstrate his technique for "nailing" a broken hip. On this occasion, however, his well-known showmanship got the better of him. He began to describe the importance of "feeling" the position of the nail in the various parts of the bone from just the sound of the blows of the mallet. He struck the nail, then looked up at his audience.

"I am entering the neck of the femur now," he said. He struck another blow. "Now I am in the head of the femur. The fracture is fixed."

He turned around and ordered an X ray to confirm the good reduction of the fracture and the proper placement of the nail. When the X ray was brought into the room, we all discovered that the nail had bypassed the fracture altogether. The X ray image of the nail was crystal clear. It lay underneath the bone, having entirely missed the fracture itself.

Dr. Moore laughed out loud and said, "I guess I can no longer nail a broken hip. Gus, you finish it." He left the room, and the visitors followed him.

This end of the episode provided a rare show of humility. Dr. Moore was not a humble person. He rarely admitted to any mistakes. Quite the contrary, he was an extremely proud man who was totally convinced of his superior capabilities and judgment. Usually, he refused to allow anything to interfere with that image. He could not even accept the thought of knowing that his surgery schedule was not always filled for two days a week, far in advance. He used to submit fictitious names to the operating room, anticipating that within the next few days he would find real patients to replace the fictitious ones. He simply could not stand having anyone else know that his schedule was not always filled to capacity.

I have a bad habit of expecting my heroes and teachers to always demonstrate godlike perfection in everything they do. Inevitably, of course, they eventually disappoint me in some way. Then I become angry with them for letting me down by demonstrating their human limitations. That pattern held true with my relationship with Dr. Moore.

On many occasions, Dr. Moore told me that patients with symptoms of herniated discs should be given a reasonable period of "observation and exercise" before contemplating surgery. One day, in his office, I saw him examine a woman in her late forties, who was complaining of back pain with sciatica—back pain that radiates down the leg. He instructed her on a program of exercises and told her to await the results from that approach. He then left the room and went directly to his secretary. I was standing behind him and heard him tell his secretary, "Schedule her for a laminectomy and spine fusion four weeks from now."

For the first time in more than two years, I had reason to doubt his integrity. I wished that episode had never taken place; it spoiled my image of him forever. But I continue to believe that he was a great surgeon. There can never be any doubt that he was also a great (if imperfect) man whose influence in my life was enormous.

GETTING MARRIED

In the middle of the third year of my four-year residency program in South Carolina, I decided to make some changes in my life. The most important of these: I decided to get married to a wonderful woman who I had been courting since my arrival.

Barbara Kitchings was a nursing student. Her parents were deeply religious Southern Baptists. They regarded her marriage to a Catholic as a tragedy, and we married without their consent or knowledge. Our marriage did not stress my own religious beliefs so severely, because Barbara willingly converted to Catholicism. Her family eventually recognized our love and devotion to each other. They became very supportive, and Barbara's stepfather, Jack Gawler, became a close friend. He turned out to be one of the most inspirational men I would ever meet.

Barbara and I have now been happily married for nearly fifty years. Barbara has been a wonderful wife and an outstanding mother to our three children. I wish that I could claim to have been as successful a husband and father. I must confess, however, that I allowed my career to interfere. By today's standards, I probably did not hold up my end. Certainly we had nothing approaching the "50/50" relationship that has become the contemporary ideal. I must admit that the success of our marriage and our family is due to Barbara's devotion and hard work. I have come to wish that I had spent more time with my family. My children are wonderful people; I wish I knew them better. I have often counseled them to follow my advice, and not to imitate my deeds.

At the same time that Barbara and I decided to marry, I concluded that I should not continue my orthopaedic residency in South Carolina. I had learned that good residency programs included strong academic components. At higher-quality teaching institutions, lectures, conferences, and seminars were a regular part of the educational process. Columbia Hospital had not offered any such programming. I decided that for the sake of my future as an orthopaedic surgeon I had to get the missing experiences elsewhere.

During my residency in South Carolina, I did not know any residents at a higher level than I was at with whom to discuss the matter. In fact, during my entire residency training of five years, I never worked with a senior resident above me, supervising my activities and helping to show me "the ropes." That was unfortunate. It deprived me of the opportunity to learn from a colleague and of the healthy camaraderie that I later observed among residents. It also kept me from learning to be more of a "team player."

CREATING PROBLEMS

You might have thought that I had learned from experience. It was Simon Bolivar, the liberator of the Andean countries, who said that "judgment comes from experience and experience from bad judgment." You would expect that my chagrin at the American consulate in Bogota a few years earlier, or the shocking disappointment at Dr. Green's office in Boston would have taught me that one simply does not resign from a job before having secured its successor. That would certainly have been the wise course of action. Instead, I announced to the hospital administration that I would not remain for my last year of residency and that I had made plans for my final year of training elsewhere.

Then, after having severed my lifeline, I began sending applications to every orthopaedic program in the country. I was applying for a senior position. I assumed that my advanced training and years of being the most senior resident in my program would make it easy for me to secure the type of position I sought. As you can imagine, the response proved just as poor as the response three years before, when I had first sought a residency position.

In retrospect, I fully understand the perspective of these programs. Most had their own residents working their way through the chain of command. They had little need to hire an outsider, much less a graduate of an "unapproved" medical school who had trained at an undistinguished program in South Carolina. My only hope came from strong references, especially the support of Dr. Moore. As the weeks passed, however, I began to fear that even Dr. Moore's support would not prove sufficient.

Then I received a letter from Dr. Ralph Soto-Hall, director of the program at St. Joseph's Hospital in San Francisco. Remarkably, Dr. Soto-Hall, an extremely well-known surgeon who directed one of the Unites States' top orthopaedic programs, was offering me a position as senior resident beginning December 1, 1956.

I was elated. I not only had a job but I would also be able to complete my residency training at an outstanding academic hospital. Better yet, Barbara and I would be able to live in sunny, romantic California. (We did not yet know the difference between Hollywood and San Francisco.)

The bad news arrived a few days later: In order for me to serve as a resident, I would first have to pass the California State Medical Licensure examination. I had never taken an examination in the United States, or any examination written in English. I knew that my medical training in Colombia was not nearly as scientifically advanced as the classes in U.S. universities. I found the prospect of taking the California State Medical Licensure examination to be totally terrifying.

I was used to taking high risks myself. This time it was different. Barbara was pregnant and my mother had come to live with us. What would happen if we drove to San Francisco, only to have the job evaporate? What would I do then? We would be stranded on the West Coast of the United States. Most of our money would already have been spent. How would we survive? I believed, however, that I had no choice. Fate had again taken the upper hand. I would have to go to California and take my chances with the examination.

Barbara, my mother, and I spent our last three months in Charleston, where I took a series of basic science classes at the Medical College. Then we left Charleston for San Francisco. We stopped in Columbia to say good-bye to Barbara's parents. While Barbara visited with her family, I went to exchange farewells with my fellow residents at the hospital.

I told of the potential problems I was facing, and my dread of the California examination. It so happened that my junior resident had just completed his internship in Orlando, Florida. He asked if I had applied for residency there. I told him that I had written, but had never received an answer. He indicated that he was a "good friend" of Dr. Newton McCollough, the chief of the program in Orlando, and that he could ask Dr. McCollough why I had not received a response.

He called Dr. McCollough on the spot. Dr. McCollough said that he had just that day mailed a letter offering me the position. I knew that I could continue my training in Florida without a state medical license. We turned around immediately and instead of heading west to California, we proceeded south to sunny Florida. So much for existential free will! I became far more impressed with the wisdom of St. Augustine!

Dr. McCollough was a pioneer in orthopaedic education in Florida. He had originally conceived the idea of establishing a residency-training program in central Florida. He recognized that orthopaedics was a growing professional specialization. He believed that the only other Florida-based orthopaedics program, the group at the University of Miami, would not be able to meet the needs of the entire state

Despite his grand plans, however, he had not had many applicants for residency positions in his program. To this day, I suspect that my application had sat on his desk while he waited, futilely for something better. He must have eventually concluded that a South American kid with three years of training at a hospital in South Carolina was better than no resident at all. That is how I think I became the first Orlando trainee.

For me, however, the move to Orlando proved somewhat disappointing. The situation was almost a complete duplicate of my situation in South Carolina. In both cities, at both hospitals, I had become a resident in the program, presumably for lack of any other applicants. In Orlando, as in Columbia, the program had no educational component. I had turned down the outstanding program at Pittsburgh to go to Columbia, because of my own ignorance. This time, I turned down an appointment to the prestigious program in San Francisco because of my fear of the state licensing examination.

MY NEW MENTOR: NEWTON McCOLLOGH JR.

We arrived in Orlando the next day. I met with Dr. McCollough immediately. He made a deep impression on me from the first. A casual and most friendly gentleman, his style was far different from the courtly formality of South Carolina. He was wearing a short-sleeved shirt and no jacket. I had never seen a medical professional dressed that way. I tried not to let my surprise show on my face as my brain tried to deal with this latest culture shock. I could only guess that many things were going to be different here in tropical Florida.

Dr. McCollough took me on a tour of the hospital and gave me instructions concerning my new responsibilities. Then he took me to a bar just down the street from the hospital, where we drank and talked. Then he looked across the table at me and said, "Son, we are going to get along very well."

At the time, I was unaware of this casual southern usage of the word, "son." I was deeply impressed and felt extremely honored by the fact that he had addressed me in this manner, and had already come to think of me as a member of his family.

I immediately sat down and wrote a letter to Dr. Soto-Hall in San Francisco, explaining that I would not be joining his program. A few days later, I received a telegram from Dr. Soto-Hall. In the angriest terms, he wrote that I was legally obligated to honor the contract with his hospital. He expected me to report to duty in one week. If I accepted another position, elsewhere, he would report me to the American Board of Orthopaedics; I would never become a board-certified orthopaedist.

I immediately went to see Dr. McCollough and showed him the telegram. He read it, and without much thought replied, "You'd better go. Soto-Hall is very influential in medical politics." He told me that he and Dr. Soto-Hall had known each other while in military service. "Soto-Hall is the type of person who would not hesitate to follow through with his threat."

Dr. McCollough quickly realized that I had probably spent whatever money I had when I arrived in Orlando. Without my saying anything, he gave me a check for 500 dollars and told me I could repay him whenever I could.

I went back home to inform Barbara of the latest events. By the time I arrived at our apartment, I had already rented a trailer and hitched it to my old Chevy. We started to pack immediately. We would have to drive more than thirty-five hundred miles, and I wanted to start as soon as possible. By nighttime, we had already loaded our possessions.

My mind was in total turmoil. I was extremely relieved that my mother had returned home to Colombia and had not been caught up in this mess. I was truly frightened by the uncertainties facing us. I was afraid of the long drive facing us. I was also incredibly angry over the situation. As far as I was concerned, I had done nothing wrong. The problem lay with California and the state policies on licensing medical practitioners. My perfectly reasonable instinct for self-preservation had dictated my decision. I was disappointed that Dr. McCollough was willing to give in so easily. Why did I have to bow to this man in San Francisco and follow his dictates? Would I allow my life to be redirected at the whim of a man I had never met, simply because he was influential and capable of being vindictive?

In a remarkable moment of almost pure epiphany, I regained control of my life. I would not yield to unreasonable threats. I would not allow myself—and my family—to confront a week of driving at least five hundred miles per day, or the dreaded examination awaiting me in California. I asked Barbara to help me start unpacking. We were going to stay in Orlando.

The next morning, I walked into Dr. McCollough's office and told him that I had decided to stay. He responded that I was still welcome, and that he had to tell me again that I was making a grave mistake. I returned his $500 check and went to work as the first and only resident in the new program.

I was treated well in Orlando, and had many opportunities to observe others at work. The orthopaedists in the community were good surgeons; some of them were skillful, but teaching, in the academic sense, was not their avocation. There were no research activities under way, anywhere in the hospital. The staff held no formal conferences to advance the training and capabilities of the interns. It was a familiar but discouraging environment. I decided to learn as much as I could from the attending surgeons, and to read as much as possible.

BACK TO MEDICAL SCHOOL

As the months went by, the old restlessness returned. What was I to do when the year was up? Where was I going to practice? The medical school where I had graduated was not recognized by the U.S. accrediting boards responsible for graduate medical education in the United States. At the end of the year, I would have completed internship and residency requirements, but I would still have no medical license, and no way to get one. I shared my concerns with Dr. McCollough. Together, we concluded that my only option was to go back to medical school and get a degree from an approved U.S. medical school.

But how would I finance my schooling? We already had a baby at home.

McCollough was well known in Florida orthopaedic circles; he was also skilled in the practice of medical politics. He contacted Dr. Arthur Weiland, the chief of orthopaedics at the University of Miami. He suggested that I be admitted to the University of Miami medical school. In light of my extensive professional experience, the school would grant credit for two years of advanced standing. I could then graduate from the University of Miami in just two years. To finance my activities, Dr. McCollough suggested that I could work at Jackson Memorial Hospital as a senior resident.

Coincidentally, Dr. Weiland had a related difficulty. The person scheduled to serve as his senior resident at Jackson Memorial Hospital, the main teaching hospital of the university, had just announced that he would be leaving to open a private practice. Dr. Weiland urgently needed a replacement, and finding a qualified senior resident on such short notice could be extremely difficult. Dr. Weiland and Dr. McCollough recognized the obvious solution to both problems. Dr. Weiland, a full-time surgeon and part-time administrator, agreed to work out the details with the chief of surgery and the director of admissions at the medical school. A few days later, I was told that the plan had been fully approved. All I had to do was to go to Miami for an interview.

I realized the next two years were going to be difficult, but I could hardly wait to begin my life as a medical student. I had left medical school six years earlier. I found the idea of competing with younger students to be an irresistible challenge. The real burden, I knew, would fall to Barbara, who was faced with raising our son, virtually alone, while I became a full-time student and a full-time resident.

In early June 1957, I drove my old Chevy to Miami. I had placed my college, medical school, internship, and residency diplomas on the back seat of the car. Somewhere between Orlando and Miami, I felt the air in the car growing suffocating. My view of the road became blurry. I decided to stop for a few minutes to rest, and pulled over to the side of the road. When I got out, I saw and smelled smoke. I immediately grabbed my documents and threw them out of the car. Then I opened the trunk. Almost instantly, flames erupted and almost scorched my face.

I took off my shirt, soaked it in a creek next to the road, and threw it over the flames. Miraculously, the fire went out. A few seconds later, I realized how foolish I had been. Nothing was worth the risk that I had just taken. The gas tank could have exploded. Any of a million other things, all terrible, could have happened. I had been extremely fortunate, but I still had to get to Miami for the scheduled interview.

I was able to restart the car, but all of the lights and gauges on the dashboard had gone dead. I was afraid to stop anywhere, because I feared that I might not be able to start the car again. I was afraid to ask a mechanic for help, because I was afraid that he would insist on keeping the car, and prevent me from keeping my scheduled appointment in Miami. So I just kept driving.

My shirt was still wet, and still smelled of smoke when I arrived in Dr. Weiland's office. Our meeting was cordial, but I sensed a chilly distance in his reaction to me. I relaxed when he assured me that my official acceptance would soon be issued, and sent me to meet with Dr. John Farrell, the chief of the department of surgery at the medical school.

My meeting with Dr. Farrell was brief, and I did not ask for details concerning the manner in which I was to divide my time between my residency responsibilities and medical school chores. I did not even ask about my salary as a senior resident. I though there would be plenty of opportunities to deal with those issues at a later day. I drove back to Orlando. I was pleased with the apparent resolution of my problems. I looked forward to a new beginning and to having my trusty old Chevy repaired.

Barbara, our new son, Augusto Jr., and I drove to Miami a few days later. We immediately found a small apartment, not far from the hospital, and quickly settled in. The next day I started work as the chief resident. Again, I would be the only senior resident on staff. The other four residents were at lower levels of training. I was excited over the new position and found the other residents competent and friendly. I had the feeling I was going to have a great time. I could only assume that somehow I would have sufficient time to attend classes at the medical school.

Jackson Memorial Hospital was the largest hospital in the state of

Florida, and one of the busiest in the country. It handled an enormous number of cases. In those days, it was still segregated into "white" and "colored" wards. The "colored" wards were in a separate building, which was known as "The Colored Hospital." I still found the custom odd and distasteful. I had been in the South for four years, but I had never become used to this peculiar kind of institutionalized racial prejudice.

I must, in defense of Jackson Memorial, note that except for the different complexion of the patients, the "colored" wards did not look any different than the "white" ones. And in my years at Jackson Memorial, I never had any cause to believe that any of the residents or any member of the medical staff ever deliberately provided a lower standard of care to patients in the "colored." wards. The same "separate but equal" standard of care had been maintained in South Carolina.

Outside the hospital, there was gross and flagrant discrimination against the African American residents of Miami. I could not avoid comparing the treatment of the black by the white in the United States with the way the low classes were discriminated against in my native Colombia. In Latin America, we had none of the official, institutional segregation that was practiced throughout the southeastern United States. In Latin America, however, the wealthier classes typically discriminated against the poor in ways that were, to me, far more offensive.

On one occasion, I remember seeing our elderly maid carrying a huge basket full of groceries to supply my mother's store. I told my mother that I thought we were being cruel. The old woman could barely walk at the end of the twenty blocks of labor. My mother turned and faced me almost with anger. I cannot forget the expression on her face. She seemed to be saying, "That is the way things are. What do you expect? If she doesn't carry the heavy basket, who is going to carry it?"

In her way, she was right. If the maid did not do the job, there was no one else to do it. But even to this day, I am deeply disturbed by the rampant social injustices that I see throughout the world. The growing gap between the rich and the poor is not right. Unless we find a simple, peaceful remedy, we may someday face a major upheaval of universal propositions.

The collapse of the communist movement of the twentieth century does not mean that Marx was completely wrong. History continues its unending march. To me, the Hegelian dialectic seems to be a continuing force for change. The creation of synthesis has not been cancelled but only postponed. The "end of history," which Fukuyama has defined as having taken place with the apparent acceptance of liberal democracy throughout the world, may not become a reality. Though I agree that liberal democracy should be the most desirable among of all systems thus far tried, it may not prove to be successful in the long run. History has managed to disappoint generation after generation, despite the most optimistic expectations. Samuel Huntington, in book *The Clash of Civilizations*, quotes Arnold Toynbee and makes reference to the English historian's remarks about the "mirage of immortality" that made previous empires suspect that theirs was the final form of human society.

To avoid a violent upheaval, the world's wealthiest classes and nations—not just in the United States, but everywhere—must find a peaceful path to a more equitable distribution of wealth and health care. The current sweeping interest in globalization may be in the final analysis nothing more than an aggravation of the existing problem of inequality. The realization of the pervasive trend that continues to exploit the poor has made me lean over the years to the few politicians who appeared to be sincere in their desire to change the status quo; Robert Kennedy was one of them.

A few days after beginning my work at Jackson Memorial Hospital in Miami I asked when my classes would begin at the medical school, and requested a list of appropriate subjects. I received no answer. In response to my further inquiry, the admissions office denied any knowledge of having seen an application on my behalf.

I soon discovered the issue concerning my entering medical school training had never been officially addressed; worse yet, well-established university policies prevented the school from approving the plan that allegedly had been worked out for me. Dr. McCollough and I had been cheated. Dr. Weiland needed a senior resident for his program, so he had led us to believe that our plan for me to enter the medical school had been consummated. In fact, Dr. Weiland had made no effort on my behalf.

I never raised the issue again. As the medical administrators had anticipated, I feared that any protest on my part would cause them to terminate my residency. They knew that I could not afford to have that happen.

So, once again, I found myself working as a hospital resident, although I had already met all requirements necessary to practice my profession.

Despite repeatedly finding myself in the same trap, I was also always extremely fortunate. Repeatedly, I found outstanding orthopaedic surgeons who, for whatever reason, took a liking to me, helped and guided me, and taught me what they could. A few remarkable, highly talented, devoted professionals like Bill Vargas in Bogota, Samuel Yachnin in Passaic, Austin Moore and Barney Freeman in Columbia, Newton McCollough in Orlando, and several others in Miami gave those years great value. It was these men, together with my own instinct to rise to any challenge, that kept me from becoming another victim of a damnable system.

As a past president of the American Academy of Orthopaedic Surgery, I must say that I understand the concerns that led the United States to close its doors to foreign trainees. Many of these trainees, like me, end up permanently residing in this country. We represent a competitive threat to native-born citizens who attend established medical schools at great cost. Yet, surely wealthy nations such as the United States have some degree of responsibility toward residents of other, less fortunate lands.

I suspect that if the great political thinkers in the United States really sought to solve this problem, they could find a way to do so. Surely, there is a way to provide high-quality advanced education and training to graduates of medical schools in developing nations. The United States may have an overabundance of physicians, but the rest of the world does not. I do not believe that it is right for my adopted homeland, the United States, to simply close its doors to those seeking medical knowledge and training.

The issue is complicated. It will not be easily resolved; as H. L. Mencken said, "For every difficult question there is a simple answer, and it is wrong." The U.S. medical organizations have worked to control the number of physicians practicing in the United States by controlling the number of medical school graduates. At the same time, foreign-educated doctors find themselves drawn to the United States by high wages and outstanding medical facilities.

I must also recognize sins of physicians like myself, who choose not to return to our native countries. We have deprived our own countrymen of our acquired skills. We have contributed to the ills of our nations rather than to their amelioration. Over my career, I have contributed to my profession and to the science of orthopaedics. I have helped thousands of patients to a better quality of life. But I must always feel the guilt of not fulfilling my personal responsibility by failing to return to my family, friends, and countrymen in Colombia so they could benefit from my medical skills.

chapter 12.
light at the end of the tunnel

"Men have been born for the sake of one another. Either teach them or bear with them."

—Marcus Aurelius

In the late 1950s, the babies who eventually constituted the "baby boom" were making their appearances all over the United States. State health authorities began to realize that students were not coming through the medical school pipeline rapidly enough to meet the needs of growing populations. They began to rethink laws designed to protect the existing medical establishment, and a few states, including Maryland, began to allow graduates of foreign medical schools to sit for medical licensure examinations.

I had finally accepted the reality that I had no possibility of obtaining a medical license in Florida. I applied for a license in the state of Maryland, and drove to Baltimore where I sat for the examination. My old nemesis, chemistry, did me in. Because of my weakness in the chemistry exam, I scored one point below the passing grade.

A few months later, I returned to Baltimore and sat again for the medical licensure exam. This time I passed. I returned to Florida with the knowledge that when I finished the year in Miami, I could, hopefully, win employment as a fully licensed staff orthopaedic surgeon at a hospital in Maryland.

During my two trips to Baltimore my father-in-law, Jack Gawler, had accompanied me. (Jack was actually Barbara's stepfather). He had just turned fifty. He was a remarkable man and a delightful companion. He was also one of the most inspirational people I have ever met.

Jack had discovered that he was afflicted with a serious condition in his right eye while in college, most likely macular degeneration, a condition that usually produces gradual damage to the eye leading to complete blindness. Realizing that the loss of his other eye was inevitable, he took advantage of the brief window of opportunity to learn braille. He also began an intensive study of blindness, and practiced functioning without his remaining sight. By the time his left eye failed, he had read everything available and taught himself everything possible about the art of functioning as a blind man. He sharpened his remaining senses remarkably. I remember that when we drove to Baltimore, he demonstrated that he could tell how fast I was going just by the feel of the car and the sounds of the wind and the road. He would say, "Now you are going 60 miles an hour." He was just as accurate as the car's speedometer. He also had a remarkable memory, and carried an accurate mental map of every city or town he had ever visited.

As you might suspect of someone who would rise to a desperate situation with such remarkable class, wisdom, control, and foresight, Jack has led a fulfilling and productive life. He was already blind when he married the divorced mother of three young children, the youngest of whom would one day become my wife.

His favorite recreational activity was listening to baseball games on the radio. I can only imagine his distress when, later in life, he began to lose his hearing. For his last ten years, he was totally deaf and blind. He still refused to give in to adversity or to see himself as a victim. He retained his sense of humor and continued to make self-deprecating jokes about the problems he encountered in his daily life. Voltaire could have gotten inspiration for his *Candide* from Jack's remarkable example.

As he aged, Jack continued to enjoy a daily swim in the public pool near his home. One day, however, he was notified that he could no longer use the facility. Other people had complained that his lack of vision had, on occasion, inconvenienced them. The authorities felt that his swimming had become "a threat to the safety of others." Our species' remarkable capacity for cruelty continues to amaze me. Man's insensitivity to man, as Erich Fromm said in his book *The Anatomy of Human Destructiveness*, is limitless.

Jack's wife, Barbara's mother, stood unflinchingly by his side. Now in her late eighties, she had developed Parkinson's disease. That made it difficult for her to help her ninety-year-old husband. I believe that only their lifelong deep and sincere Christian faith made it possible for them to endure and thrive despite their incredible ordeal. When, on occasion, I find my own faith flagging, I seek and find inspiration in the faith of this remarkable couple.

After getting my medical license in Maryland, I began to send letters to orthopaedic offices in Baltimore offering my services at the end of the year. There were no takers. I wrote to the hospitals and public health agencies in West Virginia. A clinic in Morgantown, heavily involved in the care of miners, requested my curriculum vitae. Our negotiations progressed satisfactorily. I began to prepare my family for our coming journey to West Virginia, and to think about the year that I was just completing.

My year at Jackson Memorial Hospital had provided many highly memorable opportunities and experiences. As chief orthopaedic resident at one of the largest teaching hospitals in the United States, I had a wealth of clinical material at my disposal and received valuable training in medical, surgical, and administrative skills. I took advantage of the situation. I also did my best not only to increase my own knowledge but also to function as a role model for the other residents.

The younger residents were fine people. Many of them proved to be bright and enthusiastic. Every day, at 6:30 A.M., we began our rounds. Every day, we visited every patient on the service. Because of the pressure of other duties, our rounds had to be conducted quickly. By 8:00 A.M., some of the residents had to be in surgery and others were due in the outpatient clinics. I always made sure that our visits with the patients were effective and beneficial from an educational point of view.

Sometimes, the lessons we learned on rounds could be extremely discouraging. One morning, a resident who had just begun his senior year, was proudly telling us about the busy and productive night he had. He had performed several surgical procedures. Everything had gone well. When our group reached the bedside of an elderly lady whose hip he had replaced (following a broken hip resulting from a fall), he called loudly, "Miss Blain." He awaited her response. Assuming she was asleep, he touched her shoulder and called even louder, "Miss Blain." Miss Blain did not move. Miss Blain was dead.

We moved to the next room. At that moment, we heard the loud noise of a large metal object on wheels moving on the hard surface of the floor. A large black man appeared to be carrying a hospital bed on his back. Then we saw that he was fastened to the frame of the bed by a rope that connected his skull to sand bags. The man had broken his neck the night before. His doctors had drilled holes in his skull and had inserted tongs connected to weights. This type of traction was the standard procedure used at the time to prevent damage to the spinal cord.

Apparently, the patient was suffering from alcohol withdrawal symptoms. The man was extremely strong, but totally helpless in the grip of delirium tremens, irrational behavior that often affects alcoholics when alcohol is suddenly withdrawn. Because the bed did not fit through the door, he inadvertently slammed it into the doorframe. With one last Herculean attempt to smash his way through the doorway, he applied so much force that he dislocated his fractured cervical spine. He instantly dropped to the floor, dead. He had effectively hanged himself.

Despite such episodes, work at the hospital filled me with enthusiasm. Although I was not attending medical school classes, the academic environment became more and more attractive to me. That attraction became even more powerful with the arrival of a newly assigned full-time division head, Dr. Wallace Miller.

Dr. Miller was barely ten years older than I was, but he had received outstanding training. A graduate of Harvard Medical School, he completed his residency at Indiana University, where he had also served as a full-time member of the faculty. He appreciated the fact that I was very much interested in helping out with the education of the residents. He took an active interest in my activities and my work.

I had become a good surgeon who was not afraid to tackle any problem that came along. The residents began to depend upon me a great deal. I made myself available to them around the clock—days, nights, and weekends. I had remained a good student and read every available journal and book dealing with orthopaedic surgery. I also discovered that I thoroughly enjoyed sharing my knowledge with medical students and residents.

Just before the end of the year, as I was completing preparations for my move to West Virginia, Dr. Miller offered me a faculty position in the division. Since I did not have a medical license in Florida, I would not be able to have my own practice. I would only be able to assist others perform surgery on indigent patients. As an instructor, my salary would be only $5,000 a year. In West Virginia, I would have been fully licensed and able to start a private practice in addition to my hospital responsibilities. I would have been an attending physician, and would have been paid substantially more money. Yet, I found the prospect of becoming a member of the faculty at the University of Miami to be irresistible. I had fallen in love with academic medicine; I accepted Dr. Miller's offer.

Living on such a small salary was not easy. As usual, the burden fell primarily on Barbara, who handled it with her usual quiet strength and grace. Because she was working as a nurse at the hospital, we took our son, Gus Jr., to a preschool during her working hours. I am sure that Barbara found it extremely difficult to be parted from Gus, and to place him under the care of others.

Barbara scheduled her work in such a manner that both of us could take turns being with our son, and we thoroughly enjoyed the child and our life as new parents. I created as much time as I could to be with him, though I was always on call at the hospital. Happily, we lived only a few miles from the beach. That made it easy for our family to enjoy the tropical life of Florida.

Many residents of the university lived in the same small apartment community located just two blocks from the hospital. (Sadly, it was equally near the city incinerator.) Two doors down the street lived Tom Starzl, a surgical resident who later became the "father" of liver transplants in the United States. Newton McCollough III, who would precede me as president of the American Academy of Orthopaedic Surgeons, also lived nearby. It was an active, stimulating academic community.

It was there that our daughter, Janette, was born. We named her after the popular singer and actress Jeanette McDonald, who performed with Nelson Eddy. Only years later did I discover the spelling error. Janette has grown to be a marvelous person. It appears, however, that she has inherited her singing ability from me, rather than from her namesake.

With the birth of our second child, my mother returned to the United States. Barbara went back to work, and my mother took care of the two children during our absence from home. Despite my low income, we were comfortable and happy. Eventually, however, problems associated with my low salary began to emerge. I watched enviously as my own formerly junior residents graduated and began lucrative private practices. Barbara, too, had to look on, as their wives were able to quit working, become full-time housewives, and moved

to better neighborhoods. We knew that there was no way we would
be able stretch my meager academic income so far. Even with our two
incomes, Barbara and I were barely able to make ends meet.

Then, although I continued to enjoy academic medicine, my formerly close relationship with Dr. Miller began deteriorating. Gradually, he seemed to be rescinding opportunities and authority. I could
not understand why, because I thought I was doing a good job.

Anxious to develop an area of expertise that would not infringe
on Dr. Miller's territory, I proposed that he permit me to start a hand
surgery program within the division. He agreed, and I proceeded to
see patients with hand injuries and to follow them on a scheduled
outpatient clinic day. Clifford Snyder, an excellent plastic surgeon in
town, offered his support. Soon, residents from both general surgery
and orthopaedics were calling me with hand-related problems. I
studied the relevant journals and literature, even as I acquired clinical
experience. I was beginning to think that I could become a top-flight
hand surgeon when, without warning or explanation, Dr. Miller took
the program away from me and decided to run it himself.

I accepted the change with equanimity and set out to find a different opportunity. I had enjoyed spine surgery since my earlier days
as a resident of Austin Moore. (The national orthopaedic community
regarded Dr. Moore as a stellar hip surgeon, but I knew that he actually preferred to work on the spine.) I organized and managed a spine
clinic.

My career as a spine expert ended in much the same way as my
work on hands. Dr. Miller decided there was no need to separate
patients with spinal complaints from the other orthopaedic patients.
Philosophically, I agreed with his position. Even then, I was beginning
to feel uncomfortable with the idea of exaggerated subspecialization.
My philosophical understanding, however, did little to prevent my
growing resentment of Dr. Miller's actions.

This time, I chose to start a hip and knee clinic. Unlike the spine,
problems of the hips and knees typically seem to exist in relative isolation from the rest of the musculoskeletal system.

At first, Dr. Miller left me alone in this new endeavor. In fact, he
seemed supportive of my efforts. Then he announced a new policy,
under which he would personally direct all future activities of the
participating faculty. I was the only individual member of the full-
time faculty. All others were voluntary faculty. He informed me that

my time in the operating room with the residents would be limited to every other Tuesday afternoon. This policy change took away both my close relationships with the residents and curtailed my ability to continue exploring a new surgical specialty.

Then in 1960, two years after I had completed my residency and become an instructor, Florida fell in line with other states: it changed its law regarding the licensing of graduates of foreign medical schools. With the stroke of the governor's pen, I was suddenly eligible to sit for the examinations of the Florida Medical Board.

I knew that by obtaining my Florida license, I would not only be able to increase my income substantially but would also significantly increase my freedom of action. I would no longer be totally at the mercy of the University of Miami or of Dr. Miller. I took the exams at the earliest opportunity; again my lack of advanced coursework in basic science proved a handicap; I flunked bacteriology. I passed on my second attempt, and finally secured the right to practice my profession.

Later that year, I swore allegiance to the United States and became a naturalized citizen of my new country. At last, I was able to expand my horizons. I knew that I would allow nothing to impede my success as an academic orthopaedist. Had I been a better student of my own life history, I would have known that the real struggle was just about to begin.

chapter 13.
a full-fledged practitioner

"Errare humanum est."

"It is sobering, humiliating and tragic to realize that in all we do all suffer from the limitations of the knowledge of our time."

—John Silber

In 1960, eight years after graduating from medical school, I finally held a license to practice medicine in the state in which I resided and in which I was employed. I was delighted that, for the first time, I would be able to treat patients on my own. My family was thrilled that I would *finally* begin to earn a respectable income. All of us took great pleasure in knowing that, at last, I would assume my place in the community as a full-fledged professional.

To my added delight, the hospital provided me with my own private office. It was located behind the office of the chief of urology, and was barely big enough to accommodate a desk, but it was mine. I had no secretary, but Doctor Miller's secretary kindly volunteered to type correspondence for me, and to provide other necessary clerical assistance.

My first private patient was an older man who was referred to me by a radiologist at Doctors' Hospital in Coral Gables. He arrived with what appeared to be a simple fracture of his upper arm. I ordered the appropriate X rays and proceeded to treat the fracture with a cast and a sling. The case seemed simple, but it marked my transition to a full-fledged physician.

The patient, however, continued to have more pain than I expected. Two weeks later, I ordered a second set of X rays. To my surprise and chagrin, I realized that the fracture had taken place over an area where cancer had extended and destroyed the surrounding bone. In those days, the prognosis for such pathology was extremely poor.

While I had treated the fracture itself correctly, I had missed a serious, fatal pathology. I would have to tell the patient what had happened. Then I would have to inform him about his true condition. It was not such a simple case after all, and proved to be a memorable introduction to the private practice of medicine. The man died a few months later.

My next patient was a young man who was experiencing wrist pain after an injury sustained and treated a year earlier. I ordered X rays and made the diagnosis. The pain resulted from an ununited fracture of the young man's navicular bone, one of the small bones in the hand. I assured him that I could correct the problem, and took him to surgery to repair the defect.

I had spent two years assisting the orthopaedic residents, but had not been permitted to do surgery on my own. The residents were well aware of the significance of this occasion. The two senior residents on duty followed me into the operating room, loudly proclaiming that I was likely to need a great deal of help since I had probably forgotten how to operate. They enjoyed their little joke immensely.

Happily, the procedure went well. At the end, I joined in the humorous spirit of the moment and turned the tables on them. I jokingly pretended to be an important surgeon who was too busy with other duties to handle routine tasks myself. I said to them, as solemnly as I could, "You close the wound and report to me later." I left the room smiling at my success and at the good-hearted kidding.

Later that evening, before going home, I stopped at the X ray department to look at the films of my young patient's wrist that I had ordered taken shortly after the surgery. Much to my amazement and incredible embarrassment, I discovered that I had placed the metallic staples incorrectly. The staples are used to immobilize the nonunited bone fragments. The fragments should have been stapled to each other. The X rays showed, however, that instead of bridging the bony fragments of the ununited fracture, I had tied a fragment of the broken bone to the next normal bone. I would have to do the operation over.

My first thought was to go home and have a drink or two while I considered how to tell the patient about my mistake. Instead, I decided not to postpone the inevitable. I went straight up to his room where he lay, still in pain from the day's surgery, and gave him the bad news. I told him that I had made a mistake and that I would have to correct it. I would be taking him to surgery, again, the next day.

Needless to say, he was deeply disturbed, but he allowed me to continue with his case. I performed the second surgery without difficulty or complications. The patient went home a few days later, and moved to Louisiana a few months later. I would have understood fully had he never wished to hear my name again. Instead, we kept in touch and exchanged Christmas cards for several years.

The experience taught me an extremely important lesson: I have always been totally honest with patients, and have never hidden anything from any of them. I have always adhered to that premise, and never deviated from it. I have also sought to teach all my students that we must acknowledge errors as soon as they are discovered. Prompt disclosure of the truth is, by far, the best medicine, the best medical policy, and the only ethical way to manage this kind of difficult situation.

The young man with the ununited fracture could have litigated against me and probably would have won. He had good grounds. I had no defense. I believe that my candor with him made him realize that the mistake had been innocently made. I know that he understood that his welfare had been my first concern. He knew that I had done everything possible to correct the mistake, and to make sure that his arm healed fully and completely, as quickly as possible.

Not long after that the episode involving the young man with his broken wrist, the wife of a well-known rabbi from Miami Beach came to see me. She was suffering from an uncommon disease that had caused major damage to her hips. She was probably in her mid-forties, but so severely incapacitated that she was not just bedridden, but totally incapable of any movement while in bed. Any attempts to spread her legs to clean herself produced excruciating pain. Her condition was demeaning and pathetic.

The family had come to me because the surgery, which involved replacement of the hips with prosthetic joints, had been widely publicized and was becoming popular. Their own physician had told them about the procedure but seemed unsure about the extent to which it would help in her case. They also knew that hip surgery was still somewhat experimental. They had also learned that Dr. Austin Moore in Columbia, South Carolina, was the nation's leading hip surgeon, and that I had studied with him.

After my examination, I knew that the chances of successfully restoring the woman's mobility and eliminating her pain were extremely slight. The damage caused by the disease was simply too extensive. The family, however, pleaded with me to try. The patient assured me that she was willing to take the risk. Despite my reservations, I agreed to go ahead with the hip replacement.

As I scrubbed for the procedure, I looked through the window into the operating room. The woman lay on the table. I watched the anesthesiologist doing his job. I watched the nurses preparing the equipment and completing preparations on my patient. I looked at her face as she slept on the table. I thought about her desperation. I thought about her family's hopes.

I then remembered the day in South Carolina when I had challenged Dr. Boyd's authority under similar circumstances. Suddenly I was seized by self-doubts. I questioned my ability and the ethical legitimacy of the decision that I had made. I cancelled the surgery and instructed the anesthesiologist to awaken the patient.

I then headed toward the waiting room where her husband, the rabbi, was waiting to be informed of the outcome of surgery. I sat down next to him and said, "I have canceled the surgery. To continue would have been to abuse the trust that you have placed in me. There is too small a chance of success, and too high a risk of complications. This case is beyond my powers as a surgeon. Had I operated under these circumstances, I would have been playing God."

The rabbi's face filled with great disappointment, but he said nothing. After a few minutes of silence, he turned to me. He said that he understood the meaning of my remarks and thanked me for my honesty. I suggested that the family consult a neurosurgeon and consider a different procedure. I told him about an operation with a high likelihood of ending her pain. It would, however, mean that she would never walk again.

The family followed my advice to consult a neurosurgeon, and agreed that the alternate procedure would be the best course of action. The woman had that surgery. She became confined to her wheelchair, but free of pain. My professional relationship with the family remained good. I know that they appreciated my actions that day in the operating suite.

As you can see, building a private practice did not come easily. The slowness of the process, however, did not bother me. I was enjoying the new opportunity. I knew that sooner or later, I would find success. I was willing to wait.

My main preoccupation remained the growth of my academic career, which seemed to me to be moving far too slowly. I believed that my division head, Dr. Miller, was preventing me from pursuing expanded clinical and research interests. I decided that I needed to become more assertive; the relationship between the two of us continued to worsen. It appeared that nothing I could say or do would please him.

I grew increasingly uncomfortable and began to question myself. I remembered our initial close relationship and thought that I must have done something wrong. It became an obsession. I was spending every free moment reviewing the history of my relationship with Dr. Miller. Finally, I reached the inevitable conclusion. I had done nothing wrong.

What can I say? I was still a young man. I could not, at the time, see that my own approach to the situation, rather than being reasonable and compromising, had become rigid and stubborn. With crystal-clear hindsight over the last four decades and then some, I can see that I had not matured enough to handle this delicate relationship in a reasonable way. At the time, however, I began to tell myself that Dr. Miller's unreasonable rigidity must be the result of fear and jealousy.

I was a young man, barely getting started in the academic world. He was a full professor and chief of a division. I had graduated from an unknown medical school in Colombia. Dr. Miller had graduated from Harvard. Virtually no one in orthopaedics knew my name. Dr. Miller had already established a substantial reputation, and was well on the way to becoming known around the country. I guess, perhaps, that he was not jealous of me. I can now see that to the extent that he was aware of my activities, he probably found my immaturity irritating and annoying. Apparently, however, he valued my work sufficiently to continue putting up with me.

SEEKING ADVICE

At the time, of course, I remained convinced that Dr. Miller needed correction. I decided to meet with Dr. Arthur Weiland, the former chief of orthopaedics. I knew Dr. Weiland was highly regarded in Miami, and I had already tried to forget that just a few years earlier, he had orchestrated the plan that had brought me to Jackson Memorial Hospital. While that plan had solved Dr. Weiland's need for a senior resident, he had not been able to deliver on the promise that I could earn my medical degree from the University of Miami. As a result, I had almost left Miami for West Virginia. I had not forgotten that Dr. Weiland had been instrumental in bringing Dr. Miller to Miami.

Dr. Weiland received me in his office, and I presented my view of the growing chasm between Dr. Miller and me. I said, "Our relationship is very tense and I feel incapable of making any progress in my work. What should I do?"

Dr. Weiland knew exactly how to handle an ambitious young foreigner who did not know his place. He knew just how to manipulate an overgrown ego. His voice crackled with authority as he looked directly at me and replied, "Leave town. There is no room for the two of you in Miami." This was not the response that I had been eagerly anticipating. I stood up, thanked him, and went back to work.

During my more than twenty years as a department head at the University of Miami and at USC, I have frequently thought about that conversation. As you can imagine, a medical school department head must frequently mediate conflicts between staff members. I was also often consulted by young physicians in the department, ambitious, energetic young doctors who thought themselves unappreciated or unfairly treated by others.

I have always taken my conference with Dr. Weiland as an abject lesson in poor personnel management and bad administration. Delicate situations such as the one I was experiencing must be handled more sympathetically. I never forgot my brief meeting with Dr. Weiland. It took him less than ten seconds to instill an indelible lesson that has lasted ever since.

Successful surgeons in general and medical administrators in particular seem especially vulnerable to arrogance. They find themselves with power over other people's lives and careers. They yield to the temptation of hubris.

Hubris, the Greek concept that resembles our own sin of pride, is the "fatal flaw" that destroys the central figures of most classical Greek tragedies. Heroes such as Oedipus become infected by a Promethean hubris. They come to believe that they can defy fate and challenge the powers of the gods. Inevitably, their hubris brings them to a tragic end. Our culture has restated the concept in other, more familiar words: "Pride goeth before destruction and a haughty spirit before a fall."

In our everyday lives, humdrum administrators all too often find themselves overcome by what was once a flaw of heroes. Hubris overpowers many people who find themselves in authority before they have learned enough to use that power wisely. They justify their acts as expressions of forcefulness, leadership ability, and "willingness to make the hard decisions." Without second thoughts, they consciously, often deliberately, hurt many of the people under their control.

I must admit that I did not recognize those flaws at the time, and I didn't realize the danger that Dr. Weiland's narrowmindedness represented to me personally, to many of my colleagues, and to our patients. Only later did my eyes open sufficiently to recognize that even physicians could possess grossly flawed characters.

Dr. Weiland probably thought that he had made his point and that I would soon be leaving town. He came close to being right. I began to look for a job. I let the local orthopaedists know that I was available and would like to take a position in a private office. I found their response gratifying and encouraging; I received several offers to join established, lucrative practices.

The prospect of leaving the university and going into private practice delighted Barbara. She had grown increasingly dissatisfied with the low salary and with my frustration with the deteriorating relationship with Dr. Miller. She happily looked forward to a future of shorter hours, more pay, and less anxiety. She probably also hoped that a change to private practice would enable me to spend more time with our growing family.

I came close to accepting a job that would have instantly quadrupled my income. The generous offer even included a guarantee of rapid future financial growth. The surgeon who made the offer was highly respected, ethical, and successful. I would have enjoyed working with him. Yet, I continued to search for a way to improve my position and income, but to stay in academic medicine. I finally decided to stay with the university, and work through my current difficulties.

With a somewhat delayed flash of brilliant insight, I also decided that it was not Dr. Miller's responsibility to accommodate me but my responsibility to do whatever was necessary to persuade Dr. Miller that I could be an asset to his program, rather than a hindrance. It had become obvious to me that my questioning the rationale and wisdom of some of Dr. Miller's comments and attitudes was not conducive to improvement of a difficult and awkward situation.

I began to stay away from division conferences and meetings. When I attended meetings, I tried to remain quiet. I also tried to make myself indispensable by volunteering to assist in areas where others were not anxious to participate, rather than seeking out highly visible, exciting activities. I accepted my assigned responsibilities without complaint, and stopped attempting to assume authority beyond my position. In short, I stopped playing the prodigy and became a team player. This newly acquired wisdom eventually paid off at the University of Miami, just as it does in most organizations.

chapter 14.
in love with academia

"The greater the hubris the greater God's punishment."

—Plato

The University of Miami, in the early 1960s, had a nationwide reputation. Unfortunately, it was known not for academic rigor but for parties, beach sports, and football. It was popularly referred to as "Sunshine U." At the same time, the city of Miami was known primarily as an adjunct to Miami Beach, a winter resort for wealthy refugees from northern snows, and as the jumping-off point for the Florida Keys. We faculty members at the medical school found ourselves bound together by a mutual determination to win respect for ourselves and an identity for our medical school.

Only now, in thinking back about those early years on the faculty at the University of Miami, have I realized that they comprised my first true experience with professional "colleagues." In Passaic, New Jersey, I had been isolated by language and my recent arrival in the United States. In South Carolina and Orlando, Florida, and even during the first year at Miami, I had been virtually alone—the only resident with senior responsibilities yet no hope of advancement. Only when I received my Florida medical license and won appointment as a university instructor did I finally move into a status that I shared with others.

Our research experiences at the University of Miami were of a rather unsophisticated nature. In orthopaedics, we had no financial resources for research at all, and no significant physical resources. We would have been grateful for the opportunity to work on a shoestring, but there were no strings to be had.

We were, however, young, creative, and imaginative, so we did not allow such minor concerns to keep us from trying to carry out some investigative studies. Since the fractured hip had fascinated me since my earlier days under Dr. Moore, I attempted to conduct my own crude experiments with hip joints.

Over the years, we had built up a close and mutually supportive relationship with the chief coroner and medical examiner for Dade County. He was a remarkably knowledgeable and forceful individual. He facilitated our research by helping us obtain autopsy material. Whenever a patient died following hip surgery, the coroner allowed us to remove the entire hip joint. The directors at various nursing homes in the area also notified us upon the death of any indigent patient with a history of hip fracture.

From the bones we had obtained in the hospital morgue, I managed to collect a large number of specimens. We then designed and built a set of homegrown devices to help us compare the different surgical techniques of the day. James Hobbs, a professional engineer later to become a friend, converted an automobile jack into one of our first laboratory devices. It allowed me to subject bony specimens to mechanical loading. We did not have a lab, so I conducted the studies in the X ray department of Jackson Memorial Hospital's emergency room. Whenever the X ray technician had time, he would take pictures while I held the broken bone together and used the converted automobile jack to apply load to the joint.

The bone I had removed from the deceased patient was secured to the modified automotive jack with plaster of paris. A gauge would record the pressure I applied to the head of the bone. After I applied a few pounds, the technician took an X ray. I then added a few more pounds and requested another X ray. This was repeated several times until we heard the noise of the collapsing bone, indicating that the nail we had used to fix the fracture no longer held the pieces of bone together.

Remarkably, regardless of their crudeness, the experiments proved to be extraordinarily valuable. We published the results, which advanced understanding of how surgical procedures help stabilize broken hips. These experiments with our "Rube Goldberg" laboratory equipment earned the first professional recognition for our small team at Jackson Memorial—and for me.

About thirty years later, my engineer friend who helped our team's research career came to my office. He was suffering from advanced arthritis in one of his hips. We joked about the old apparatus that he had built for us by modifying an automobile jack. We talked about the many changes that had taken place in both of our careers. Then I replaced the diseased joint. The operation alleviated his pain and restored his mobility. I wonder how often anyone becomes such a direct beneficiary of a past accomplishment!

My discovery of perceived benefits of becoming a team player brought not only a new peace of mind but also a substantial improvement in my relationship with Dr. Miller. Coincidentally, it also brought more rapid growth of my reputation beyond the walls of the university, and a new relationship with an old friend. I was deeply moved when Austin Moore, my mentor from Columbia, South Carolina, approached me with an offer to join his practice. Dr. Moore had developed a keen interest in my career and had a very high opinion of me; he probably felt that practicing together would be mutually beneficial.

Many states were becoming increasingly aware of their growing shortage of physicians, even nearly a decade after the Korean War. Because of that shortage, young physicians found themselves actively sought after by employers throughout the nation. That, in turn, created an administrative nightmare for state medical authorities, as physicians began seeking licensure in many different jurisdictions.

Most of the states moved to adopt the obvious solution—reciprocal licensing of physicians. Because I had passed examinations in Florida and Maryland, I could now be licensed in South Carolina as well. Austin Moore wrote to me and promised that if I would return to Columbia and join his practice, he would personally handle the paperwork with the state medical office. He also offered to guarantee a salary far higher than what I was earning at the University of Miami.

I went to Columbia to renew our acquaintance and discuss the offer in more detail. I took great pleasure in seeing him again. He, too, must have enjoyed our visit. He promised to make me a full partner in just in three years, and offered to lend me the money I would need to make a down payment on an "appropriate" house. I almost agreed to the generous terms expressed by my old mentor, but I returned to Miami without making any kind of commitment. I told Dr. Moore that I wanted to discuss the move with Barbara, although I knew that she would be thrilled by the prospect of returning to her hometown. I was right about her reaction, but, much to my amazement, I discovered that I had been wrong about my own feelings. I remembered that Dr.

Moore's relationships with his colleagues in Columbia were not always smooth. I wondered how some of them would react to my return. As the days passed, my second thoughts grew to become serious reservations.

Mostly, I found myself increasingly concerned that I would be smothered by Austin's outstanding reputation. I knew that I would always be known as "Doctor Moore's assistant," and never for my own accomplishments. The practice would always remain as he had built it. It would never take off in new directions. Finally, I feared the loss of the "team" feeling that I had developed at the university; I also feared losing the intellectual stimulation of the academic community. I wrote Dr. Moore a long letter expressing my concerns.

Much to my amazement, Dr. Moore made every effort to change my mind. He had promised that from the beginning he would introduce me to society as his associate, not as his assistant. He reiterated the financial advantages of the promised arrangement, and wrote eloquently about the freedom of private practice. I was tempted, but again, I chose to stay at Miami. Our relationship became quite tense for a while, following my decision. I realized that I had disappointed him deeply. He also probably felt betrayed. After a while we regained the friendliness of earlier years, and he continued to offer me the benefit of his wisdom and advice. Less than two years later, he died, suddenly, at the age of sixty-three. I had often heard him say that he wanted to die while performing surgery, assisted by someone who could take over without difficulty. That is precisely how his life ended.

I immediately flew to South Carolina; I felt orphaned. In a letter of condolence to his wife I presumptuously referred to myself as the "heir to his intellectual heritage." I felt no one had learned as much from him as I had; no one else had continued to promulgate his philosophy and teachings as much as I had.

I found the funeral to be more than I could bear. I have never been good at handling emotional stress. The art of maintaining outward strength while experiencing inner turmoil is beyond me. I told myself that I would never again subject myself to such an experience. His funeral was the last one I attended involving a person especially dear to me. That is why I did not return to Colombia for the funeral of my own mother. I am not good at handling the emotional intensity of such final good-byes.

Some years later a neighbor of ours I had gotten to know and appreciate a great deal called me at the office suggesting we meet late in the day, but privately. He told me that he had been diagnosed with cancer of the liver. He had been told that chemotherapy was his only option. He wanted my opinion. I responded that I needed a day or so to consult with others before I could make my suggestions. Two days later we met again. I had found out that the prognosis of his condition was dismal. In those days, chemotherapy would have extended his life by a few months at best and would impose a great price of extremely unpleasant side effects accompanied by a great deal of pain. I advised my friend to get his spiritual and financial affairs in order. "If you have pain," I assured him, "I will not let you suffer much." He died less than six weeks later. Despite everything that I could do, his death was painful because the cancer had reached his lungs. I did not go to his funeral, either, although my family did attend the ceremonies.

I saw Dr. Moore's widow one more time, a few years later, when I returned to South Carolina for my induction into the Columbia Orthopaedic Hall of Fame. We spent a few minutes talking about the pleasure that the great man had brought to both of us, and his tremendous impact on his community.

ACADEMIC POLITICS

Among the faculty at the University of Miami at that time was Dr. John Farrell, chief of surgery. Farrell applied his intense dedication to developing a strong academic program. Despite his involvement in the "plan" that brought me to Miami, I made him my first academic role model. I admired his intensity and his single-minded dedication to academic quality. I thought he was doing an outstanding job, but in just a couple of years he found himself under attack by a large segment of the surgical department for an alleged lack of organizational ability and lack of vision. They eventually brought about his academic demise.

A surgeon, formerly from New York, masterminded the rebellion. He was a smart but manipulative individual who wanted to climb the academic ladder in the shortest possible time. He missed no opportunity to quickly carve his way through any opposition. I found him a dynamic, stimulating leader. I resolved to learn as much as possible from him.

One of his projects was the treatment of certain cancers, using a technique known in those days as isolated extremity perfusion. The new technique had been developed at Tulane University, in New Orleans. It consisted of connecting a heart-lung machine to the patient's major arteries and veins of the arm or leg, after applying a tourniquet at the top of the limb. Drugs that were too toxic for vital organs such as the kidneys, brain, or liver were then circulated through the cancerous limb while protecting the vital organs.

One day, as I was admiring the aggressive procedure in progress, I realized that the system might be applicable to the treatment of bone and joint infections. I knew that no one had attempted such a use of isolated extremity perfusion. With great enthusiasm, I prepared my first grant application for the National Institutes of Health (NIH). The chief of research, the same physician who had ended Farrell's career, helped me assemble the proposal. I won the grant and immediately began to carry out my first major basic scientific research project. The first step involved experimentation with animals. Only if those experiments proved successful would we be able to advance to the next step and try using the technique on human subjects.

The animal studies went well. We injected a variety of antibiotics in dosages that under ordinary circumstances would have been extremely toxic. With the successful completion of the animal studies, we began our search for human candidates. It was not difficult to find them; osteomyelitis, a serious bone infection, was still far too common.

We performed the experimental procedure on nine or ten patients. In some instances, we combined the procedure with removal of infected bone; in others, we did not. I prepared a report on the experiment for presentation at a forum on research at the annual meeting of the American Medical Association.

When I presented the abstract to the chief of research, he made a few changes. I had initially thought that our experiment had produced mixed results. The suggested changes, however, eliminated some of the bad results "because we had not followed protocol appropriately." Once those results were eliminated from consideration, I discovered that our results were far more encouraging that I had originally perceived. We received an award for the study. That pleased both the chief of research and me a great deal.

I began to prepare the manuscript. I presented my draft to the chief of research, who began to remove additional failed surgeries from the series. He argued that these, too, should be eliminated because of failure to follow protocol.

By that time, I was beginning to emerge from my naïveté. I realized that the manuscript, if completed, would not reflect the truth of our scientific investigation. I refused to associate myself with it. When I informed the chief of research of my decision, he controlled his anger only with great, visible difficulty. He argued that I was inexperienced and unaware of the proper way to conduct and evaluate basic research. He assured me that if I did not follow his advice, I would never again be able to obtain another grant from the agency. He threatened that as chief of research, he could never again support a grant proposal from me. That was the end of our relationship. A year later he was asked to leave the University of Miami.

At the time, I considered this kind of "fudged" research to be an aberration. Previously, I had foolishly assumed that all scientists and all physicians behaved with irreproachable intellectual integrity. Forty years in the academic trenches have shown me that the manipulation of research results is not unusual. While most scientists and physicians are honest, far too many are not.

Years later, I saw people within my own faculty at the University of Southern California inappropriately manipulate results in order to win acceptance of articles submitted to major journals. One such colleague, whom I had recruited and later asked to resign, was obsessed with the idea that he was destined to win recognition as one of the greatest surgeons in the land. His residents loudly and openly referred to the "fudge factor" in his reports. While he is no longer on the faculty at USC, he remains a successful surgeon who has managed to impress a broad spectrum of the public with his flamboyance.

The Miami episode was not the last experience concerning dishonesty in medical research. I saw it several more times and I suspect it is more common than we are willing to acknowledge. The pressure to publish and the desire for promotion prompt some people to indulge in unethical practices. That, of course, is precisely why the medical and scientific professions require that research results be independently reproduced before anyone takes them seriously. Now that medicine's dependency on industry's support has reached a previously unimagined degree, the problem has become a very serious one.

The medical research industry is marred by other forms of fraud as well. One of my earlier research applications for NIH support had to do with a proposed method to induce osteoarthritis in dogs by artificially traumatizing the knee join. I described the methodology in detailed drawings and explained the appropriate steps. The grant was not funded. Two and a half years later, while serving as visiting professor at another institution, I visited their research laboratories. I was stunned to find researchers executing an experiment identical to the one that I had submitted to NIH. I was even more stunned to discover that the lead researcher had been a member of the panel that reviewed my application, and had voted against it. (I do, however, take comfort from knowing that while the initial results were received with great enthusiasm, the process eventually failed to prove scientifically important.)

Several years later, after that particular individual had become head of orthopaedics at another institution, I again sought to cooperate with him. I had been impressed with a piece of equipment they had in their research laboratory. I showed them how their equipment could be readily used to investigate the motion that takes place at the site of a weight-bearing fracture, and suggested the possibility of a shared grant proposal. They responded enthusiastically, so I proceeded to write out the goals and methodology of the proposed investigation. I never heard from them about the progress of the applications. Later, I found out that the research proposal had been approved and funded without any mention of my work, or of cooperation with my department.

Those of you with your own experience with research and research institutions are probably wondering how I could have been so naive. I sometimes ask myself the same question. Usually, I ask myself that question just after I have done something else that is equally foolish.

I once recruited a young scientist (a Ph.D., not an M.D.) who had impressed me favorably. Shortly after his arrival in California, he asked me to lend him 5,000 dollars to facilitate his relocation to Los Angeles. I provided him with the money, and he agreed to pay me back "as soon as he could."

Quite a bit of time passed, and I still had not received any repayment. I assumed, however, that he had not yet had time to establish a financial base. One night, he invited Barbara and me to dine at his home, and we had a pleasant evening. During the course of the conversation, he made reference to the timely loan I had given him and apologized for the delay in beginning its repayment. To me, such a discussion seemed highly inappropriate at that time and place. I said, "Please, don't worry about it," and ended the conversation. Three years later, he had not yet attempted to honor his financial commitment to me. In the interim, I had also become concerned over various aspects of his academic performance. I began considering the possibility that we would have to terminate his relationship with the university. Then he announced his departure from the department and his move to another center.

Prior to his leaving, I asked him to repay the 5,000 dollars I had loaned him. He responded that I had told him earlier that I had decided to make the loan a gift. When I expressed surprise at such a claim he said, "That night at my house, when I apologized to you for the delay in initiating payments, you said, 'forget about it.' That meant, to me, that you were excusing me from any payments." I was extremely startled by his interpretation of that dinner-table conversation.

During his tenure with us, he had been investigating the effect of the cement used in total hip replacement surgery upon the surrounding bone. The findings that he had described in preliminary reports appeared to be interesting and informative. I urged him to prepare the material for publication, but he ignored my plea. He insisted that he was too busy. He assured me that soon he would find the time to put the material together for publication.

When the time came for his departure from the university I insisted that he repay my 5,000 dollars, and that he also deliver to me both his raw experimental data and a completed manuscript reporting on his study. I reminded him that because he was a university employee, the research belonged to USC. It was not his property. In response, he said that if I would forgive the debt, he would give me the paper, ready for publication.

I expressed my anger at his outrageous proposition, and reminded him again of his financial obligation to me and his professional obligation to the university. He left town a few weeks later. When I threatened him with litigation, he sent a check for 5,000 dollars along with a shoebox full of photographic slides depicting the surgical experiment. He had neither labeled the slides nor placed them in any order.

This researcher subsequently became well known in the field. Today, he is highly thought of in orthopaedic research circles. I am not familiar enough with his work to evaluate his current reputation. I hope that professional and personal responsibility came with maturity and a fresh start. He had always had the potential to be an outstanding researcher. I trust that he finally realized that great promise.

In more recent years I have had the opportunity to observe the rapid deterioration in the medical professionalism. It appears that for the sake of fame and profit, many physicians are acting in ways that not too long ago everyone considered entirely inappropriate. Vivid examples of inexcusable behavior I have seen displayed by orthopaedic surgeons marketing surgical techniques and devices. In spite of lack of evidence to justify the use of new materials for total hip implants, they openly state that they can be guaranteed for life, even when performed in the very young.

Though the dishonesty that seems to steadily creep into our profession is most often motivated by financial greed, other times it takes a different face. A colleague of mine saw nothing wrong with intellectual dishonesty. A few years ago I prepared a study dealing with the prevention of blood clots following hip surgery. I was ready to submit the manuscript for publication. I asked my colleague if he would be interested in adding his own material to my study. I felt the total number of patients in the review needed to be higher, and this would also give him the opportunity to add his name to the literature in an important subject.

He immediately responded that he had kept very accurate records of his patients and assured me he would give his data to me within the next few days. I provided him with a copy of my manuscript.

Accordingly, three days later he presented to me a hand-written list of nearly twelve hundred "surgeries." The number of patients in his report was slightly less than in mine. There were no names or initials, only final tabulations. The figures included in his report dealing with results and complications were almost identical to mine. Suspicious that he had fabricated the data, I asked him to give me information on a few other parameters and suggested that it would be better if he could give the raw data, since there was a probability that the editors of the journal where I was planning to publish the paper would request it. He agreed to do so. He never did, and I am glad he never delivered it, for I knew it did not exist.

chapter 15
creating an opportunity

"All life is an experiment. The more experiments you make, the better."
—Ralph Waldo Emerson

"All things come to those who wait," they say. Of course they also say, "He who hesitates is lost." In any case, after several months as a loyal team player, I finally succeeded in persuading my division head to allow me to develop a rehabilitation program at Jackson Memorial.

In the late 1960s rehabilitation was still unexplored territory in Florida. While Florida waited, however, the new medical discipline was attracting attention in other states. Howard Rusk, director of the Rehabilitation Institute in New York City, had recently visited Miami as a guest of the Dade County Medical Association. I attended the lecture, which illustrated his technique with slides of patients with spinal cord injuries. His work seemed fascinating and extremely valuable.

Clearly, I thought, this would be a good time for the University of Miami and Jackson Memorial Hospital to start a rehabilitation program. Such a program would solve many of the problems that I had been having with Dr. Miller. And judging by Howard Rusk's presentation, it would provide great benefits to our patients. There was only one problem with this plan. I did not know exactly how to manage such a project, since I did not have a clear idea of just what "rehabilitation" was all about.

I recalled that a few years earlier, while serving as a resident in South Carolina, I had accompanied a young paraplegic on a plane to the Rusk Institute in New York City. That initial exposure to the institute had almost cost me dearly. The young man was one of Austin Moore's patients, and I agreed to accompany him as a favor to my mentor. Inadvertently, I forgot to notify my own chief, Dr. William

Boyd, where I was going, and why. There was no love lost between the two orthopaedists, and as soon as Dr. Boyd learned of my whereabouts during those two days, he became infuriated. He told the other local orthopaedists about the incident, which added to my reputation of insubordination and irresponsibility. It played an important role in my subsequent decision to leave South Carolina.

Unfortunately, that visit to the Rusk Institute had been brief. I did not see or learn enough to appreciate the true nature of its work. When I heard Rusk's talk a few years later, however, it revived old memories and convinced me that I could become interested in the subject.

In retrospect, it is hard to believe that in 1963, the University of Miami and its main teaching hospital, Jackson Memorial Hospital, still had no rehabilitation program. One noncertified physical therapist and two orderlies with no formal training administered all physical therapy treatments. They had virtually no equipment.

A few days after Rusk's speech, I approached David Reynolds, the chairman of our neurosurgery department, and asked what, in his opinion, could be done for paraplegic and quadriplegic patients. His response was brief and to the point. "We can do nothing at all. We sometimes do laminectomies, trying to decompress the spinal cord, but they don't really provide much relief. These poor people develop pressure sores and kidney infections. Sooner, rather than later, they die. It is a tragedy."

I told him about Rusk's lecture and about Rusk's positive and dynamic approach to those unfortunate individuals. Reynolds smiled sardonically to express his skepticism. I continued to be intrigued by what I had heard at the Rusk lecture. I must admit, however, that Reynolds's pessimistic outlook significantly dampened my enthusiasm. Events would soon conspire to reignite my interest in rehabilitation.

A few days later, I was called and asked to consult in a matter involving two young people, both victims of spinal cord injuries. They were in the hospital with associated fractures; large draining ulcers covered their sacrum. The physicians requesting the consultation were urologists. They needed help concerning the paralysis and pressure sores of the two young men.

I was deeply depressed by what I saw. It brought memories of the second day of my year of internship at the Central Army Hospital in

Bogota. On that day, more than a dozen years earlier, I was walking toward the orthopaedic ward when I heard someone call my name. In a small, dark room, I found a bearded man, whom I did not recognize at first, lying in bed.

The man was a former classmate of mine, from our early high school days together in Bucaramanga. We had not been especially close friends. He had left the Jesuit school and moved to a public school. We saw each other on occasion, particularly during fiesta days, when the two schools competed against each other in sports. He and I were the drum majors of our respective schools. He was tall, good-looking, street-wise, and a better drum major than I was. Now he was in the Central Army Hospital in Bogota, paralyzed from the waist down. There were huge, rotting pressure sores on his back and legs. He was also incontinent, and his room had the terrible smell produced by the combination of urine, feces, sweat, and pus. The stench must have been similar to the intolerable one the old Greek mythology describes emanating from the ulcerated leg of their hero, the possessor of Heracles' powerful bow, whom they found necessary to abandon in a deserted island. I had never before spoken to a paralyzed man.

We talked about the accident that had paralyzed his lower body, and about the visiting French surgeons who had operated on his spine. They had promised him eventual recovery. He said he was expecting to be able to walk again "one of these days." I visited him frequently during my tour of duty at the hospital.

It did not take long for me to realize that he knew that he would never recover. He was extraordinarily bitter that the team of French surgeons was traveling through South America, performing useless operations. He cursed his luck that they had been in Bogota when he was injured. He was furious that his family had gone into debt to pay for their so-called services. He wished that he had been allowed to die and that his family had saved their money.

There are ethical and dedicated physicians who often volunteer to help others in countries lacking financial resources. They provide invaluable services for which we all should be grateful. However, at that time, I did not know about the hypocrisy and dishonesty of those itinerant peddlers of false medicine. Later, I learned that such occurrences are common, particularly in underdeveloped countries. These visiting doctors prey on the unfortunate and demean the profession just to make a fistful of dollars. At the time, they came primarily from Western Europe and the United States. The poverty of many Latin Americans and their blind faith in authority makes them easy prey for such vultures. So, too, does the lack of uniform high-quality medical care.

Jairo Hinostrosa, my paralyzed friend, had not left the dark room since his admission to the hospital. He just lay on his bed in the dark room, watching people walk by and cursing the unjust tragedy that had befallen him. In my mind, I saw him trapped in a living parallel to Plato's allegory of the cave. In *The Republic*, Plato describes a dark cave filled with people who are chained to their places, unable to turn their heads or move their bodies. Their only concept of reality is based on shapes that they see only as shadows cast on the wall of the cave by the light of a distant fire. The residents of the cave have no *real* lives. They have no *real* experiences. They perceive only shadows of images.

I left Bogota and moved on to the United Sates. I do not know how much longer Jairo lived. I suspect, and hope, that it was a short time.

From that time on, I have felt that quadriplegia is the most terrible condition to affect a human being. I visualize the innermost circle of hell as a huge room full of quadriplegics with exposed, infected sores, swimming in pus, feces, and urine; the stench overwhelming. There is nothing that frightens me more than permanently losing my ability to move freely, control bodily functions, and be completely independent. Heaven, if there is one, must be graceful place of perpetual motion.

I had not been able to help my friend Jairo in Bogota; there was equally little that I could do for the two young accident victims in my own hospital. The memory of Rusk's recent words, however, prompted me to seek Dr. Miller's support for developing a rehabilitation program at Jackson Memorial. Dr. Miller agreed that it seemed like a good idea. He even agreed, at my request, to allow me to run it without major interference from him. (He may simply have thought that it would provide a good way to keep me out of his hair.)

I immediately flew to New York to visit the Rusk Institute again. I wanted especially to learn about the rehabilitation of patients with spinal cord injuries. I was most impressed with what I saw. They had a number of paraplegics and quadriplegics who received intensive care. These patients also received highly committed attention from an extremely competent staff. It was the first time I heard the term "comprehensive rehabilitation team" and saw the concept skillfully applied.

In the physical therapy area, I observed several young victims of paraplegia learning to walk with the aid of crutches. Their therapists told me that before they were discharged from the center, they would have to demonstrate their ability to cross a busy street at the traffic light. I was amazed that these paraplegics had learned to handle themselves so well. "What an extraordinary accomplishment!" I said to myself. I immediately saw that the opportunity to duplicate this performance at my own university would be a demanding and intriguing challenge.

I was again filled with enthusiasm as I returned to Miami. The next morning, I approached the administration, seeking support for my plan to develop a program like the one in place at the Rusk Institute. At the time, there was no spinal cord rehabilitation program in our entire state, but the hospital's medical director, Dr. Kermit Gates, a retired military physician, would promise only to "look into the matter." Days passed, but I did not receive an answer. That meant, of course, that nothing was going to happen without further prodding. I developed a more devious stratagem.

I asked one of the two physical therapy orderlies, Leroy Collier, a man in his late thirties, to accompany me, after working hours, on a visit to nursing homes in the community. We rode together in my car. At the nearest nursing home, I introduced myself and asked to see any paraplegics or quadriplegics they had in their facility.

Mr. Collier and I were taken to the most isolated room in the building, where three young paraplegics were lodged. All three had major pressure sores. All three were febrile from chronic skin and kidney infections. All were less than twenty years old. They had been in the nursing home for at least six months. The stench from the mixed bodily secretions was the same one I had experienced in the military hospital in Bogota ten years earlier. I offered to take them to Jackson Memorial Hospital to see if we could do something to help them. They and the nursing home administrator happily agreed to my request.

I called the orthopaedic resident on duty and asked him to go to the emergency room and prepare to admit three young men. Since elective admissions were not permitted without prior approval, I told the resident to record a diagnosis of "acute injuries." I placed newspaper on the seats of my car to keep their body fluids from staining the plastic. Mr. Collier and I picked them up, one at a time, and bodily put them in my car.

We repeated the process several times during the next few days. Each time, we brought additional patients to the hospital. Within a few days, we had nine paraplegic patients in the orthopaedic ward. We had no equipment and no space in which to set up any kind of rehabilitation program. Worse yet, no one on the medical staff had any knowledge of how to begin their rehabilitation. I was the only one who had attempted to study the subject, and I had spent just a few days in at the Rusk Institute. My knowledge of rehabilitation barely qualified as a "modicum." In other words, we had rescued these patients from the horrors of the nursing home, but so far we could provide them with little more than a healthier environment.

At first, I pretended to the administration that our patients had been in the hospital for various periods of time. I returned to the medical director and again sought his help in establishing some capability for rehabilitation. I requested that he assign me an area in the hospital where we could treat these patients. Anticipating that he would claim that there was no suitable space, I told him that I had found a vacant ward on the third floor of the Colored Hospital. He responded that the third-floor ward had been condemned because it had no air conditioning, was termite-ridden, and the entire building was scheduled for demolition within the next two years. I argued that the lack of air conditioning would not be a problem to those patients, because the nursing homes where they had been living did not have air conditioning either. I told Gates that termites were preferable to the giant cockroaches that all of the patients had seen feeding on their open ulcers at the nursing homes.

Gates had realized by then exactly what I had done, and how I had created this sudden need for rehabilitation facilities. I confessed that he was right. I told him that I had brought nine paralyzed patients into Jackson Memorial because the conditions in their nursing homes were inhumane and totally deplorable. I invited him to accompany me on a visit to one of these homes, where he could witness conditions for himself. Instead, he not only allowed us to use the ward on the third floor of the Colored Hospital but he also assigned a full-time licensed practical nurse, and nurse's aides during evening hours.

We had opened the door. The rest would be up to us. If we could demonstrate the value of rehabilitation, the door would open all the way. For the time being, we had successfully created a rehabilitation program at Jackson Memorial Hospital, the heart of the University of Miami Medical School. We had indeed established the first comprehensive rehabilitation program in the state of Florida.

Jackson Memorial's rehabilitation program eventually earned a distinguished reputation throughout the country. It became a source of enormous satisfaction to me, and a program in which the entire university has taken great pride. I have come to believe that many rehabilitation programs are subject to abuse by hospitals and patients, but I still regard my fight with the administration and our days spent creating the unit as some of the most rewarding days in my entire medical career.

Dr. Gates became one of our strongest advocates and soon came to play an influential role in the growth of the rehabilitation center. A little more than two years later, he suffered a severe stroke and became aphasic and paralyzed on one side of his body. His family wanted me to outline his physical therapy. If life imitated Hollywood, this story would have a happy ending. I could report that our rehabilitation unit—*his* rehabilitation unit—was able to restore most of his function. But life rarely follows such cheerful scripts. Dr. Gates refused to participate in any form of therapy. He suffered a second episode just a few months later and died shortly afterwards.

chapter 16.
appreciating
the physically impaired

"In the mountain of truth, you never climb in vain."
—Friedrich Nietzsche

In the early 1960s I became interested in amputation surgery and prosthetic rehabilitation. I had first learned the intricacies of that field under the tutelage of Dr. Newton McCollough during my year as resident in his program in Orlando. He had run a juvenile amputee program in central Florida, and had achieved some remarkable results. I wanted to organize a similar program in Miami.

During the previous year, I had taken several courses dealing with amputation surgery and prosthetic rehabilitation at Northwestern University, University of California at Los Angeles, and New York University. At one of those programs, I heard that a Polish surgeon had begun fitting amputees with prostheses immediately after completing the amputation, while the patients were still anaesthetized. The Polish surgeon was reporting significant successes. I had witnessed the problems associated with late prosthetic fitting, particularly in the elderly, and found the new concept extremely appealing.

I had no firsthand knowledge of the Polish procedure; the only information I had came from a few brief comments made by a physician from New York at one of my courses. I did, however, have a firm vision of how such a combined procedure *should* be done. So, I began my own experiment by applying a plaster of paris artificial leg to an amputee who was still in the operating room. My crude plaster prosthesis somewhat resembled the Patella Tendon Bearing (PTB) permanent prosthesis that was popular at the time.

I later learned that my experiment constituted the first time that such a technique had been tried in the United States. I also discovered that my technique marked a substantial advance over the Polish procedure. The Polish surgeon had simply been wrapping plaster over the stump to immobilize the knee joint and constructing a temporary appliance to function as a prosthesis. His cast that extended above the knee obviously prevented motion of that joint, making ambulation more difficult. Our temporary prosthesis left the knee free. Patients found walking with the artificial appliance a great deal easier.

Serendipitously, I found myself pioneering a procedure on the world stage. The best news came with our discovery that the patient did amazingly well. Just one day after surgery, he was already capable of walking and bearing some weight on the new prosthesis. We had some concern about the impact of the prosthesis on the newly stitched stump. One week later, however, when we removed the temporary prosthesis and inspected the stump, we found the suture line to be in good condition. Perhaps best of all, we discovered that the rapid rehabilitation brought with it a rapid improvement in patient morale.

We reproduced this experiment more than 100 times within the course of the next year. People from all over the United States visited our program to learn about our new technique. We emphasized the importance of preserving the knee joint during amputation surgery, since the rehabilitation potentials of the above-the-knee amputee were limited in the older age group. Others, of course, had made that plea in the past, but we found that adoption of our new technique brought an unexpected bonus. Within the year, we succeeded in reversing the ratio between above-the-knee and below-the-knee amputations. The reports of our clinical results brought acclaim and widespread adoption of our techniques. It also brought us many interesting patients.

Once, I saw a man in his late twenties, whose right hand had been bitten by a rattlesnake a few years earlier. The man lived, but the poison almost destroyed his hand, which retained only two fingers, both with severely limited motion and almost no sensation. For all practical purposes, the two remaining digits were useless. The patient had come to us hoping that we could somehow restore the use of his mangled hand.

I quickly concluded that a good prosthesis would serve him better than his remaining natural digits, and convinced him that amputation was the treatment of choice. I removed the hand at the wrist joint, seeking to preserve as much rotation of the forearm as possible.

Surgery went well; we recorded the entire procedure on film. At the end of surgery, working primarily with William Sinclair, the first prosthetist hired by the hospital, we molded a plaster prosthesis over the stump. Sinclair attached a hook and harness to the end of the cast. Much to my amazement, the patient was able to operate the hook skillfully just twenty-four hours later. Using his "hand," he was able to feed himself and to carry out most common daily activities. I planned to leave the plaster prosthesis in place for two weeks in order to minimize the swelling that I anticipated would develop if the cast were removed too soon.

Coincidentally, the hand surgery chapter of the American College of Surgeons was meeting in Miami Beach at that time. Our medical school was hosting many of their sessions. I asked the meeting chairman to give me a few minutes to present an interesting patient, and he graciously made time available.

First, I displayed slides that depicted the grotesque hand of the snake-bitten young man. Then I asked the group for opinions concerning the most appropriate treatment; the group quickly came up with several creative ideas. One surgeon suggested transplanting the man's big toe to the hand; that opinion received great support. Finally, I then told the group that I had already completed surgery and wanted to share the result.

We brought our patient into the auditorium. He had undergone the amputation just five days before. The plaster prosthesis was heavily stained with dry blood. I asked the patient to demonstrate what he could do with his artificial arm. He reached into his back pocket and withdrew his wallet. Holding it with his good hand, he opened the wallet and one by one removed his credit cards and a few dollar bills. The jaws of the hand specialists dropped, and for a few seconds their mouths remained wide open.

It was an entertaining and wonderful experience. A few days later, we split the cast and inspected the stump. Happily, it proved to be clean, and we were able to fit the patient with his new, permanent prosthesis. The patient returned to his previous activities a few days later. We published the result of this experience without realizing that we had carried out the first immediate postoperative prosthetic fitting of an upper extremity amputee in the world. Twenty years later, after I had become department head at USC, the man called just to say "hello." He was traveling through California, and had seen my name in the USC directory. He was still delighted with the success of the amputation.

My experience with this young man shed light on the true meaning of the disability that follows the loss of a limb during the productive years. From that case, I have developed a firm belief that far too often we refuse to amputate mangled extremities and subject patients to a multitude of surgeries because of *our* difficulties, not because of *their* best interests. We picture an amputated limb as being a great problem and disability. We see having to amputate as an admission of defeat. Foolishly—sometimes to the great detriment of the patient—we become fascinated with the form and ignore the function.

We must learn to view our cases from the patients' perspective, not from our own vantage point. To the patient, it may be far more important to maximize the *function* of a limb than to save vestigial appearance. Amputation may well be preferable to other available options—including skin grafts and reconstruction of nerves and vessels. Amputation becomes especially appealing in cases involving limbs that are partially anaesthetic, and have stiff, deformed, and frequently painful joints. If the surgeon can preserve the knee or elbow joint, the amputee has a relatively minor disability. He or she can carry out basic activities with less disability.

In the foreword to the book on management of open fractures by Charles Court-Brown and Associates, I wrote:

> Sometimes heroic attempts to preserve limbs are the result of the natural desire on the part of the surgeon to do every possible thing and not to give up, as well as a lack of clear understanding of the true disability associated with amputation surgery. It is not widely recognized that the disability of a below-knee amputation can be minimal, particularly when compared to that created by a shortened and deformed limb with partially ankylosed and painful joints. Economic and psychological factors also need to be considered, particularly at a time when our society finds itself burdened with financial problems not anticipated even in the recent past.

Six months after our pioneering hand amputation, a middle-aged man arrived in the emergency room with a terribly mangled arm. He was a butcher; his arm had been caught in a meat grinder. The paramedics brought him into the hospital with the machine still attached to his body. The remnant of his hand and forearm were readily visible in the depths of the machinery. One expects to see this kind of accident on television, not in one's own hospital.

We took some photographs of the damaged tissues and proceeded to complete the amputation that the machine had begun. Unfortunately, we had to amputate above the elbow. We made a temporary plaster prosthesis and attached a harness and a hook.

Again, the results proved extremely rewarding. The patient quickly learned to operate the terminal device. A few weeks later he returned to work as a butcher. We took great pride in our part in his rapid rehabilitation and return to employment. We, *and he*, should have been more cautious; perhaps we did not stress enough the need to master the use of his artificial arm before returning to work.

Tragically, he was later brought back to the emergency room with his other arm mangled by another meat grinding machine. I was out of town at the time. In my absence, another surgeon carried out the amputation. This time, they chose the more traditional procedure, and fitted the prosthesis several weeks after the stump had healed and the tissues were well conditioned. Perhaps they hoped that the extended recovery required would give the patient time to think more clearly about the dangers of meat grinding machines. Unfortunately, we lost touch with the patient and were not able to follow up on this outstanding opportunity for a comparative study.

With growing global interest in our techniques, we began to present courses on amputation surgery and prosthetic rehabilitation at the Americana Hotel in Miami Beach. We held the first one in 1964. I had never organized or run a continuing education course. In fact, I had never attended one, either, unless you count the few annual meetings of our American Academy of Orthopedic Surgeons.

I did not let this minor inconvenience slow us down. I prepared the scientific program and issued invitations to several of America's best-known experts in amputation surgery. We asked them to present case studies and demonstrate their techniques. We presented our own experiences and demonstrated some of the new techniques we had learned or developed.

One of those techniques dealt with a modification of what is known in orthopaedic circles as the Syme's amputation, an amputation performed just above the ankle. This amputation, performed in the traditional manner, had the disadvantage of requiring a rather bulky and unsightly prosthesis.

I modified the surgery in order to make possible the fabrication of a more cosmetic appliance. The amputation-prosthetic innovation was the product of a joint effort between the prosthetist and me. My presentation at the course was met with reservations by some of the members of the visiting faculty. One of them, a surgeon from Los Angeles, openly criticized my proposed modification and warned the audience about its possible complications, such as pressure sores and ulcers at the end of the stump.

Two years later, my critic reported in a major medical journal, and as an original contribution, the technique that he had heard me present in Miami. He never gave us credit for the initial concept, or acknowledged that he had been an outspoken critic. Without saying anything about his unethical and unprofessional conduct, I sent him a copy of the tape recording of our Miami presentation, complete with his comments. The two of us met on several occasions over the next few years, but neither of us ever mentioned the Miami meeting, his article, or the tape.

Our conference taught me a great deal about continuing education. It also caused me deep embarrassment. When I issued invitations to speakers, I assumed that they would pay their own traveling and hotel expenses. Shortly after the meeting, I began receiving itemized requests for reimbursement. In my ignorance of the usual and customary professional practice, I had not budgeted such reimbursement. Furthermore, the initial course had been poorly attended by paying customers. (We had filled the small auditorium with medical students, residents, and various employees at Jackson Memorial Hospital.) We were already operating at a loss.

I had to write to my most distinguished colleagues, apologize for my innocent and naive mistake, and accept responsibility for the problem. Then I had to tell them that we did not have the funds to reimburse expenses. Happily, not one of them objected to my news; several wrote gracious letters stressing their pleasure in participating; a few suggested that we repeat the program the following year. We followed their advice. We repeated this educational conference not just the following year but every December for the next fourteen years.

These continuing education programs became my introduction to the national orthopaedic community. Largely because of our program in Miami, I was later selected to chair the American Academy of Orthopaedic Surgeons committee on Continuing Education, a major and prestigious position that I held for several years. My work on that committee became a great pleasure and a most rewarding experience. It brought me great visibility within the academy, and eventually, no doubt, contributed significantly to my selection as president.

My work with continuing education and our conferences had one other side effect that took on disproportionate importance to my life and career. During preparation for the 1968 conference, our clerical support staff unexpectedly collapsed. Happily, a young woman named Ann Karg was looking for a job at the time. Ann, a surgeon's daughter from Akron, Ohio, had little clerical experience but was clearly bright and seemed willing to work hard. We hired her as continuing education coordinator on the spot, and she performed admirably.

I did not know it at the time, but Ann would be with me for thirty-two years. Throughout my years on the board of the academy and my career at the University of Miami, USC, and Health Care International, Ann took on a bewildering variety of responsibilities. She took care of many responsibilities that were beyond her title but never beyond her abilities. She often represented me at faculty and staff meetings, and routinely assisted me with budgets and other financial matters. She also managed my departmental private practice plans and my surgical practice. She freed me to think in broad, conceptual terms by taking care of the constant flow of organizational detail and follow-up.

Our experimental program on the treatment of amputees proved equally successful and began growing rapidly. It seems amazing in these days of multimillion dollar research grants, but in those days, we were working on a frazzled financial shoestring. We depended on the generosity of local prosthetists who regularly donated old, discarded prostheses. I also received frequent calls from nursing homes notifying me of the deaths of patients with history of hip trauma and surgery. I used to drive around the Miami area to pick up their donations at their respective facilities.

Over the years, I conducted simple research using implants and bones I had removed from patients who had died after having sustained either fractures of the hip or had a hip joint replaced. At first I brought the specimens to my house and saved them in the refrigerator. My wife objected strongly, but I managed to convince her that the specimens were important to me and that they would not be kept there very long. When the number of specimens became large she put her foot down and threatened to throw them away. Eventually, someone took mercy on Barbara and donated a large, old freezer to our "lab."

On one occasion, I found myself out of town for four days. Upon my return to the office, I found out that the entire building had been evacuated the day before. The old freezer had failed, and the rancid stench of decay had filled the building. I suppose that I should have been more understanding and more concerned about my coworkers. Instead, I only wanted to know what had happened to my specimens. They had been thrown away, of course. I could have cried.

Many of our other activities were almost as primitive. I used a hacksaw to cut used wooden legs to accommodate the stumps we were fitting in the operating room. Once I ran out of right prostheses and had nothing left but left feet. Several bilateral amputees ended up being fitted with two left prostheses; henceforth, they had to wear two left shoes. It seems strange, and it may even seem cruel. From our perspective, however, we were doing some exciting things, advancing the state of medical knowledge, and helping a lot of poor people. Our patients could not afford to purchase new prostheses. In those ancient days before Medicare and Medicaid, they would have had to make do without. We never asked what they thought of our treatment.

Not all of our patients were poor. One day, I treated an elderly gentlemen afflicted with severe arteriosclerosis who developed gangrene of one of his legs. It had progressed to the point where an amputation had become necessary. I carried out the surgical procedure and applied a temporary prosthesis in the operating room. The patient did well and eventually went home. Someone (I have never been able to remember exactly who it was) told me that this elderly gentleman was "one of the wealthiest men in Miami Beach."

When he came for a follow-up visit, I mentioned to him that I was in the process of drawing up plans to build a major center for orthopaedics and rehabilitation at the University of Miami. I explained the nature of the project and told him that contractors had estimated that its construction would cost $15 million. I probably trembled, slightly, as I asked if he would be interested in helping us with a donation. It was my first experience seeking this kind of high stakes philanthropy.

The gentleman responded that he needed to think about it; he promised to give me an answer the next time he came for a visit, and I anxiously awaited his return. At his next visit, he informed me that he had decided to help. I told him how happy I was; his generosity would make it possible for us to begin construction in the near future.

He then preceded to hand me a check. Could he possibly be financing the entire $15 million? I looked at the check. It was for $25. I could not help myself. I began to laugh. Then I had to explain the reason for my laughter.

He apologized profusely, and told me that he was a poor man living on Social Security. I could have strangled whoever it was who had told me that this man was wealthy. I was looking out a window that overlooked our parking lot when the man left the building. I continued watching, as his chauffeur opened the door of his black limousine. I never did find out how rich he really was.

In many ways, I deeply regret that I did not continue my involvement in amputation surgery and rehabilitation. The pleasures and sense of accomplishment of those days were enormous. Unfortunately, when I became chairman of the department of orthopaedics I elected to limit my work to hip surgery. My administrative responsibilities and busy practice left little time for other activities. I also reasoned that my younger associates deserved freedom from my direct involvement in all areas of orthopaedics. After all, I did not want them to seek out other department heads and move away from Miami. I did not want them to feel blocked at every turn. I did not want them wondering how best to "handle Sarmiento." I wanted, instead, to maximize their freedom to grow, explore, and to build our department into an outstanding, world-class program.

I am extremely gratified, however, that my work in amputation and rehabilitation was not totally forgotten. Twenty-five years later, I was honored by the American Academy of Orthotists and Prosthetists with honorary membership in the society in recognition for my contributions to the field. My induction took place in San Francisco in 1997. It was all the more memorable for the Sarmiento family because at that same meeting, our youngest son, Gregory, became a member of the same organization. His older brother, Gus Jr., came up from Los

Angeles to join us on the occasion. Rarely do the gods grant us mere mortals the kind of extraordinary pleasure that was given to Barbara and me that week. We were so proud of them and of each other.

chapter 17.
understanding
the spinal cord injured

"In our sleep, pain which cannot forget falls drop by drop upon the heart until, in our own despair, against our will, comes wisdom through the grace of God."

—Aeschylus

Within a year of the arrival of our first patients, the spinal cord injury unit at Jackson Memorial Hospital blossomed with a unique form of macabre, tragic beauty. Paraplegics, quadriplegics, and amputees filled the termite-infested third-floor ward of the Colored Hospital. Ugliness and depression filled all available space, but hope, too, was always present in the ward. I remained inspired by my visits to the Rusk Institute in New York, where I had watched paraplegics learn to walk. I remembered that in order to "graduate," these patients had to demonstrate their ability to cross a New York street.

As arriving patients filled our facility, our staff was also growing. The administration authorized me to recruit a registered therapist. Among the people who came for an interview was Bella May, an unusual young lady who seemed self-possessed and knowledgeable. She also seemed forceful enough to survive the emotional onslaught that is always present in rehabilitation wards. She was the daughter of a French physician who had practiced in Indochina (Vietnam) prior to the 1954 defeat of the French at Dienbienphu, the battle that led to the departure of the French and the subsequent arrival of the Americans.

Bella May impressed me in many ways, but my inquiries to former supervisors brought nothing but critical comments. According to those who wrote, she was a difficult person to deal with. They accused her of being demanding and impatient. They told me that she seemed incapable of accepting directions from others. At first, I was disappointed; then I realized that while others may resent those attributes, I believed them to be assets. I asked her to return for a second interview. By the end of the day, I had come to believe that she probably would prove difficult to work with. I also recognized that I needed somebody who was committed to making things happen and would challenge the status quo. For me, she would be precisely the right person in the right place at the right time.

Bella May turned out to be an astonishing individual and a loyal associate. We ended up working together for several years. Together, we recruited a group of highly motivated nurses and therapists. Before long, we had built a first-class program and expanded it beyond our initial dreams. I found myself increasingly troubled, however, by our inability to restore practical function to many of our patients, no matter how hard they and we worked at it. We still anxiously awaited for the first paraplegic patient who would reward our efforts by demonstrating a restored ability to walk. We spent many hours working with custom-designed braces. Some of our patients learned to take a few steps (with a great deal of help); none learned to walk without major assistance. We were even more discouraged to learn that when they left the hospital, they discarded their braces and crutches and accepted the fact that they were confined to their wheelchairs.

In the wake of our initial success by all other measures, however, we began to treat patients with head injuries and victims of strokes. We initiated a pediatric rehabilitation unit with family education programs for their relatives. We transformed our "chewing gum and bailing wire" unit into a widely admired facility that not only brought great benefits to patients but also enormous intellectual satisfaction to us. We brought new prestige and influence to the University of Miami Medical School and began to outgrow our dilapidated physical plant.

The administration took due notice of our success, acquiesced to our requests, and offered us a possible move to larger quarters in a building occupied by the medical department. The chairman of the department of medicine immediately raised serious objections. The resulting dispute might still be going on, had it not been for acute personal problems he suffered. At the height of the debate, he was involved with a major community scandal, arrested, and charged with public intoxication and other, more serious offenses. The incident ended both his academic career and his ability to resist our move into his building. Happily, after extensive rehabilitation, he became a highly skilled and successful researcher at a major pharmaceutical company. In the meantime, we were able to build a leading, state-of-the-art rehabilitation facility.

We did not realize it at the time, but our efforts at Jackson Memorial Hospital were part of a broad-based national phenomenon that made those years the golden era of rehabilitation. That may well have been due to the influence of television, an adolescent industry that was actively seeking ways to create a brave new world. The drama of physical rehabilitation proved to be ready-made fodder for TV news. You could not turn on a TV news show without watching a story about the rehabilitation of victims of spinal injury and other musculoskeletal conditions. One station would show a story about a high school student, injured in an automobile accident, who desperately wanted to walk to the stage at his graduation. Then we would watch him, covered in steel and leather braces, struggling in crutches, walk to front of the auditorium as his classmates cheered.

Another station would broadcast the story of a young woman who had been seriously injured just before her wedding. The families had postponed the nuptials because the bride insisted that she only be married when she could walk to her new husband, without help. Then, with the organ playing Wagner or Mendelssohn, and the bride, wearing a lovely white gown along with her steel and leather braces, walked, assisted with metal crutches, down the aisle. The camera moves from close-up of proud parents to close-ups of the tearful friends, family, and guests in the audience.

Dr. Rusk and other experts became welcomed guests of television talk shows. The federal government, charitable organizations, and, above all, the Easter Seal Foundation opened the doors to their treasuries. Making people walk again—restoring the full independence—became almost a national obsession.

Curiously, despite all of our experience and knowledge, that obsession is stronger than ever today. Celebrities and politicians still flock to the cause of restored ambulation. The only problem is that, over the years, the medical community has learned that we do not know enough about the nervous system to restore our patients' independence.

As the rehabilitation center at Miami grew, we learned more and more about the art and science of rehabilitation. Because of our initial optimism, however, much of what we learned proved extremely discouraging. Initially, we all sought to restore our patients' ability to walk. We were willing do anything necessary to achieve that goal. We designed new rehabilitation equipment and medical devices. We worked with neurologists and neurosurgeons to learn more about the spine and its functions. We learned that we were not gods.

One evening, Bella May and I spent several hours discussing the growing professional crises in medicine and its relationship to the function of rehabilitation clinics around the country. We found that we agreed on a number of issues. We had both become increasingly concerned that our respective professions—rehabilitative medicine and rehabilitative therapy—were guilty of having, unwittingly perhaps, precipitated the problems and contributed to their perpetuation. We were both starting to question the real, enduring value of rehabilitation.

Bella May left some time later and moved to Augusta, Georgia, where she became a successful professor and director of the School of Physical Therapy at the Medical College of Georgia. Nearly twenty-five years later, she was invited to deliver the commencement address at the School of Physical Therapy at the University of Miami. I had the honor of introducing her to the audience. I congratulated her for a brilliant career and for many outstanding contributions to rehabilitation, acknowledged her hard work for me and for our rehabilitation center, and thanked her for having done so much for our profession and our community.

I was beginning to see rehabilitation of the musculoskeletally impaired under a different light. I began to question many of the things we were trying to do for these patients. I knew that all of our services were extremely expensive, but, in those days, we physicians had still not yet become actively concerned about the rising cost of health care. The physician was the exclusive arbiter of patient care. A new national program, Medicare, ensured that even elderly patients without other insurance would be able to pay for their treatment and rehabilitation.

REFLECTING

My other concerns were much more serious; I began to wonder if our rehabilitation activities were effective. I began to question our goals. My first doubts arose with long-term follow-up studies of stroke patients. In our efforts to teach stroke victims how to use affected extremities, we typically provided intense and prolonged physical and occupational therapy. Therapists worked with them several hours per day, often for months. We knew that some patients responded and some did not, but no one wanted the responsibility of declaring a condition hopeless and of terminating a patient's program of therapy.

We eventually concluded that one does not need months to determine whether the function of a partially paralyzed spastic or flaccid arm can respond to therapy. All it takes is a few weeks. Dr. Newton McCollough and I reported those experiences in an orthopaedic journal. We reported that patients who do not respond in the first few weeks are highly unlikely to respond at all. We argued that the incidence of spontaneous recovery was higher than the incidence of positive response to prolonged treatment occurring after the first few weeks of therapy. We expressed our continued concern for these patients who did not respond to therapy. We suggested that the best thing to do for them is to concentrate on teaching them how to function despite their disabilities, i.e., without the use of one hand or with only limited use of one leg. We also noted that patients and physicians could continue to hope that some spontaneous improvement of function in the affected side take place. Our results were duplicated by researchers throughout the United States, but politicians, insurance companies, celebrities and foundations chose to ignore the truth. Demands for more therapy and longer therapy continued to dominate the health care debate. Despite the national commitment to cutting health care costs, we continued to spend a phenomenal amount of money on unnecessary and ineffective rehabilitation.

Our findings did, however, lead to my discovery of what you might call "Sarmiento's First Law of Medical Economics." As long as some agency—be it an insurance company, Medicare, Medicaid, or other federal, state, or charitable program—is willing to pay for unnecessary rehabilitation services, patients will receive continued physical and occupational therapy. It does not matter if the services are useless and inffective. They may even be painful and unpleasant. The only variable in length of rehabilitation therapy is the term of treatment "approved by the agency." The advent of managed care, which should have corrected this pernicious trend, has not made matters better; quite the contrary, they have gotten worse. "For-profit" medicine seeks financial advantages in all possible areas. Thus far, abusing rehabilitation has proven a fertile ground.

In recent years, there has been no growth in the proportion of the population requiring physical and occupation therapy. The *rate* and *extent* of successful rehabilitation have also remained constant. There has, however, been a tremendous growth in the number of physical and occupational therapists, and the number of centers or institutes of physical and occupational therapy.

In order to maximize revenues, many of these therapy businesses offer a variety of "modalities of therapy," typically involving a new practice known as separate billing. Traditionally, therapists billed a set fee per timed treatment session. Under separate billing, the therapist presents an invoice for, let us say ten minutes of hydrotherapy, fifteen minutes on one specialized machine, ten minutes on another machine, and, perhaps, the balance of the session for massage. The total, as you might imagine, is significantly higher than the traditional per session bill. The separate billing practice also allows one therapist to treat several patients simultaneously.

These abusive practices seem to be growing more excessive every day. At first glance, the situation makes no sense. How can it be that the insurance companies and Medicare authorities in Washington have not recognized this obvious ploy? Why have they not done something about it? Why, to the contrary, do they seem bent on encouraging the perpetuation of the farce? How is it that they continue to authorize unnecessary, ineffective, and expensive therapy? Is it possible that they really do not know about the abuses being committed in the name of "good care"? I suspect the powerful lobbying and influence of insurance companies and manufacturing companies of medical-related equipment are partially responsible for the continued trend. Often, trustees representing the two groups sit at the same tables where corporate planning is done. Ignoring the role patients' advocate groups play in this field would be a mistake. Their input is needed to better identify their needs.

Admittedly, I am no longer responsible for managing a major

rehabilitation center, and no longer spend every day watching the progress of many patients. I am, however, up to date on the literature. I continue to read the major journals. I continue to attend national and international conventions. I see this great nation frightened into many serious errors of policy by its effort to restrain the growth in medical costs, while continuing to tolerate the most egregious abuses under the guise of rehabilitation.

I see elderly victims of arteriosclerosis or diabetes who have a leg amputated above the knee. They spend weeks and months desperately trying to learn to walk with new and expensive artificial prostheses. Only after they have suffered months of frustration do they discover that their goal was unrealistic from the beginning. Only after their therapy "benefits" have finally run out do they learn that use of a wheelchair is the most effective and practical means of locomotion. While new developments in prosthetic fabrication do offer improved potential to help above-the-knee amputees, it will be a long time before a substantial number of elderly patients can be successfully rehabilitated. The energy and strength necessary to operate even the lightest prosthesis may no longer be present in many elderly people.

That story is repeated over and over for many different pathologies with the same ending. Only after the "benefits" end does false therapy end. Only after occupational or physical therapy "benefits" run out are patients equipped with the wheelchairs that will help them maximize the quality of life remaining to them. Even then, many never discover that their inability to rehabilitate themselves was always inherent in their condition and was never a personal failure.

I adopted a similar philosophy about the care and rehabilitation of the spinal cord injured patient. Restoring ambulation to complete paraplegics is a totally unrealistic goal. It was unrealistic when Dr. Rusk attempted it. It was unrealistic when I sought to achieve it. It is unrealistic today.

I experience astonishing personal fury when I see injured celebrities heartlessly exploited by people who seek only to extend rehabilitation "benefits" to increase their personal fortunes. Naive, good-hearted people are easily seduced by these stories of personal tragedy and superheroic individual effort. Well-intended politicians and other celebrities line up for opportunities to lend their own fame and status on behalf of further extensions of uncontrolled "benefits." TV producers love film of heroic patients struggling to walk, unassisted, toward a glorious tomorrow. Rehabilitation industry leaders readily and happily abuse them all.

The heroism of the patients is truly inspirational. These amazing people are totally worthy of our culture's highest accolades, although within a few days after the cameras depart, they will angrily discard their braces, forever, in favor of wheelchairs. By the same standard, those who exploit them for publicity or political advantage—those who market programs and equipment that promises the impossible—are guilty of the grossest human depravity. I can only hope that they condemn themselves to one of the innermost circles of Dante's *Inferno*. I call for them to spend eternity chained to one of their own machines, constantly seeking freedom that will never come, desperately working to achieve goals that can never be reached; replicas of Sisyphus, forever trying to roll the rock to the top of the mountain, and never succeeding.

I am convinced that if the abuse of rehabilitation and the unnecessary use of technology were brought under control, many of the problems created by escalating health care costs would be reduced without resorting to the damaging, draconian measures that we experienced in the 1990s.

On one occasion, the president of the American Paraplegic Association came by to visit me at Jackson Memorial Hospital. He had become aware of the growing presence and influence of the Rehabilitation Center. He had heard that Jackson Memorial "refused" to help patients learn to walk. A paraplegic himself, he came into my office in a wheelchair. I do not know if he believed that his failure to restore his own ambulation had been his own fault.

I told him that as a matter of policy, my department would not use braces or seek to ambulate paraplegics. I told him that our policy was the result of several years of study and our own experiences dealing with paraplegics. At Jackson, we concentrate our main rehabilitation efforts on the prevention of skin and bladder complications, on working with the psychological aspects of total or partial paralysis, and on teaching prompt resumption of active independence as wheelchair-bound individuals.

I told him that Jackson Memorial would not emphasize bracing and ambulation training since we knew that ambulation for complete paraplegics was a demanding exercise in futility. I acknowledged that some patients with low spinal injuries eventually learned to ambulate themselves sufficiently to cross a street. In every one of those highly publicized cases, I reminded him, the patients invariably discarded their braces within days and began their lives in wheelchairs. I argued that the most humane policy was to inform them early, and in the must sympathetic manner, that their disability was permanent.

We taught our patients that the permanent loss of the ability to ambulate is not the end of the world, that life in a wheelchair can be totally compatible with living a productive, rewarding life. We would teach them that even the difficult issue of sexual function could be dealt with in similar terms.

I told my visitor that I was convinced that the overwhelming majority of patients with spinal cord injuries would learn to accept their disabilities more quickly and more easily if everyone would approach them honestly and with integrity. I asked that he work with us to end the public exaltation over cases that spread false hopes by presenting artificial, misleading outcomes. I talked about the thousands of patients who end up bitter and disappointed with a system that denies them the courtesy of a prompt explanation of the true prognosis of their injury.

I made it clear that I was not implying that such an approach was easily carried out with all people. Every physician must always remember that individual considerations are essential, and must constantly keep in mind many factors concerning each patient. The personality and individuality of each victim of paralysis becomes paramount. It is too tempting to regard all paralyzed patients the same, because they are suffering from the same condition. It is vital to remember that every individual victim of paralysis remains, first and foremost, an individual. It is the arms or legs that become paralyzed, not the personality.

At first, the visiting president of the American Paraplegic Association argued with me vehemently. He took issue with every point that I raised. Then he became quieter; it seemed to me that he was listening more carefully. He courteously listened to everything that I had to say. Then, after hearing me describe to him my philosophy of rehabilitation of the spinal cord injured patient, he stormed out of my office. As he furiously propelled his wheelchair out of my office, he said, "You are the worst medical doctor I have ever met in my entire life."

I hated to hear that judgment, particularly because I had just described to him an attitude that made me feel that I was being creditable, honest, and forthright. Throughout my tenure, my program at

Jackson Memorial remained dedicated, exclusively and totally, to the welfare of our patients. We often ignored administrative procedure, cultural dictates, and other "minor impediments" to our patients' best interests. Our success came not because we worried about "the bottom line" when planning treatment programs but because we cared about our patients as much as we cared about ourselves. We built a world-leading facility because all too often, we cared more about our patients than they cared about themselves.

I recall that once we admitted a young man to the unit. He had become paraplegic after being shot in the back at a dance. He was a schoolteacher and I could tell from the outset that he was bright. His wife was attractive and flirtatious. Allegedly, someone had made amorous passes at her, and an argument had broken out. The events of the moment that followed changed several lives.

In this case, the patient virtually immediately accepted the fact that his paralysis was permanent. We told him that he could return to the classroom in a short time, but that he would be confined to a wheelchair. He expressed interest in doing everything possible to accelerate his recovery, and rapidly learned to transfer from bed to chair, and to propel himself with minimal difficulty. He knew how to regulate his bladder function; he quickly learned how to prevent the development of pressure sores and the importance of turning over frequently while in bed. We were all extremely proud of his progress. Less than twenty-five days after his admission to the Spinal Cord Unit, he was ready to go home.

Just before his discharge, I discovered that he had developed a small pressure sore over his sacral region. He and I were both surprised by the complication. Our patient appeared to be concerned and unhappy about the fact that his discharge would have to be postponed. I found his explanations less that satisfactory, and decided to probe further into the matter. Before long, he admitted that he had deliberately provoked the complication by remaining in one position over several hours. His reason was rather simple: He did not want to go home because he had realized that he was not going to be able to have an erection. He told me that when his wife came to visit him, he had initiated sexual advances and suggested that she perform oral sex on him. Her attempts to stimulate an erection had failed. He feared that impotence would end his marriage. He concluded that he needed to stay in the hospital until his sexual function returned to normal.

During subsequent conversations with him and his wife, I found out that he had questioned several people on staff concerning his sexual prognosis. He had received different, sometime contradictory answers. He did not realize that many people are afraid to discuss sexual issues; they believe that the best thing to do is to give false hope, and to end the conversation quickly. I immediately issued instructions that henceforth, I would be the only staff member to discuss sexual performance issues with victims of spinal cord injuries.

I, in turn, enlisted the aid of a psychologist and specialized urologists. Instead of ignoring the issue, we focused on treatment options, which have increased exponentially in recent years. We were not able to restore the injured schoolteacher's potency. I do not know how that eventually affected his marriage or his life. I hope that he and his wife were able to adapt to the change in his sexuality as successfully as they had accepted the loss of function of his legs. If not, I hope that they were able to take advantage of some of the surgical or pharmaceutical options that later became available.

The experience with the teacher was repeated a number of times. Once, I brought a young man from a nursing home to the center with terribly debilitating decubiti. We eventually had to amputate his legs. His problem was so severe that the amputation included his pelvis. In order for him to sit erect, we designed and built a special bucket-like device. Only his skin separated his abdominal content from the walls of the bucket.

Despite his extreme disability, he developed an amorous friendship with one of the secretaries in my office. I was always keenly aware of the patients' loneliness and their need for friendships. I encouraged everyone on our staff to visit them as often as possible. I soon noticed, however, that this particular friendship seemed well on the road to becoming a serious relationship. One night, I saw them kissing behind the closed curtains around his bed.

The next day, I spoke to the secretary and broached the subject. I told her that I would be upset if I found out some time later that she was giving the young man false hopes. I reminded her that he was our responsibility. I hoped that she did not intend to summarily drop him from her life at some point. I did not want him hurt. I did not want to see him suffer more than he had already suffered over the years.

The next day, when I made my rounds, he was red with anger. He proceeded to tell me in no uncertain terms that I had no business getting involved in his personal life. He forbade me from ever again discussing his relationship with my secretary. I apologized, and admitted that he was right. Their romance continued.

Two months later, my secretary failed to report for duty. She had left town without a word to anyone in the office—let alone to the unhappy and now bitter paraplegic. Sometimes, there is simply no proper way to handle a difficult situation. Fortunately, this remarkable young man continued to pursue happiness. He later married a practical nurse from the center. When I last heard from him, a few months after he left the center, they were still happily married.

On another occasion, the head nurse on the Spinal Cord Unit requested an urgent meeting concerning a young quadriplegic who had been found by one of the other nurses smoking marijuana. His friends had brought it to him.

His given name was Wayne. I forgot his family name many years ago, but I have never forgotten his face. He lay in his hospital bed twenty-four hours a day, totally incapable of moving his arms or legs. He had to be fed, cleaned, and turned by others. He had no hope for recovery. He would remain in bed for the rest of his life.

His "drinking buddies," the friends who had been with him on the night of the car crash, visited him with some frequency. Friends visit our patients quite often, especially in the dark days immediately following an accident, shooting, or other tragic event. I knew from experience that within a short time, the frequency and duration of their visits would decline. Before long, the visits would end entirely, and the "friends" would disappear from the scene. Few friendships can survive paraplegia without outside assistance.

The nurse was appalled when I told her that rather than prohibiting Wayne's friends from bringing him marijuana, I wanted to encourage it. In fact, I was willing to make a deal with Wayne's young visitors. If they would promise to visit him at least once a week, for a solid year, religiously, no one in the hospital would become aware that they were smoking marijuana and I would personally pay for the weed. The nurses may have disapproved, but they kept their silence and helped us carry through on our end of the deal.

Wayne was eventually taken to surgery, where the hand surgeons performed a tendon transplant on one of his hands. They hoped to give him the ability to hold an object or turn on a television switch. In the midst of surgery, he went into cardiac arrest. It appeared that he was dying. The surgeons fractured Wayne's ribs in their heroic attempts to resuscitate him. I was watching the residents' efforts and fervently hoped that they would just give up. I prayed that their resuscitation efforts would fail. Instead, they successfully demonstrated their remarkable skills and brought Wayne back to life.

I have asked myself a thousand times why should we, under those circumstances, believe that we have a responsibility to carry out heroic measures of that nature. Why is it that the surgeons could not accept the fact that the cardiac arrest was the best possible thing that could have happened? Instead, Wayne survived and was later discharged from the Rehabilitation Unit. We also lost track of him, although I am sure that he is now dead. He probably died in a nursing home, soaked in pus, urine, and feces, with no friends to bring him marijuana cigarettes and hold them to his lips.

chapter 18.
the abuse of rights

"The practice of medicine, the profession of providing health care, is a sacred calling, not a for-profit enterprise"
—Joseph Califano

As a young man entering medical school, I was convinced that almost without exception, all physicians, everywhere, were dedicated, selfless, and committed citizens who acted as professionals at all times. Perhaps the Jesuits who ran my high school and college taught me too much about ideals and too little about reality. Perhaps it was because the idealistic professors at my medical school in Bogota instilled in me the belief that my patients' needs must always be my first priority. Whatever the source of this naïveté, I never doubted that doctors always subordinated their personal interests to the interests of those they served.

Only slowly, after many years in the United States, did I come to realize that some physicians have been known to ignore their responsibilities. They abuse their prerogatives, making the practice of medicine little more than a means to enrich themselves as much as possible. For them, the care of patients is secondary. If they believe anything, they believe that the providing care and dealing with sick people should inconvenience them as little as possible.

I hold the advent of Medicare in the early 1960s primarily responsible for this sad transformation. In Mark Twain's short story "The Man That Corrupted Hadleyburg," the leading citizens of a fictional town are extremely proud of their "incorruptibility." A visitor to the town realizes, however, that while they had never been corrupted, they had also never been tempted. He lays a trap, and all of the town fathers tumble into it.

Medicine before Medicare was like the good citizens of Hadleyburg before the stranger came to town. Extreme financial rewards were few. The pride and self-respect of physicians were more precious than available incomes. Even as recently as the early 1960s, most physicians maintained middle-class lifestyles. Most hospitals were public, charitable, or philanthropic institutions. Medical devices and pharmaceuticals were manufactured and sold with modest profit margins. The profession had a reputation for extraordinary integrity although perhaps, like Hadleyburg, it was incorruptible only because of the absence of sufficient temptation.

With the advent of Medicare in the early 1960s, the practice of medicine and the attitude of many physicians toward their work changed dramatically. For the first time in the history of medicine, doctors began to earn high, previously unimaginable incomes. Huge numbers of elderly patients, once treated at city or county hospitals at no charge, now had their care paid by the federal government. Doctors doubled, tripled, or even quadrupled their incomes. They began to move from middle-class communities into neighborhoods previously reserved for wealthy businessmen. They became part of the nouveau riche.

The federal largesse, intended to satiate the medical community's need for more income, only generated more greed. A few physicians began abusing the system by providing unnecessary treatment or surgery, by submitting bills for services that they did not provide, or by inflating prices. Worse yet, the prospect of astounding financial rewards brought a new type of individual into medicine. Financially ambitious young people who would once have sought careers in law or business, now flocked to medical schools. Young idealists, who once sought careers in medicine out of their desire to help people live healthier, happier lives, increasingly went elsewhere. Consequently, a growing segment of today's medical students has little in common with the older generation of practitioners.

The counterargument given by some to justify these practices is that medical students, upon completion of their studies, are deeply in debt. Although there is some merit to this claim, it is not enough to offset the end result. After all, the mechanism that exists for the repayment of debt is reasonable, and many have done so while remaining ethical and committed physicians.

At the same time, the rising financial rewards of the health care industry brought about a pharmaceutical and technological revolution. The giant pharmaceutical companies began producing new drugs almost on a daily basis. The inventive genius of American industry discovered the health care gold mine. Inventors began creating the new machines that dramatically improve our capability for accurate diagnoses and facilitate many forms of treatment. The computer revolution played an extraordinary role in reshaping clinical laboratories and diagnostic imaging. Computers also dramatically increased the ability of hospitals, insurance companies, and even private medical practices to maintain patients' medical and financial records.

In orthopaedic surgery, major developments took place with enormous speed. The successful replacement of arthritic joints and the use of the arthroscope for the treatment of damaged structures inside of the knee came first. Many new technologically assisted surgical techniques followed. As new, young physicians discovered the psychological and financial rewards of the surgical disciplines, they began abandoning nonsurgical methods even when surgery was not necessary. Upon completion of medical school training, the new graduates began to seek additional training through subspecialty fellowships. Each new subspecialty emphasized surgery as if nonsurgical treatments were no longer part of the arsenal of the orthopaedic physician.

Individually, each of these developments offered some promise of improved care, along with a modest measure of increased cost. Together, they conspired to aid an inflationary spiral that has made the cost of health care one of the most critical social issues in the United States. Many "cures" have emerged to break the pattern. One of these so-called cures, managed care, has become a social illness that is far more threatening to our patients than the original disease.

When I returned to Miami in 1994, after nearly twenty years in California and a short stint in Scotland, the managed care system had made deep inroads in Florida. The hospital where I went to work was a for-profit institution run by a corporation that controlled a large number of hospitals and rehabilitation facilities throughout the country.

During my initial negotiations with the administration, I candidly expressed my views about my experiences with hip replacement surgery performed expeditiously, followed by immediate rehabilitation and early discharge from the hospital. Apparently they liked what they heard from me; they promised to support my efforts to build a comprehensive Arthritis and Joint Replacement Institute.

Those plans and my hope to make the institute a model of patient-oriented financial restraint would not survive my encounters with Medicare, managed care, and nobody-seems-to care.

During my first week back in Miami, I discharged my first patient from the acute ward to the rehabilitation area. At my hospital, we call the rehabilitation area the Skilled Nursing Unit. In theory, the Skilled Nursing Unit administered intensive physical therapy. I soon learned, however, that there was nothing skilled about the services provided in the unit. In fact, there were few nurses and many were poorly trained. For that matter, I soon learned that there was less rehabilitation provided in the rehabilitation area than on the regular surgical wards.

The physical therapists assigned to the area spent a large portion of their time "treating" elderly individuals suffering from terminal conditions. Such patients deserve quality care, but should not be undergoing wasteful physical and occupational rehabilitation. Often these people are unaware of their whereabouts. Their memory spans only a few seconds; they wish only to rest and sleep.

Instead, the Skilled Nursing Unit subjects them to its brand of "intensive" physical therapy modalities. Once or twice a day aides take them to the therapy area. There, a therapist or an assistant ranges their arms or legs for a couple of minutes, and suggests to the patients that they actively repeat the motions for a few seconds. Medically, such treatment is a total waste of time and may be distressful to the patient. It is, however, unusually profitable to the hospital. Under managed care, the more "therapy" the staff provides, the more revenues they manage to generate.

My patient, in the new environment, improved as expected, in the manner in which most patients recover following hip replacement surgery. By the end of the fifth postoperative day, she was independent in transfer activities and capable of walking with the aid of a walker. She could also climb steps and use the toilet facilities. I therefore initiated procedures to discharge her, and made plans to see her in my office a few weeks later.

Within the hour, my patient called and angrily told me that according to her social service administrator, Medicare "entitled" her to stay in the hospital for a total of twenty days. She would then be able to choose either to go home, or go to another rehabilitation facility.

My attempts to dissuade her from staying in the hospital proved futile. She knew her "rights" and she wanted to exercise them. On the twenty-first day, she went home.

She probably would have recovered more quickly at home. She certainly gained little from her extended stay. The hospital, however, gained a great deal financially. After that introduction to managed care, I had a number of similar experiences. I learned that in our brave new world of modern health care, most patients now miraculously get well on their twenty-first day of rehabilitation. Though the approved length of stay may be shorter today (but I doubt it), the principle I have addressed remains firm.

On another occasion, I sought to discharge a rehabilitation patient who, in my opinion, had already improved as much as possible from our facilities and care. I had plans to leave the city the following day; I wanted to discharge her before my departure. I was at the nurse's station, writing the discharge orders, when my beeper went off. It was a moderately urgent call that required my prompt response. Inadvertently I left the ward without signing the discharge. The next day I left town. I returned four days later.

Two weeks after my return, I found a message on my desk inquiring as to when I was planning to see this patient. The question had come from the Skilled Nursing Unit. To my amazement, the patient had never left the hospital. As I apologized to my patient, I trembled with mixed fury at the nurses and with embarrassment over the entire situation. My patient, however, was unconcerned. She was quite content, and pleased that she had used her full twenty-one day rehabilitation entitlement.

In one of the regular hospital units, such incidents would be inconceivable. Five days after surgery I would have been approached by a clerk ordering me to discharge the patient because further hospitalization was not authorized. That kind of needed vigilance, however, occasionally produces its own problems.

Not too long ago, one of my patients traveled from California to Miami so that I could revise a failed total hip prosthesis that I had performed fifteen years earlier. She did well after surgery. On the fourth postoperative day, I wrote on her hospital chart that she had walked that day, with the aid of the therapist, approximately two hundred feet.

The same afternoon, a hospital/insurance clerk wrote a note indicating that the patient should be discharged the next day because her insurance company would not approve additional time in the hospital. I immediately called California, where the doctor on the insurance company staff repeated to me that additional hospitalization was not necessary and refused to authorize payment. His rationale: "If the patient is capable of walking, it means that hospitalization is not needed."

I informed him that the patient was able to walk two hundred feet, but that she could not get out of bed without assistance, could not use toilet facilities; could not get in and out of a car, dress herself, or go to the airport and sit in an airline seat for five hours. He insisted that the rules of the company were clear and that in his "medical judgment" the woman had recovered sufficiently to leave the hospital. He steadfastly refused to approve extended care. My patient had to finance her extended stay in the hospital with her own funds. She eventually forced the insurance company to reverse this obscene decision and reimburse her, but only after spending a great deal of time and effort.

Following discharge, the social service department of the hospital assigns, if requested by the treating physician, visiting nurses and physical therapists to visit the patients at home for whatever period of time is necessary. I used a similar system in California, but only for those few patients who needed such extended support. In the case of patients recovering from total hip surgery, only a small minority fall into that category. I can only speculate that to Medicare and Florida Medicaid, the cost may not be justified by *medical necessity*, but is required for the welfare of lawyers, lobbyists, and politicians.

Many rehabilitation centers subject all patients, even those who are transferred for simple therapeutic measures, to a number of evaluations. Private insurance, Medicare, or Medicaid pays for these procedures. Medical consultants evaluate these patients' concerns with vague, often unimportant or unrelated problems, even as the staff is already providing physical and occupational therapy.

A bill for physical or occupational therapy often lists separate treatments such as massage, electrical stimulation of muscles, application of heat, passive exercises, active exercises, and gait training. Imagine if nurses were allowed to unbundle their services and charge separately for every single task they perform: answering the bell, bringing in a bedpan, changing a dressing, taking the patient's temperature, making the bed, administering meds, and so forth. Their bills would be astronomical. The system would crash and burn within days. Recently, third-party payers have begun to appreciate this waste and abuse. Many are attempting to correct the situation. In the process, unfortunately, they have begun to deny payment for *necessary* rehabilitation.

I was once approached by a physical therapist at the hospital's Skilled Nursing Unit who requested that a patient of mine, a woman recovering from a hip replacement operation, be prescribed upper extremity occupational therapy. I pretended not to understand what she was trying to tell me. I said that my patient required only learning how to get around with crutches. The patient had been fully independent at home prior to surgery; she did not need any upper extremity treatments. The physical therapist, however, insisted that the musculature of my patient's arms was weak, and it would be "important" to strengthen her muscles. I initially declined, but the patient later requested the additional therapy to which she was entitled. The physical therapist then suggested that the upper extremity rehabilitation be provided by an occupational therapist since she was not qualified to provide it. That was a specious attempt to increase revenue for the rehabilitation facility.

In Miami, the undisputed capital of medical fraud in the United States, a plethora of clinics and health care facilities are egregiously abusing the system and stealing millions of dollars from Medicare and Medicaid. The media regularly uncover and report their crimes, district attorneys indict the perpetrators, the courts slap their wrists and new clinics sprout up the next day. If we are serious about controlling health care costs, we need to attack heath care fraud and abuse with the same focus and intensity (and hopefully with more success) that we have devoted to the war on drugs.

I became a careful student of the situation during my tenure on the board of directors of the American Academy of Orthopaedic Surgeons for eight years—and particularly during my year as president of the organization. I find the medical profession guilty to a degree much greater than I would like to admit. Medicine's concern with profit has transformed our once proud profession into just another business; far too many medical professionals have become little more than greedy businessmen. Physicians who once managed their own practices have become employees of giant health care corporations, and are now becoming interested in unionization. I can hope that lev-elheaded physicians will prevail, but I cannot be optimistic.

It would be an awesome undertaking to even partially dismantle a system that went awry. It would take a commitment of enormous magnitude. Robert Kennedy, a hero of my younger, more restless days, once said: "The best way to guarantee the success of evil is for good men to do nothing." Robert Kennedy was also fond of quoting George Bernard Shaw's lines from *Pygmalion*: "I know of people who see things that happened and say why. I dream of things that never happened and say why not." I have not stood idly by as our national health care crisis has developed. I have been working throughout the last three decades to convince the medical community that it must rehabilitate its own professionalism.

In 1991, I participated on a panel discussion at a meeting of the American Orthopedic Association dealing with ethical aspects in entrepreneurial activities of physicians. I found myself passionately arguing that doctors must continue to subordinate their own interests to those of their patients. I argued that we have to restore a commit-ment to true ethics that endure, rather than adapt to pseudoethics of convenience. I pointed out that the agenda of medicine is totally at odds with the agenda of industry. "The care of patients is the corner-stone of our profession. Industry has no patients—only customers."

Since then, I have raised the volume of my attack on the growing power of the orthopaedic industrial complex. I have spoken out in lec-tures at medical schools, conferences, and other forums around the world. I have never proposed that financial incentives be forbidden to any health care professional. I suggest simply that we seek some rational way to balance the untamed, uncivilized entrepreneurial engine that currently seems determined to mow down our entire national economy.

Some would argue that in today's environment, patients are health care consumers who are expected to be aware of the services being provided to them. Awareness of those services is a healthy pat-tern that probably has helped in better education of the American people. However, the resulting connotation that "patients" are "cus-tomers" emphasizes a cold commercial transaction that diminishes the unselfish relationship that should exist between doctor and patient.

In 1997, I spoke to the incoming class of the American Academy of Orthopaedic Surgeons. I told them that if they succeed in restoring the ethical and professional underpinnings of medicine, they would reduce today's crisis to a footnote in history. "This is the real crisis in medicine: the declining professionalism of its practitioners; the lowering and anesthetizising of ethical standards; the belief that everything is okay, which eliminates the possibility of being morally wrong."

chapter 19.
a changing profession

"The fear of being wrong is a disease."

I have often lamented the absence of liberal arts education in pre-medical and medical school curricula in the United States. Medical students elsewhere, especially in Europe, make time to study history, literature, and philosophy. I am firmly convinced that such a lack of learning in the liberal arts is partially responsible for the current national health care crisis.

Today, medical schools and residency programs seem determined to drive their students even further from global questions. At one time, physicians studied the whole patient, body and mind. The Roman ideal, *mens sana in corpore sano*, a sound mind in a sound body, endured for almost two thousand years. With the explosion of scientific learning in the late nineteenth and early twentieth centuries, physicians found it necessary to create such specialties as orthopaedics, psychiatry, pediatrics, gynecology, and ear-nose-and-throat.

I was, and still am, a participant in orthopaedic subspecialty societies. I was among the founding members of two of them and became president of the Hip Society, one of the world's most prestigious subspecialty organizations. You may be surprised, therefore, that I now regard some of these organizations not only as superfluous but also as harmful. Their proliferation has trivialized specialization itself and weakened the glue that keeps "organized medicine" organized.

I do not deny the obvious benefits that subspecialization has produced. To do so would be blindness of the worst type. My criticism is
with the modern trend toward excessive glorification.

Today's orthopaedists have increasingly become technicians first,
and only then, medical practitioners. In the case of fracture care, they
are often more concerned with cosmesis than with function and the
biological approach to medical care of musculoskeletal disorders.
They do not seem to find time for learning about the body and the
healing process. These trends are threatening the foundations of the
orthopaedic profession. I am sure that parallel developments are
affecting other medical specialties.

During my tenure as president of the American Academy of
Orthopedic Surgeons (AAOS), I realized that any attempts to persuade the board of directors of the pervasive and growing dangers
associated of excessive subspecialization were futile. Most of the
directors were, like me, subspecialists themselves. Many were deeply
involved in the affairs of their own subspecialty societies. They were
not anxious to rock their own boats.

In addition, the academy believed that its own creation, the
Council of Musculoskeletal Societies (COMSS), would effectively prevent a serious and permanent splitting of the discipline into independent societies. A few years earlier, the American College of Surgeons
had experienced the rebellion of many specialists into organized
autonomous academies, such as orthopaedics, neurosurgery, ophthalmology, urology and many others. AAOS believed that the establishment of COMSS would prevent orthopaedics from traveling the same
road, and would effectively "keep the family together."

On the day that he assumed leadership of AAOS, Dr. Charles
Rockwood spoke eloquently about the orthopaedic family. During his
address, he showed photographs of his wife and their nine children.
Their togetherness was to be a good example to orthopaedists.

At the time, I, too, thought COMSS was a good idea. Unfortunately, its formation actually fostered the creation of several new subspecialty societies, which, through membership in COMSS, gained
the full prestige of the parent organization. Several superfluous societies sprouted almost overnight. Each has its own officers and its own
national or international meeting and many of them, of course, publish their own journals. This astonishing proliferation of journals is
but one more part of the growing threat to medicine. According to a

report provided to me by a professor at Oxford University, as recently as 1996 there were thirty thousand medical journals worldwide; three thousand new medical articles were published daily; and one thousand of them entered Medline (the major medical component of the Internet). One can't help but wonder how much this information really contributes to the growth of knowledge.

I cannot speak for other specialties, but I know that our own residents in training no longer read the leading orthopaedic research journals the way residents in earlier days read them. On several occasions, I have interrupted regularly scheduled continuing education conferences to ask if anyone had read a given article in the previous month's edition of the leading orthopaedic scholarly journal. Most of the residents immediately raised their hands. I then asked specific questions, drawn from the article under discussion. One by one, I questioned the residents who had raised their hands, only to learn that most of them had not read it after all. Most of them do, however, glance at the highlights of various throwaway publications provided, at no charge, by equipment manufacturers and pharmaceutical companies. Tabloid journalism now sets the pace in orthopaedics. These publications, not subject to peer review, often publish results from unproven treatments and techniques. Believing the information is based on solid data, many orthopaedists apply these techniques to their practices, with obvious harmful consequences.

The publication of too many journals has greatly weakened the overall quality of medical publishing. In order to remain profitable, many of these publications have more pages committed to advertisements than to scientific papers. To fill their scientific pages, they are increasingly willing to accept manuscripts that would never pass the traditional peer review process.

Because orthopaedics is a subspecialization, many medical professionals outside of orthopaedics have concluded that orthopaedics no longer represents a readily identifiable body of knowledge. Many general practitioners, podiatrists, neurosurgeons, and even plastic surgeons now believe that anyone with a modicum of manual skills can learn to execute orthopaedic technology. As managed care cuts into their established practices, they maintain their incomes by expanding their territories. Physicians with no orthopaedic training now perform orthopaedic surgery. To learn the "technology," they simply contact the manufacturers of surgical instruments and devices.

The manufacturers demonstrate the technology. One would suspect that such a pattern would have created by now a field day for malpractice attorneys. It has, but not to the degree I anticipated. It shows that as long as a surgical procedure has been used to treat a given condition, and the technique has been properly carried out, it is difficult to prove the commission of malpractice. What often constitutes the inappropriateness of care is the performance of surgery unnecessarily, for the wrong indication, or performing it incompetently.

In the late 1970s, when I was head of orthopaedics at the University of Miami, I had a long and difficult dispute with a local podiatrist, who wanted full privileges at Jackson Memorial Hospital.

Traditionally, podiatrists were not considered doctors and confined themselves to caring for minor problems of the foot: removal of ingrown toenails, the prevention of foot sores in diabetic patients, and the prescription of arch supports. The podiatrist who wanted hospital privileges felt that he was qualified to do much more. He explained that podiatric education and training had improved and expanded dramatically over the years.

I was chief of the department of orthopaedics at the medical school, as well as at the hospital. It was my responsibility to establish guidelines regarding privileges to be granted to podiatrists. The applicant considered himself a physician and demanded surgical opportunities to perform surgery of various types. My orthopaedic medical staff and I regarded the procedures he wanted to perform as the purview of our specialty. We felt that orthopaedic surgery required a clear understanding of the anatomy, physiology, and pathology not only of the foot but also of the body as a whole. The guidelines would clarify exactly which procedures would be opened to the podiatrist.

I prepared guidelines and presented them to the administration of the hospital. I had consulted with other academic orthopaedists in various parts of the United States in an attempt to give my submitted guidelines additional credibility. The guidelines I prepared were indeed restrictive. The podiatrist characterized them bluntly: "Doctor Sarmiento has ruled that I should be allowed to perform any surgery I wish, providing only that I do not go below the skin." His characterization of my guidelines was close to the truth. Our proposed limits proved unacceptable to him.

His peers across the country anxiously awaited the outcome of his application. They looked forward to breaking the barrier that had kept them from entering the mainstream of medicine in the United States. When the university accepted my guidelines, the podiatrists appealed to the board of trustees, which granted them a formal hearing.

That hearing became extremely personal and acrimonious. The podiatrists charged my department with neglecting the welfare of our patients by denying them needed services. I charged the podiatrist with performing large numbers of unnecessary surgeries. I added, "With all due respect, I suspect that the main reason for the large numbers of surgeries performed by the doctor is pure, unadulterated greed." The hospital attorney representing me kicked me under the table and quietly instructed me never to make statements of that nature.

We argued over various compromises at different meetings. The podiatrist proved a brilliant, well-educated, articulate opponent. Asked how he would handle one difficult medical complication, he responded that he would do "exactly the same thing doctor Sarmiento does under similar circumstances," he would call in additional consultants. He was right.

At several times during the hearing, I thought that my cause was lost. At the end, however, the board decided to uphold my recommendation. We would fight the next round in the state courts. Fortunately, the podiatrist not only thought he was a fully qualified doctor but also believed he was a qualified attorney. He forgot the old legal adage: "He who acts as his own attorney has a fool for a client."

When the court published the final verdict in 1978, my family and I had already moved to Los Angeles, where I had just been appointed to serve as professor and chief of the orthopedic department the University of Southern California. The news of the outcome of the trial was delivered to me via telephone by the lead attorney, while his group celebrated the victory at a noisy bar. He said that they wanted me to join them in a toast to "Doctor Sarmiento's unshakable commitment to principles."

As I look back at my stubbornness and unwillingness to compromise, I remind myself of the harm as well as the good that such attitudes have done to many causes over the years. In retrospect, I am not proud of my actions in the affair of podiatry at the University of Miami in the 1970s. I was unreasonable in my demands and abused the power of the office I held.

During my tenure as president of the American Academy of Orthopaedic Surgeons in 1991, the president of the American Academy of Podiatry asked to meet with me. He wanted to discuss the possibility of joint ventures between his organization and ours. At the end of the meeting, I stated to him that I would be happy to deliver the message to our board of directors. I added, however, that in order for me to do so I needed to hear from him the philosophy of his profession regarding to the scope of his discipline. I asked how his group went about determining the boundaries and scope of their specialty. Did they expect to confine themselves to problems involving the foot? Did they believe themselves qualified to treat the ankle joint? Did their expertise extend to the knee?

In fact, his association had recently explored just that question. They had resolved such an important issue not by evaluating their training and the curriculum provided to student podiatrists, but by a vote of the membership. To me, that seemed to indicate that the podiatrists did not understand their own limitations. The issue ended our discussion, but I knew that podiatry would continue to seek greater freedom and professional privileges.

The more things change, however, the more they remain the same. When I returned to Miami after an absence of nearly twenty years, I discovered that my colleagues at the local hospital were still facing the same questions. This time, however, the administration did not side with the orthopaedists. They granted privileges to the podiatrists that include major surgery of the foot and leg "all the way up to the knee." The hospital is a for-profit institution. From their perspective, the fees earned by the podiatry business are just as welcome as fees from any other source.

The podiatrists in Miami had also made it clear to the hospital committee that they were willing to litigate until they achieved their "rights." The hospital granted the podiatrists the privileges they requested without litigation. The managed care industry would like to bring podiatry and others into competition with orthopaedic surgery. They see such competition as a way to lower the fees paid by managed care and, therefore, as a way to raise insurance company profits.

Many forms of quackery and borderline medicine are also flourishing in the current health care environment. Medical clinics have sprouted all over the town. Most are small, poorly equipped, and inadequately staffed facilities that often take advantage of the uneducated and the large immigrant population living in the city. Though there are many foreign physicians practicing first-class medicine in south Florida, there are also many foreign-trained physicians who have not acquired the additional education and necessary experience to become skilled doctors. These doctors staff most of the street corner clinics. While their medical skills may not be first-rate, their business acumen and promotional skills are world-class. I recently watched a program on one of the major broadcasting networks that discussed the "well kept secret" of the excellence of medicine in Miami. According to the network, wealthy citizens from all over Latin America are traveling to Miami for medical care. Among the factors the program discussed was the tremendous advantage of having its doctors be able to speak Spanish.

I, of course, had long been aware that financially well-off Latin Americans often sought medical care in the United States. I had believed, however, that these patients came to the United States in anticipation of being treated by American doctors who had been trained in American medical schools. I thought they were willing to tolerate the inconvenience of having to communicate with their doctors through interpreters, that they accepted inconvenience as part of the price for receiving the best of care.

Amazingly, I have only recently realized that many Latin American patients prefer Spanish-speaking doctors, no matter where they were trained. They probably assume that all physicians who practice medicine in the United States are equally qualified and deliver top quality care. I never realized that so many of my Latino compatriots were so naive.

chapter 20.
the big break

"There is nothing as powerful as an idea whose time has come."
—Victor Hugo

*"It matters not how strait the gate
How charged with punishments the scroll
I am the master of my fate
I am the captain of my soul."*

—William Ernest Henley
Macmillan–London

My work with amputees and their rehabilitation continually provided my most rewarding experiences. On one occasion it opened the door to opportunities far beyond my wildest dreams. One day, I was studying an amputee functioning with a below-the-knee prosthesis. He was walking on a treadmill in front of a cineradiography machine, a piece of equipment that makes it possible to take X rays of moving objects, a procedure that I had conducted several times before. This time, however, as I watched the limb in motion, I had a flash of intuition, a momentary insight that would eventually challenge longstanding beliefs and orthodox treatment of fractures.

That day, as I watched the filmed images moving on the screen, I questioned, for the first time, the time-honored principle of immobilizing the knee and ankle joints of patients who had sustained fractures of the lower leg. I watched the way that the artificial prosthesis effectively transferred the weight of the body from the ground to the proximal end of the stump. If a prosthesis could be so effective, I thought, then a cast, molded like the prosthesis, should enable a patient with a fractured tibia to bear weight on the fractured extremity without experiencing shortening of the leg. Furthermore, I reasoned, since the amputee's stump did not experience contact with the bottom of the socket, the patient with a fractured tibia should also be free of such shortening. It seemed to me that the proximal fragment of the fracture would, under those circumstances, function as the equivalent of the amputee's stump.

All of these thoughts passed through my mind in an instant. I almost dismissed them just as quickly. I knew that this theory ran contrary to all existing practices. Orthopaedists had always assumed that proper treatment of a fracture required immobilization of joints adjacent to the fracture. A thousand years of medical orthodoxy taught that broken bones would heal most quickly and most securely only when treated with the greatest possible immobilization. Could that really be wrong?

European orthopaedic surgeons had recently perfected surgical techniques that enabled totally rigid immobilization of broken bones. They made improved, sophisticated plates and screws to maximize compression between bony fragments. Their concept, which is still popular today, had only recently gained worldwide acceptance. Even as my own theory began evolving in my mind, I realized that it would be politically unwise not only to question traditional thinking but also to go against a widely accepted contemporary school of thought. To do so would be to risk alienating not only the most traditional authorities, but also some of the profession's most influential practitioners.

I left the radiology room, where I had been admiring the effectiveness of the amputee's prosthesis, in search of a patient with a fractured tibia. In the orthopaedic ward, I found a young boy who had been injured in an automobile accident a few days earlier. His leg was wrapped in a cast that extended from the toes to mid-thigh.

I took him to the plaster room where I sedated him, removed the cast, and proceeded to apply a new cast, which I molded in a manner that resembled an amputee's prosthesis. I left his knee free, wrapped his lower leg and ankle, and added a walking heel to the plaster. As soon as the plaster dried, I helped the patient to his feet and suggested that he bear as much weight on his leg as his symptoms permitted.

The results of this impromptu experiment were extraordinary. Much to my surprise, I discovered that he was able to bear almost his entire weight on his leg. He began learning to use his crutches that afternoon. To check on the possibility of the leg shortening under this new stress, I ordered that X rays of his leg be taken every day. The fracture healed without any shortening, beyond the mild shortening that he had experienced at the time of the injury.

This simple, one-patient trial convinced me that my theory was worthy of further exploration. I became quite enthusiastic about the new idea, and the residents shared my excitement. We began to seek out as many patients with tibia fractures as we could find. I treated all of them in my new way. The initial results seemed to be consistently good.

Coincidentally, Professor Lorenz Bohler, from Vienna, happened to visit Miami a few months after I had begun working with the new method. At the time, Professor Bohler was perhaps the best-known and most respected orthopaedist in Europe. His reputation, skill, and knowledge influenced orthopaedics throughout the world. He had published extensive research studies advocating the treatment of fractures using casts that immobilized all adjacent joints but that permitted and encouraged weight-bearing ambulation.

During his visit to Jackson Memorial, I presented to him a few of the patients I had treated, or who were under treatment, with the new method. He observed the patients and casts carefully. He did not say anything in front of the group. At the end of the meeting he took me aside and in a low voice, so no one could hear his remarks, he said: "Young doctor, do not continue on your efforts to treat tibial fractures in this manner. Your idea will not work. It is contrary to all basic principles of trauma care. Give it up. I have treated over 15,000 tibial fractures with my long leg cast, and the results have been very good. The knee must be immobilized."

I attempted to explain to him again the rationale of my proposed treatment to no avail. He had made up his mind, probably fifty years earlier, that the foundation upon which his treatment was based was supported by centuries of tradition. His mind remained unshakable. He could not, however, find any fault with the healing of any of the subjects I had presented to him.

I was disappointed by his lack of support, but could not let myself be dissuaded from continuing my experimentation. Professor Bohler retired soon after his return to Vienna. In 1965 I traveled to Poland as part of a group of U.S. physicians and prosthetists. Our group spent several days with Professor Marian Weiss in Warsaw. Professor Weiss was a remarkable man who possessed a fertile and highly organized mind. He seemed unconfined by traditional thinking. His rehabilitation center was far ahead of any rehabilitation center in the United States. His work had first popularized the immediate postoperative prosthetic fitting of the amputee. His vision had led directly to my own work on postoperative prosthetic fitting, and, indirectly, to my work on the functional below-the-knee cast for fractured tibias.

On my way home from Warsaw, I stopped in Vienna to visit Professor Bohler, who graciously received me in his home. His wife served us tea while I discussed my experiences with my functional below-the-knee cast. To document my theory, I had brought many photographs of fractures that I had treated. It was a memorable afternoon in an old, classically lovely Austrian apartment. While I did my best to convince Dr. Bohler that we had made important progress, the proud old man reminisced about his experiences in medicine and continually referred to his own contributions to the treatment of tibial fractures. He was especially proud of the Austrian celebrities who had sought his care.

"During my career I treated several professional skiers with broken tibias, who went on later to win Olympic medals," he said. Almost as an afterthought he added, "I have recently heard that a young man won a medal after having his leg treated with a plate." He paused for a couple of seconds. "However, it was only a silver medal." Unfortunately, I could not convince Bohler that functional, below-the-knee casting was worthy of further exploration. Perhaps he would have been more impressed if I had conducted more experiments in Aspen, and fewer in Miami!

The rest of that trip to Europe proved more enjoyable and intellectually useful. It provided my first opportunity for a close look at the practice of orthopaedics in the Old World. I met several giants in the fields of orthopaedics and prosthetics, and was able to observe them in their own environment. It also provided the first opportunity for me to visit some of the great cities of England and continental Europe. I was thrilled to finally experience the remarkable beauty of these countries, which I had read about all of my life, but which, with the exception of Italy, I had never seen for myself.

In Warsaw, we attended the Opera House to watch a performance of Verdi's *Aida*. I was totally captivated by the grandeur and elegance of the production. The "Triumphal March" included elephants and other large African animals from a local circus. I had never seen anything like it.

Throughout our stay in Warsaw, we had been eating at modest restaurants. After the opera, we went to dinner at a luxurious restaurant, an experience that seemed out of place in Communist Poland. Despite the grandeur and opulence of the evening, our hosts seemed to be extremely reserved and quiet. In retrospect, their somber demeanor seemed to have overtaken much of their country. I could only believe that it reflected their response to the Russian occupation of their proud land. Thirty-five years later, when I visited Lublin and Warsaw, I was amazed at the free and gay behavior of Poland's new generation.

When we returned to Miami, I continued my work with renewed enthusiasm. Perhaps because of my inability to convince Professor Bohler, and perhaps because I remained uncertain about some aspects of my treatment, I had a functional cast applied to my own leg. (I did not, however, go so far as to have my own tibia fractured.) For three days, I walked around with the cast on my leg. Even though I did not have a fractured leg, the experience changed my understanding of the way in which the cast functioned. First, I realized that I had experienced neither pressure nor discomfort over the areas where the cast had been firmly molded. Second, there was no redness, even over those parts of the leg where, theoretically, weight-bearing stresses concentrated. Third, I distinctly felt increased pressure over my calf muscles.

I had originally suspected that my cast functioned by transferring the patient's weight to the patellar tendon (the structure that connects the kneecap to the thigh muscles) and the flares of the bone just below the knee. Only after experimenting with the cast on my own leg did I began to suspect that the new cast, which was applied snugly against the flesh and muscles of the lower leg, transferred the weight to these soft tissues. This observation supported the theory that further shortening of a broken leg could be effectively prevented.

This latter observation rapidly led to a radical and significant modification of the original concept. I proceeded to free the ankle joint, which, until that time, I had immobilized. In search of a good way to connect the cast to the patients' shoes, my colleagues and I experimented with various metal and plastic artificial joints. I also sought a new plastic-based material to replace the traditional but heavy plaster of paris cast. I even traveled to Johnson & Johnson research facilities in New Jersey to propose research concerning new casting materials. A team of engineers received my ideas enthusiastically and promised to start work on the concept immediately.

A few weeks later, they asked me back to their laboratories, where they shared their research into various materials and demonstrated a few experimental products that could be used to manufacture casts and braces. I immediately tried the products—wrapping them over the legs of the engineers. While they recognized a distinct need for improvement, they remained convinced that they were close to developing a practical product.

I never heard from them again. At a later meeting of the American Academy of Orthopedic Surgeons, I ran into one of the engineers whom I had met at Johnson & Johnson. When I inquired about the status of "my" project, he told me, "confidentially," that they had developed a product, but that someone high in the organization had ordered cancellation of clinical trials. He and his team had been told, "off the record," that there was no need to challenge their successful plaster of paris business with another product. Apparently, the executives had decided to keep the new product on the shelves. They would release it only when another company challenged their domination of the plaster casting technology.

A few years later, another company produced a new plastic-based casting system. Within a remarkably short time, Johnson & Johnson released its own new plastic-based system as a substitute for plaster casts. Plastic and fiberglass casting systems are now used throughout the world. That change should have taken place much sooner.

Meanwhile, back in the hospital, we conducted our own search for substitute casting systems. At one point, we experimented with a synthetic rubber material that was then popular for the fabrication of hand splints. The material was available in stiff sheets that, once heated, became soft and malleable. In the softened condition they were wrapped over the injured leg. A few minutes later the material again became hard. The method was a definite improvement, but the application technique proved difficult and subject to many possible errors. Realizing that there was a need to make the system more foolproof, we began experimenting with prefabricated braces that the surgeon could select "off the shelf." We measured the legs of over 100 volunteers—mostly students, therapists, nurses, and even a few members of the faculty. We used that data to manufacture the world's first prefabricated functional fracture braces.

Shortly after the onset of my investigations with the use of fracture bracing, and during the process of recruiting others to become part of the new rehabilitation program, I was fortunate enough to meet two people who became key to the many developments that subsequently took place in the fascinating project: William Sinclair, a prosthetist-orthotist (brace and artificial-limb maker) and Loren L. Latta, an engineer. Both were young and extremely talented. Both proved highly committed to excellence and totally loyal. Together, we have conceived and discussed hundreds of ideas. Their support has been extremely valuable for many years. It was with their help, and with the help of many of the residents in training, that we first realized that my original concept, which we had, at first, applied only to tibial fractures, could and should be applied to other bones. Enthusiastically, we began experimenting with fractures of the arm, thigh, and wrist.

It was then that I realized that contrary to long and widely revered belief, motion at the fracture site could be an important aid to the healing of fractures. The more we studied and explored the essential nature of the healing process, the more this concept made sense.

We were reminded that, for example, animals cannot immobilize their broken bones. The wolf that breaks a leg refuses to walk for a short period of time, then it manages to hop to the nearest puddle of water to quench its thirst. Little by little it begins to touch the ground with the broken limb. It steadily increases the amount of weight until finally, all four legs again enter in the normal gait cycle. Animals in the wild behave in a similar manner. In fact, naturalists, museum curators, and anthropologists agree that evidence of nonunited fractures is extremely rare. To the contrary, skeletal remains provide irrefutable evidence of healed (though often deformed) fractures.

We also know that many fractures in the human that cannot be immobilized heal readily. Many of you will have learned that already, from the painful experience of a broken rib. There is no way to immobilize this bone, yet it heals, and often heals extremely rapidly without treatment. The collarbone and several other bones are also treated without immobilization when fractured. Yet we have continued to immobilize all other bones, simply because we can. Currently, a very large percentage of fractures are treated by surgical means, as a result of sophisticated metallurgical, imaging, and surgical techniques not available four decades ago. With increasing frequency the surgical treatment has become, without any doubt, the treatment of choice.

Many medical dogmas are nothing more than pronouncements once made by someone with bestowed authority. They remain unchallenged because they have the imprimatur of tradition. Physicians continue to assume that they are valid, only because they have never been challenged. These medical dogmas are the functional equivalent of other inherited truths: thunder and lighting are expressions of God's wrath; the sun rotates around the earth; time is an inflexible absolute. The real problem is simply that medicine had not, until recently, had its fair share of skeptics.

Our suggestion that minimizing immobilization could actually accelerate healing met with a great deal of professional skepticism. Professor Bohler proved to be just the first of many staunch defenders of the old faith. We found our research and our teachings subjected to vicious attack, not only locally but also throughout the national orthopaedic community. The attacks often came from some of the profession's most respected leaders.

Despite the setbacks, I remained determined to prove my point. My enthusiasm and dedication took on almost pathological proportions. I began to experiment with similar treatment for many other fractures.

The results proved somewhat humbling, with success rates that showed a wide range of variation. My attempts to treat fractures of the femur (thigh bone) and the forearm produced unacceptable numbers of complications, such as excessive and unsightly angulation of the fractured bones. The results from bracing the humerus (upper arm bone) and fractures about the wrist yielded almost consistently good results.

We carefully recorded and photographed the clinical results obtained with our new method of treatment. We were increasingly anxious to report our findings to the orthopaedic community, but we knew that we would face opposition. Because our concept ran contrary to firmly established beliefs in the orthopaedic world, I delayed reporting until we had irrefutable data.

Finally, I submitted an application to the American Academy of Orthopaedic Surgeons' annual program committee. The committee rejected my application. I tried again the following year with the same result. Only many years later did I discover that Dr. Miller, my own department chief, had informed the program committee that it would be "dangerous" to allow me to present my work, as it was too radical and unconventional. A few months before his death, Dr. Miller sent me a file in which he had saved all records of correspondence with me and about me. His "Gus file" included his letters to the AAOS program committee.

Even as he was privately revealing the facts to me, Dr. Miller was publicly proclaiming his pride in my accomplishments, and the accomplishments of my colleague in his department, Dr. Newton McCollough III. At the time, both of us had become presidents of the AAOS—within just a few years. I have since been told that Dr. Miller frequently bragged about the fact that he had launched my academic career. He had a right to say so. I will forever be in his debt for inviting me to join his department at the University of Miami. He seemed to have forgotten, however, that he also threw a continually changing variety of hurdles in my path. I remember both the good and the bad. Dr. Miller was a good physician, a very good educator, and a complex human being.

I remember that I was an instructor in Dr. Miller's department at the medical school when a friend requested permission to nominate me to become director of education and head of the orthopaedic residency program at a small hospital in Cooperstown, New York. I was honored, but I could not picture myself holding such a position. My skills with English had improved, but I was still extremely self-conscious about my remaining accent. I had published only a few papers, and I did not think I had a chance. I decided to seek the advice of Dr. Miller.

"Dr. Miller, I have been with you for several years and you know how much I enjoy academic medicine. Do you think that some day I will able to run a residency program?"

He hesitated for a minute and then said, "Gus, sit down and let me tell you something that no one would have the courage to tell you. What I am about to say will be painful to you and that is the reason why no one else would say it. I only want to be helpful, but with your name, accent, and background you have no future in American academic medicine. Don't set your sights too high. You will do well in practice or in academic medicine but the position of chief you will never get. This is a WASP county, and academic medicine is even more so."

It was the first time I heard the acronym WASP. Dr. Miller explained that WASP meant "White, Anglo-Saxon, and Protestant." I was shocked by his willing acceptance of the deeply ingrained xenophobia of American medicine.

I left Dr. Miller's office after thanking him for his candor. I also swore that day that I would never accept his verdict. That night, I wrote to the hospital in Cooperstown and told them that I was not interested in the position. I did not tell them that I had resolved to become chief of orthopaedics not at a small hospital in upstate New York but at a major medical center. The anger and bitterness remained with me for many years. Time eventually assuaged much of my childish ill feelings, though perhaps, a small kernel of that angst remains with me to this day. In any case, Dr. Miller had planted the seeds of a growing determination to overcome prejudice. I have devoted myself to overcoming both dogmatic obstinacy and social prejudice ever since.

When I delivered the vice-presidential address at the 1991 meeting of the academy, I dedicated it to Dr. Miller. In that address, I acknowledged my debt to him. He was not in the audience. The following year, when I presided over the annual meeting of the academy in Washington, D.C., I made every effort to recognize him. He sat with us at the president's table, something he seemed to enjoy greatly. His wife of many years, who remained ill and disabled for a long time, had died some time earlier. He dealt admirably with her illness and the resulting personal problems. During those days, he clearly demonstrated his many good personal qualities.

Among the correspondence that he sent to me in his "Gus file" was a letter that he had written to the American Board of Orthopaedics. It advised that I should not be allowed to sit for the board examinations, as I was "not as yet mature in my understanding of the basic sciences of orthopaedics." I read that letter for the first time, some thirty years after it was written. Ironically, when he wrote the letter, Dr. Miller he had put me in charge of teaching pathology to the orthopaedic residents. Pathology is basic science!

When Dr. Walter Miller died in 1993, I flew from Los Angeles to Miami to attend his funeral services. From the podium, I told the audience how uncomfortable I felt for having been responsible for many of his problems in his academic life when my immaturity may have clouded my vision of reality. It was not easy for me to make those comments on such an occasion. Nonetheless, I felt that if I did not say them at that time I would never have another opportunity to do so. His children, with tears in their eyes, thanked me for my comments.

The academy rejected my third application to present my studies on the functional treatment of tibial fractures as a scientific paper. Instead, they offered me a kind of consolation prize by allowing me to present my work as the audiovisual segment of the academy's meeting. I could have been insulted. Instead, I was delighted by the back-door opportunity and determined to exploit the opening.

In the spirit of the "audiovisual" presentation, we made a movie demonstrating the application of functional casting and illustrating our results to date. We added Sibelius's *First Symphony* as background music. Dr. Virgil May, from Virginia, was the official discussant. I had never met him, and awaited his comments with trepidation and anxiety. At the end of the movie he stood up and told the audience that they should forget all about functional casting as soon as possible. "It is contrary to all the basic principles of orthopaedics and will inevitably lead to major complications." He left the room without waiting to hear my required rebuttal. That was my first introduction of the subject at the national level. What Dr. May had done was inexcusable, but depictive of the disdain with which people like me were treated. I am certain that someone else presenting the same material would have been treated with respect.

Undeterred by the bad experience I returned home with my commitment to the project further enhanced. Apparently, someone at the academy agreed with me, and the program committee accepted my third attempt to win a full scientific presentation at the next annual meeting.

A few days later, I received a letter from the academy informing me that Dr. Relton McCarrol from Saint Louis would be the discussant. At that time, Dr. McCarrol was already one of the United States's best-known orthopaedists. He had a well-established and well-earned reputation for mercilessly destroying papers and presenters. In his sharp, staccato voice, he regularly attacked his "victims" and made mincemeat of them.

Shortly before the meeting, I received a letter from Dr. McCarrol stating that he "was honored to discuss my paper" and that he was looking forward to the opportunity. He asked to see photographic slides of the radiographs of each of the one hundred clinical patients I would be reporting on before my presentation. His request was most unusual, but I agreed to meet him in his room at the Palmer House in Chicago, two days before my presentation.

At our meeting, he indicated that he had little available time and asked me to proceed rapidly through my slides, without making any comments. In rapid succession, I displayed photographs of the X rays of one hundred patients. When I finished, he stood up, apologized for the inconvenience, and showed me to the door. He did not ask a single question.

Two days later, I delivered my paper. I have never been as nervous as I was that day. I was sure that my work, career, and reputation were about to be destroyed. Somehow, I got through my presentation. To this day, I do not remember any part of it. I remember only that I had finally presented my material.

Dr. McCarrol stood up and walked to the lectern. "When I first read the abstract of the doctor's paper, I realized that I had been asked to discuss a subject which had no merit at all. I was certain that the data were not correct, since the proposed method is contrary to everything we know about the treatment of tibial fractures. Accordingly, I asked the doctor to bring to my room, prior to this day, slides of every single patient he has allegedly treated in the proposed manner. He acquiesced and yesterday he gave me the information I requested.

"The doctor is telling the truth and I commend him on his work. He is on the right track." I know that he then asked me two questions. To this day, I cannot remember his questions or my answers. I cannot even tell you *if* I answered his questions. I know only that I returned to the microphone, thanked him, acknowledged "being overwhelmed," and left the stage. My friends tell me that I was shaking and blushing like a schoolboy who had just been highly praised by his headmaster.

Shortly thereafter, the paper was accepted for publication in the *Journal of Bone and Joint Surgeons*, a journal that has since accepted many more of my manuscripts. Eventually, the academy and the Orthopaedic Research Society honored Loren Latta and me with the Kappa Delta Award, the most prestigious award given for orthopaedic research in the United States. The Association of Bone and Joint Surgeons also presented me with its highly coveted Nicholas Andry Award for orthopaedic research.

Shortly after my presentation to the academy, I received a letter from Dr. Richard Kilfoyle, from Boston, inviting me to be the guest speaker at the Boston Orthopaedic Club. When I first received the letter, I suspected that one of the local orthopaedists was playing a joke on me. George Richards, an orthopaedic surgeon from Miami and an old friend, had recently returned from Boston where he had taken a fellowship. Richards enjoyed playing pranks; I suspected that he had forged the invitation. I finally approached him and said that my trip to Boston had been a great success, and that I wanted to thank him for having made it possible. Only when he denied any knowledge of the letter did I realize that the invitation was genuine.

I accepted the invitation at once. My lecture at the Boston Club proved to be another remarkable experience. This time, my presentation was open to questions and comments by some of the United States's best-known orthopaedic surgeons. The audience included Edward Cave, the author of the leading book on fracture management, and Otto Aufranc, the hip surgeon who ran the weekly "fracture conference" at the Massachusetts General Hospital. Their comments were polite but unequivocally expressed strong criticism of my presentation.

Curiously, the Boston experience gave me additional confidence to pursue the project with even greater fervor. I felt that I no longer had to apologize for my ideas. The critical comments I received in Boston were to be multiplied many times. The establishment did not want to be challenged. But the establishment was finally taking my ideas—and me— seriously. My theories could no longer be dismissed with casual inattention.

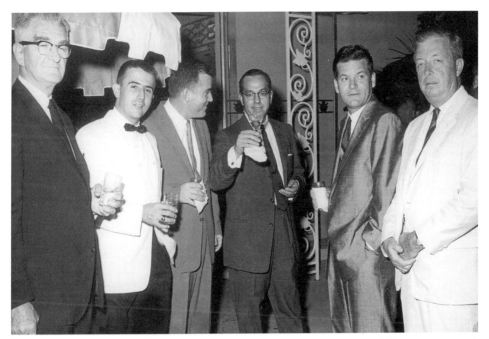

As a young academician (second from left) in 1962 with Dr. Austin T. Moore (left), my mentor and a pioneer hip surgeon in the United States, and (left to right) C. L. Wilson, Robert Keiser, Albert Wilson, and John Birch, orthopaedic surgeons in the Miami area.

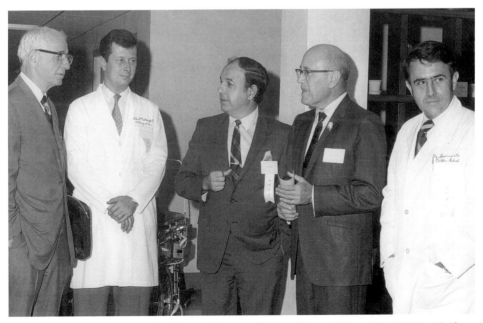

At the dedication of the new Rehabilitation Center at Jackson Memorial Hospital in 1968, with (from left to right) Dr. Clinton Compere, professor and chairman of the department of orthopaedics at Northwestern University; Dr. Newton C. McCollough III, associate director of the center; William Nordwall, CEO of the hospital; and Henry King Stanford, president of the University of Miami.

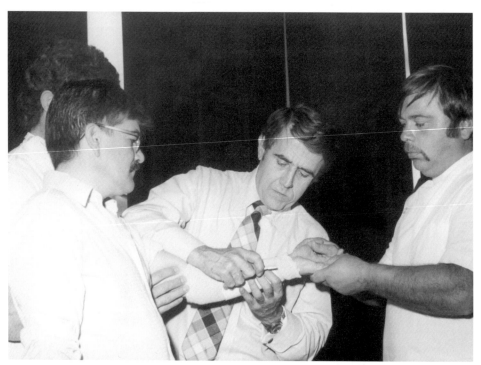

Demonstrating the application of a wrist functional brace during a trip to Latin America in the late 1960s.

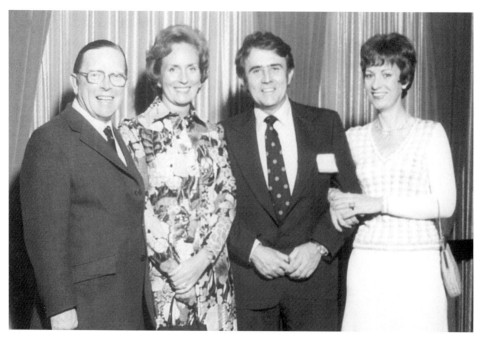

With the famed Sir John Charnley, Lady Gill, and my wife during Charnley's visit to Miami in 1974. Charnley, the most influential orthopaedist of the twentieth century, was the first surgeon to successfully perform a total hip replacement.

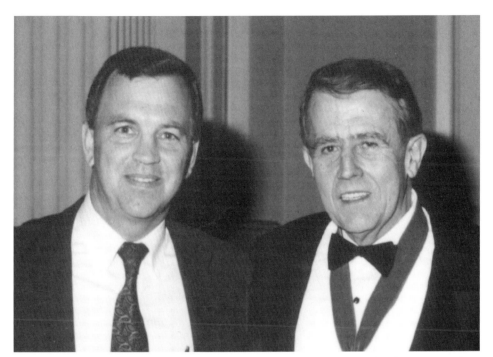

With Loren L. Latta, Ph.D., director of orthopaedic research at the University of Miami and close collaborator in many of my clinical and research activities.

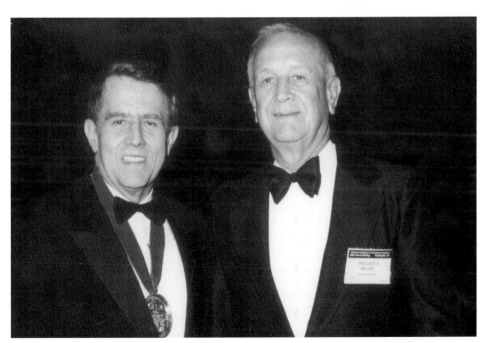

With Dr. Wallace E. Miller, my first chief at the University of Miami, during a 1992 meeting of the American Academy of Orthopaedic Surgeons. I am wearing the medallion of the academy, since I was then its president.

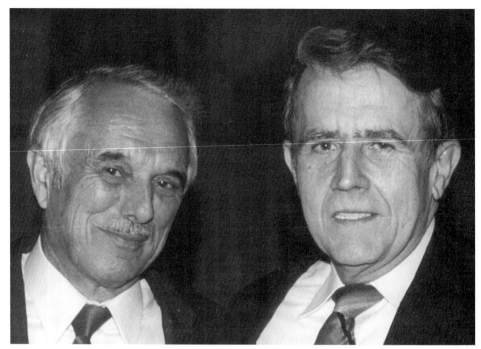

With Dr. Maurice E. Mueller, a leading trauma surgeon in Europe, at a meeting of the International Hip Society in Bern, Switzerland, in the early 1990s.

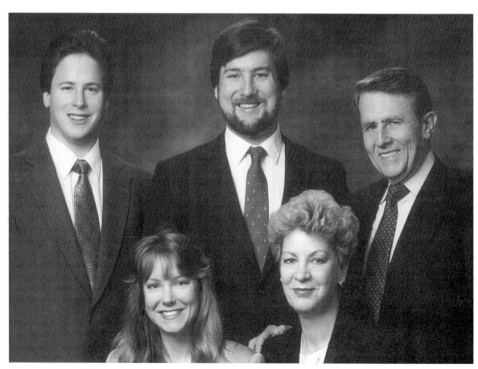

With my wife and children, Augusto Jr., Janette, and Gregory.

chapter 21.
students and friends

"We live life forward and remember it backward."
—Søren Kierkegaard

I devoted a great deal of time to my job and took seriously the many facets of it. I have often wondered what motivated me to make such a profound but selfish commitment to work, to the point of neglecting significantly my family responsibilities. I have always told myself that I was not deliberately seeking fame and recognition and that whatever I did was simply a desire to create, to improve, and to help. I am sure that, whether or not I want to admit it, the desire for fame and recognition was there, and played a far greater role than I have ever before willingly recognized.

I know that I thoroughly enjoyed teaching and learning. The intellectual rewards, whether real or imaginary, of participating in the education of others have been enormous. I like the Socratic approach to education and make it a substantial part of my own methodology. I relish the Hegelian dialectic, and love to provoke students into debate. That was never hard to do. I have always been able to create controversy without much difficulty. I believe that throughout my career, I have continuously prompted students to think for themselves. I have always sought to convince them of the need to question every assumption, and challenge the validity of any argument until logical reasoning has been fully and convincingly exercised. The rationalism of René Descartes seems to have thoroughly permeated my personal and professional behavior.

I have always been a voracious reader with an insatiable thirst for knowledge. That thirst began early in my college career. The passage of time has only increased its intensity. My library contains over three thousand books and used to be far larger. When I moved to Scotland in 1994, I gave most of my medical books to residents and fellows at

USC. I kept the books dealing with philosophy, sociology, history, politics, art, poetry, literature, and current events. I read every moment I am free and try to digest all that information. New knowledge fills me with great satisfaction. I make no claims that I remember much of what I have read. As a matter of fact, I, like Erasmus of Rotterdam, "hate a man that remembers what he hears."

I found similar satisfaction in the early success of our rehabilitation efforts and the growth of our Rehabilitation Center at Miami. I also found its success to be somewhat threatening. As the rehabilitation program grew, it required an increasing amount of my time. I knew it would continue to grow. Eventually, its growth could have forced me to abandon my research and surgery, and limit my activities to rehabilitation. I did not want that to happen.

I went directly to the dean and explained the situation. He responded (as all deans at every school instinctively respond to such requests) that the university did not have sufficient funds. He could not allocate additional resources to our division. In response, I proposed a novel scheme. I pointed out that we had always relied on the public funding that paid for our care of impoverished and needy patients. I noted that there were many prospective private patients in our area. If we could attract those private patients to the university, we should be able to generate from them enough funds to cover the salary of additional faculty. I even offered to use my own salary to guarantee my promise. I told the dean that I was willing to have my salary reduced if he would authorize two new positions and we did not bring in enough private patients to cover their cost by the end of the year. Much to my surprise, the dean agreed.

The next day I flew to California to meet with my good friend Dr. Newton McCollough III, the son of Dr. Newton McCollough Jr., who had helped me so much during my year in Orlando. Newton III had completed his medical school training at the University of Pennsylvania. He had been drafted into the military immediately upon completion of his residency. He had just returned from Vietnam.

I had first met the younger Newton McCollough at an Orlando oyster bar. I remember the occasion because prior to that time I had never even seen an oyster, let alone eaten a raw one. The sight of the slippery, shiny crustacean and the thought of swallowing it whole brought me close to nausea. My fear of embarrassment, however, proved stronger than my fear of bodily rebellion. I quickly gulped the little animal, which proved to be more satisfying and less upsetting than I had expected. (There is probably a valuable moral somewhere in that experience.) In later years, Newt III and I would consume dozens of oysters together, and chase them all with cold beer. I must admit, however, that I was never able to keep up with Newt's voracious appetite for either oysters or beer.

During his senior year in medical school, Newt took an externship with us in Miami. The friendship we formed in those years has held firm for over forty years. Our families have remained close. On more than one occasion, Newt and Mary have been of great help to Barbara, my children, and me. Newt's life in "boot camp," prior to his travel to Vietnam must have been hard on both him and the army. He had never been athletic. I still remember a postcard from him during those days of military training and indoctrination. "Gus, having a great time. Getting in shape. Doing push-ups. I am up to two."

When he left the military, Newt was planning to join his father's practice in Orlando. I wanted him to join me in Miami instead. I argued that if he came to Miami and joined the full-time faculty, we could build a first-class program. I convinced him that the opportunities for success were enormous. When he reads this book, he will learn for the first time about the deal that I had to make with the dean to guarantee his salary.

With Newt on board, we began to expand the rehabilitation program. I put him in charge of the pediatric program and made him associate director of rehabilitation. Word of our expanded program and high standards of care spread rapidly through the greater Miami community.

Remarkably, growth exceeded expectations. Every Tuesday, our amputee clinics saw as many as thirty patients. We soon found it necessary to reinforce the stroke patient programs with additional medical support personnel. Our professional results delighted all of us. The hospital administration began to cooperate with us in every respect. Within two years, our program had grown to become one of the largest and most successful in the country.

In 1969 Melvin Glimcher, the new professor and head of orthopaedics at Harvard Medical School invited me to be his visiting professor. I had met Glimcher during a National Academy of Science meeting in Washington, D.C. During the meeting, I presented some of my research on fracture healing. Glimcher asked me a few questions from the floor. He seemed quite interested in my ideas. I, of course, found his interest extremely flattering. While he was still a young man, he had developed a worldwide reputation as one of the most brilliant minds in orthopaedics in this century. Glimcher had become the prime example of sophistication in orthopaedic research and had built the most complete basic sciences laboratory in the country.

During my visiting professorship at Harvard, Glimcher suggested that I join him at the Massachusetts General Hospital. He asked if I would be interested in taking charge of the trauma program, while continuing my work in hip surgery and fracture research. I was tremendously excited by the possibility of joining the Harvard faculty.

Ever since my student days in Bogota, I had believed that Boston was the mecca of medicine. I was greatly honored by my three-day visiting professorship in Cambridge. My responsibilities as visiting professor took me to Boston Children's Hospital, where Dr. William Green was still the chief. During the coffee break following grand rounds, I reminded him of my first visit to his office many years before, and of his more recent visit to Miami, when I had experienced an embarrassing episode.

AN EMBARRASSING SITUATION

During Dr. Green's visit, I had presented the case of an approximately twenty-eight-year-old woman, on whom we had made a tentative diagnosis of cancer of the proximal tibia (just below the knee). We had taken her to surgery for a biopsy. Prior to surgery, during the discussion of the problem, we considered the remote possibility of an infection. Upon entering the bone at the level of the lesion, I had encountered a large collection of cloudy fluid, which I interpreted as being pus.

The presence of the fluid collection reemphasized the possibility of infection. A few minutes later, the pathologist came into the operating room to inform us that he had not seen anything to suggest malignancy and that the cells in the fluid were suggestive of an infectious process.

I then decided that I needed to radically remove the infection. I then decided to thoroughly remove the infected bone and to pack the cavity this created with bone obtained from the bone bank. Before the bone was packed, it was made into a paste in a blending machine. I had learned this method from Dr. Moore during my residency. I knew it was an unconventional, unorthodox method of treatment, but Dr. Moore's advocacy of the treatment led me to use it.

The surgery was uneventful and the patient had a smooth post-operative course. We sent the surgical specimen to the Army Institute of Pathology in Washington for confirmation of the local pathologist's diagnosis.

In front of the medical staff, the residents, and Dr. Green, I presented this interesting patient and described the surgical technique. Dr. Green had never heard of this treatment, and found it quite interesting. He stood up and examined the patient. While he was examining the patient, the pathologist came to the door and asked that I step outside to talk to him. He informed me that the Armed Forces Institute of Pathology had identified the specimen as osteosarcoma. At the time, that cancerous condition could be treated only by radical amputation surgery.

When I reentered the auditorium, Newt McCollough was presenting another patient to Dr. Green. I interrupted Newt's presentation to inform the group of the mistake we had made. I say "we," only because I would like to share the blame with the pathologist. In all fairness, it was mainly my fault. I mistakenly accepted the initial intraoperative preliminary report without sufficient consideration. I should have waited for a final report before carrying out the debridment and packing of bone into the area. I knew that by cleansing the cavity, I could have easily spread the cancerous cells into the systemic circulation, ensuring the rapid dissemination of the tumor. Our patient later went to the Campbell Clinic in Memphis, where the surgeons amputated her leg. She died a year later with metastatic disease to her brain.

When I left Boston my discussions with Dr. Glimcher about joining the Harvard faculty remained open. I was thrilled with the possibility but somewhat intimidated by the prospect. I was also somewhat reluctant to leave our thriving Rehabilitation Center in Miami, and worried about leaving the staff that had worked so long and hard with me on functional bracing of fractures.

The concept of functional fracture bracing continued to evolve. While we did not have sophisticated research facilities where we could carry out studies, we did have a first-class team of enthusiastic people anxious to see the program succeed. The excitement proved infectious. Even our residents in training volunteered their scarce free time to help us gather data and add to the understanding of the new philosophy of fracture care.

Within a relatively short period, we outgrew the facilities that we had finessed away from the department of medicine a few years earlier. We had as many as twenty-five spinal cord injured patients in the center, in addition to a number of amputees, stroke victims, and people with other disabilities. The outpatient programs had also grown rapidly.

Eventually we occupied the entire three floors of the building. Everyone in orthopaedics and rehabilitation worked long hours. It was no longer difficult to convince the hospital administration to give us the additional personnel we needed in order to continue providing top-quality care.

But we still wanted to do better. We wanted to have a truly comprehensive rehabilitation center. The only way to do it was by expanding. That would require us to remodel the existing facilities, build an addition, and bring on more new people. Remarkably, the new administrator at Jackson Memorial Hospital, Dr. Bill Nordwall proved to be the right man at the right time. He had vision and assisted us in looking forward toward fulfilling our dream. He adopted our cause and became our leading advocate. Before long, we learned the exciting news. The trustees of the institution had approved the expansion.

I presided over the Rehabilitation Center for several years, while still carrying out my fracture research, actively participating in the continuing educational program, and continuing my private practice in hip surgery. I was also serving as chief of orthopaedics at the Veterans Administration Hospital situated only a block away from Jackson Memorial. My family paid a high price for my success. In order to free a little time for a personal life and to recognize his contribution, I appointed Newt McCollough director of rehabilitation. Newt continued to serve as head of a new and increasingly successful division of pediatric orthopaedics. I did not fully appreciate it at the time, but I was at the beginning of the most extraordinary, thrilling, and totally rewarding period of my life.

Upon my return to Miami in 1995, after an absence of sixteen years, I was deeply disappointed to find out that although the department I had once chaired was still called "orthopaedics and rehabilitation," it no longer had any interest in rehabilitation components. Residents were no longer rotated through rehabilitation, and the department concentrated exclusively on the surgical disciplines.

In the fall of 2002 Jackson Memorial Hospital released an official announcement that it would begin construction of a rehabilitation center that would be "the first in the city of Miami." Either memory is short or the powers that be wanted to be recognized as innovators and pioneers: No mention was made of the day thirty years earlier that a previous dean announced to the community that Miami's first rehabilitation center had been opened and was fully operational.

chapter 22.
introduction to a new career

"The power of the mind is only as good as its expression."

"When the facts change, I change. What do you do?
—John Maynard Keynes

Success in my professional career seemed to follow me throughout the late 1960s and the early 1970s. My ideas about fracture healing and management continued to gain wide recognition and acceptance around the world. The American Academy of Orthopaedic Surgeons appointed me to chair its committee on continuing education, a post that brought high visibility and substantial professional prestige. I served in that capacity for six consecutive years.

During that heyday of postgraduate education, we not only managed to present as many as twelve University of Miami-sponsored courses a year at the Americana Hotel in Miami Beach but I was also peripherally responsible for an additional thirty courses across the country, under the aegis of the academy. It provided a wonderful opportunity, and made it possible for me to meet many fascinating people. It also provided a valuable way to work off the frustration I had accumulated throughout my own early years in medicine. I found myself empowered to offer continuing education programs to physicians throughout the United States. These courses attempted to keep the national orthopaedic community abreast of new developments and concepts, to demonstrate and teach emerging surgical techniques, or to review the state of the art.

I also found that I was being invited to serve as visiting professor or keynote speaker with increasing frequency. Those opportunities were gratifying to my ego and valuable learning experiences. Unfortunately, I also learned of the futility of some of those visits, and of the occasionally questionable motives behind the invitations. Industrial concerns were beginning to gain control of the education of the orthopaedist by becoming the financial sponsors of visiting professorships and lectureships. I did not suspect then the speed with which this control was to increase in the next decades. Thirty years later industry's control of education is overwhelming.

When I returned from my visiting professorship at Harvard, I told my dean that Melvin Glimcher had offered me a position on his faculty and on the staff at Massachusetts General. I had already discussed Glimcher's offer with Barbara. Despite her roots in South Carolina and my roots in South America, we agreed that the Boston area could provide many excellent opportunities for our children. There was no question in my mind; I was going to accept Glimcher's offer.

Then the dean asked what it would take to keep me in Miami. That simple question resulted in a lengthy discussion of the future of the Rehabilitation Center and the relationship of orthopaedics and rehabilitation to the other programs in the medical school. I stated my strong belief that orthopaedics should no longer be a division of surgery but a full-fledged department of its own. I also told him that in my view, orthopaedics and rehabilitation were closely related and should be managed accordingly. I strongly felt that they should be taught as an integrated discipline and administered in the hospital by one individual. I suggested that the medical school should create a new department called "orthopaedics and rehabilitation." Then I told him that while he was thinking about my suggestions, I was going to England to work at Mr. John Charnley's Hip Center in Wrightington, England.

I had been reading about Charnley's work on total hip replacement for about two years. Dr. Moore had pioneered a technique that allowed replacement of the ball portion of the hip joint, but he had not been able to create a successful replacement for the socket section of the joint. John Charley had taken Moore's work to the next stage, and created a system that allowed him to replace the entire hip joint. As you can imagine, I had followed academic reports of Charnley's work with great excitement. I had long yearned for an opportunity to go to England and see the total hip replacement for myself.

I had also taken the opposite approach, and invited Charnley to participate in a continuing education course on hip surgery in Miami as a special guest of the American Academy of Orthopaedics. He replied with a brief and pointed rejection. He wrote that total hip surgery should not be taught in an auditorium. He added that the only way to learn about his new operation was by spending a prolonged period of time at his hospital, where the only surgery done was total hip replacement. He concluded his brief note with the statement that no one should undertake total hip replacement unless they were willing to undertake the appropriate lengthy fellowship at his hospital (he thought that most surgeons required a full year of study) and dedicate themselves exclusively to the procedure.

I found his reply offensive. As a resident, I had been trained by one of the best hip surgeons in the United States. As a practitioner, I had devoted much of my time and effort to the study of hip diseases. Yet, I did not, according to John Charnley, meet the requirements to perform the surgical hip replacement he had developed. I then realized, however, that I was still intrigued by Charnley's work and wanted to learn more about it. I swallowed my pride and wrote to him again. This time, I asked him if he would accept me in his hospital for a few months. I did not expect a favorable answer. He had made it clear in his original letter that one year was the usual time requirement. Much to my pleasure and surprise, however, he wrote a gracious letter inviting me to visit his hospital for whatever period of time I wished to stay. That was good enough for me.

About two weeks later, I found myself onboard a plane taking me to Liverpool. I left behind both Dr. Glimcher's offer to join the Harvard faculty, and my dean's promise to reorganize the orthopaedic programs at Miami. It was the spring of 1970 and, as expected, northern England was beautifully green if somewhat rainy. In Miami, the weather was hot and humid. The atmosphere at the university must have been equally heavy, as the administration launched its search for someone to head the new department.

I discovered many new things upon my arrival in England. Unfortunately, the first were "right-hand drive" cars and cars with standard transmissions. To my way of thinking, there is nothing "standard" about a car that does not have the steering wheel on the left side and an automatic transmission.

Unlike Americans, who are born knowing how to drive cars, I had never driven a car before coming to the United States. In fact, I had driven for the first time in my life the year that I turned twenty-five years old.

Shortly after my move to South Carolina, I took a bus to downtown Columbia. I looked out the windows of the bus until I spotted a used car lot. I found an inexpensive 1948 Chevrolet and told the salesman that I was interested in buying it. He suggested that I try it out, and handed me the keys. I was too embarrassed to tell him that I did not know how to drive. Instead, I returned the keys to him and told him that I would prefer him to do the driving. I said that I was not all that familiar with automatic transmissions.

He must have realized that I was lying, but a sale, after all, is a sale. He drove me around the block, while I carefully watched everything that he did. At the end of the ride, I suggested that he leave the car in front of the office while I signed the appropriate papers. I was afraid that he would put it in a parking space I would not be able to maneuver out of. He completed the paperwork, and I drove off. Somehow, I managed to reach the residence at the hospital without killing myself or anyone else. As I made the last turn, however, I scraped the side of the car against a metal pole. I can still hear that terrible sound. I practiced driving around the neighborhood during the next few days, and soon ventured into the countryside.

Upon my arrival in Liverpool, nearly twenty years later, I rented a car. It was a British automobile that I was to drive all the way to Wrightington, a small village in northern England, the home of John Charnley's Center for Hip Surgery. It was drizzling and the sky was overcast. I got inside the car to find myself facing a strange instrument panel, controls on the wrong side of the car, and a standard transmission. I had never driven such a car.

The car jerked violently as I tried to get it moving; the engine died several times before I reached the parking lot exit. The rest of the trip was an equally horrible ordeal that took several hours and seemed like several days. As Joseph Campbell wrote, "Eternity has nothing to do with time."

When the light drizzle transformed itself into a downpour, I discovered that I could not find the windshield wiper control. A truck barreled directly at me, on what I honestly thought was my side of the road. I couldn't even find the horn button. I could not even begin to understand or navigate the British intersections or roundabouts. A few miles down the road, I picked up a student from Oxford University who was hitchhiking back to school. He provided me with direly needed guidance, at least until I had to drop him off just thirty minutes later.

I finally arrived in Wrightington and parked the car in front of the administration building. The next morning, I found out that the automobile had been stolen. I said a prayer of thanks, and fervently hoped that I would never see it again. I told myself that I would never again sit behind the wheel of an automobile in the United Kingdom. The next day, the police called to say that they had found my car. Some teenagers had taken it out for a joy ride. Would I please come down to the station to pick it up?

Eventually, the car, the British rules of the road, and I all came to a mutual understanding. Within a short time, I became comfortable driving the car. Over the next three months, I used it extensively to visit London and other cities in England and Wales.

My stay in Wrightington proved to be an extraordinary experience. I learned that John Charnley was a remarkable intellectual as well as a highly skilled surgeon. He was keenly aware of his superior intellect but dealt with others without attempting to demonstrate his superiority. As I watched him at work, I immediately realized that his contributions to orthopaedic surgery were profound.

During my first few days at his Hip Center, I asked him, before his large entourage, several questions concerning various aspects of his philosophy of hip replacement. Never once did he respond authoritatively or with visible annoyance. To the contrary, his responses gave the impression that he was intrigued by the question I had just asked. His responses were carefully thought out and thorough. Only later did one of his U.S. fellows suggest to me that it was possible that Mr. Charnley had already asked himself the same questions. Perhaps Mr. Charnley had even published his responses. I skipped dinner that night and spent my time in the library instead. I soon discovered that I had neglected to prepare myself properly for my trip to England.

I may not have read all of Charnley's research reports and essays, but I had devoted almost ten years to hip surgery and published several articles on the subject. I had even designed a few surgical devices that had gained some popularity in the United States. I quickly realized, however, that my small contributions and my understanding of hip disease were trivial in comparison to Charnley's. He had actually revolutionized hip surgery and, for the first time in history, had made possible the successful replacement of a diseased hip joint. I was so profoundly affected by my exposure to Sir John and his approach to hip replacement that I would follow his lead in one important respect. Upon my return to the United States, I devoted myself entirely to total hip replacements. Since my trip to England, I have never performed any other procedure.

Sir John did not always provide such a good role model. His medical staff frequently repeated the story of his surgery on his wife. When he diagnosed a ruptured lumbar disc in her back, he insisted on removing it himself. After he completed the spinal operation, he decided to operate on her foot and remove a small bunion that had bothered her for some time. He quickly completed the surgery and returned to his office. A few minutes later, he received an urgent call from the recovery room. When he arrived, he was confronted by his wife, still recovering from anesthesia, bitterly complaining that he had operated on the wrong foot! According to the story, which I suspect is still told in England, Sir John broke into loud laughter and left the room.

After nearly three months at Charnley's Hip Center, I was ready to return to the States. As I prepared to leave Wrightington, I went to Charnley's office to thank him for the three wonderful months. I also used the opportunity to invite him, again, to visit the United States and to lecture on his revolutionary and exciting operation.

> Mr. Charnley, the time I spent with you has convinced me, without any doubt, that total hip replacement surgery should not be performed by surgeons who had not had intensive training in the area, and who have not made the commitment to dedicate themselves to that type of surgery. I, myself, have decided that I will confine my own surgical practice to this procedure. However, you are wrong in believing that such a philosophy will ever find fertile grounds in America. I predict to you that within a short time there will be an 'epidemic' of total hip surgery; that surgeons everywhere will be doing the operation with little or any preparation. We in the United States have no way to prevent them from doing so.
>
> I would like you to reconsider your earlier decision and accept the Academy's invitation to lecture in the United States. Only you can convince the American orthopaedic community of the importance of special training. You are the only one with the moral authority to send that message. You will not convince everyone, but you may convince some people in the audience and prevent many complications.

He thought about my comments for a few seconds: "Gus, you have successfully twisted my arm. Your argument is sound. I will go to America."

I thanked him again in anticipation of his visit and proceeded to ask him a more profound question: "Mr. Charnley," I said, "you have changed the history of hip surgery forever. What, in your opinion, will come next?" Without hesitation, he told me that his procedure, with some improvements in the wear properties of the materials, would be the last word in hip replacement surgery. His answer took me by surprise. I thought it unbecoming of a man of his stature. It seemed unreasonably arrogant and showed an uncharacteristic lack of humility. How can anyone, I asked myself, not understand that progress is inevitable?

Unfortunately, shortly after I left England, Sir John changed his mind about visiting the United States. My prediction concerning the popularity of his operation, however, proved all too true. In the absence of moral opposition from the great man in person, surgeons everywhere began to conduct total hip replacements. Most of them lacked the most basic understanding of the hip and its diseases. Worse yet, many of them modified Charnley's procedure to suit their own purposes.

At the same time, medical equipment and implant manufacturers began designing their own devices. Over the last three decades, we have witnessed hundreds, possibly thousands of attempts to improve on Charnley's procedure and materials. I myself was responsible for several efforts to improve the system. My efforts, along with all other such changes, eventually came up short. During the last thirty years, no one has been able to duplicate Sir John's remarkable results. His operation remains the gold standard against which all other hip prostheses must be measured. Thus far, his prediction, which I found a bit arrogant, has proven accurate.

Upon my return to the United States in July 1970, I told the American Academy of Orthopedic Surgeons that I had recruited John Charnley to participate in one of its educational courses. I was at that time serving as chairman of the academy's committee on continuing education and was inordinately proud of my accomplishment. Two weeks later I received a letter from Charnley informing me of his change of heart. He stated in his letter that in a moment of weakness he had agreed to do something he strongly felt was wrong, that to teach hip replacement surgery in an auditorium was not appropriate.

Needless to say I was extremely disappointed. I wrote back to him saying that I had left England holding great admiration for him and that his letter had done nothing but further enhance that admiration.

I also had to tell him that while I admired "the courage of his convictions" the continuing education course would take place, even though he could not attend in person. Several of his U.S. students would make presentations in his place. The course was a great success. It attracted nearly six hundred attendees.

My prediction about an "epidemic" of total hip surgery in the United States also proved accurate. In no time Charnley's operation was being done throughout the land, oftentimes by surgeons who had no qualifications to do it appropriately. Many of them deviated from Charnley's methods and materials. Few of them fully understood his philosophy. The combination caused a great many serious complications. Far too many patients found it necessary to undergo a second, corrective operation, often because of improper performance of the replacement procedure. It has taken a long time for many surgeons to realize that hip replacement is not just a technique but a sophisticated philosophy that requires much study and commitment.

Many orthopaedists of course suggested changes in a sincere effort to improve on the original implant. Others, no doubt, sought only to cut themselves a slice of this lucrative market. Competition to create popular implants has been fierce. At times, there have been almost as many different hip prostheses in use as there are medical centers. Every medical facility had its own chosen candidate. The need to remain successful prompted companies to modify their own creations as fads and fashions changed. As soon as a manufacturer released a new model, they began work on its successor. In the passion to remain in front, no manufacturers had time for serious medical research.

A few years ago, the president of the Australian Orthopaedic Association commented on the "obscene" number of implants on display at the American Academy's annual meeting. I have never counted them, but I have been told that there are more than three hundred different hip prostheses on the market today.

The first dictate of the Hippocratic oath mandates that doctors "do no harm" to their patients, but a great deal of harm has been done as a result of this irresponsible proliferation of implants. Complications require additional surgeries, which are always more difficult and typically produce less desirable outcomes.

In the spring of 1996, in a presentation to the International Hip Society in Amsterdam, I stated my opinion that little progress had been made in total hip surgery since the days of John Charnley. If we had displayed an organized and unselfish approach to hip surgery, I added, we would be much further along the road. In fact we and our patients would be in much better shape if we had heeded Charnley's recommendation and followed his original theories and practices before embarking in the making of changes: "I believe that it was primarily due to our rush to gain fame and to be acknowledged as contributors to this fascinating venture. We tripped on our own egos and made the terrible mistake of permitting industry to play an overwhelmingly important role in determining the destiny of total hip replacement. Industry, almost from the beginning, gained control of total hip surgery and the education of the orthopaedist in this area."

I personally fell into the trap. My practice of total hip surgery had become extensive. I was performing approximately six surgeries a week. New patients had to wait in line for as long as one year. So, I was not surprised when a manufacturer approached me and asked me "to design my own implant." By then, I had experienced several complications with the Charnley prosthesis, such as loosening of the implant in the bone or breakage of the metal stem. I believed that some of these problems could be made preventable by using a different type of metal.

I was not alone in this belief. A few Charnley prostheses had broken because of inferior metallurgical properties—the medical literature had acknowledged the issue. Some manufacturers tried to solve the problem by strengthening the shape of the implant. Others adopted metals such as cobalt-chrome alloys that, in my opinion, could cause other problems because of their greater stiffness.

My long experience with fracture healing and my conviction that motion at the fracture site was beneficial led me to extrapolate that a more flexible material would cause stress on the bone around the prosthesis. By increasing this stress, we could eliminate the stress shielding that we were observing not only with the Charnley implant but also with newly developed prostheses. I concluded that instead of using stainless steel or cobalt-chrome alloys, we should construct an implant with a titanium alloy. While the strength of titanium alloys should be helpful, I was more attracted by the metal's flexibility. It also allowed me to preserve the geometry of the original Charnley design.

My hip prosthesis was the first one in the United States made of titanium. Before we could document a successful long-term experience, we started a new trend. My initial results proved satisfactory, and thoughts of global recognition danced, like sugarplums, in my head. I should have remembered that such pride inevitably brings its own punishment.

The first reports of complications came from other surgeons who were using their own newly designed titanium implants. They concluded that titanium was not a good weight-bearing material against the plastic cup that replaced the human socket. The resulting debris, they said, subsequently damaged the surrounding bone.

The Hospital for Special Surgery in New York had developed its own titanium prosthesis whose shape differed significantly from mine. Soon after their development, I learned that they were having complications that I had not seen. I traveled to New York to look at their problems at close hand and was surprised to see the severity of metal debris in the tissues of their patients.

By the time of my visit, we had already prepared a manuscript in which we were reporting on seventeen titanium prostheses that we had recovered after their failures. Our experience at the University of Southern California, however, did not demonstrate any evidence of the metal debris that we found in New York.

My associate Dr. Harry McKellop, whom I had appointed director of biomechanical laboratories at USC's Orthopedic Hospital, was already well on his way to becoming the leading expert on prosthetic wear in the United States. McKellop conducted the scientific investigation that led to our findings. His input enabled us to arrive at a possible explanation for the major difference between the findings of the Hospital for Special Surgery and our own. We discovered that the New York surgeons were using metal reinforcement cups to attach plastic liners in the hip socket. We believed that these metal reinforcements deteriorated and began to shed small particles into the joint. Those particles, in turn, created an abrasion that produced abnormal amounts of metal and plastic particles, which lodged in the joint. We were not using metal cup reinforcements at USC, and our own failure rate was much lower.

As a result of the New York visit, we postponed submission of the manuscript until we had a chance to review our data. When we completed the review and confirmed our initial findings, we sent the manuscript to the *Journal of Bone and Joint Surgeons*, the must prestigious orthopaedic journal in the world. The journal rejected our manuscript, allegedly because the subject was of "no interest" to the orthopaedic readership. The explanation seemed outrageous to me. Orthopaedists all over the world had heard about the New York experience. We were all concerned about the failure of titanium implants.

I was much more upset by the fact that this rejection came not from the editor in chief but from the journal's chief editor for research, who happened to be the director of research at the Hospital for Special Surgery in New York. My meeting with the various surgeons and engineers at the hospital had taken place in his office, and in his presence. A few weeks later, the same journal published an article written by researchers at the Hospital for Special Surgery that reported their own bad experience with titanium implants but did not mention our more positive findings at USC. I immediately wrote to the chief editor of the journal and stated my concerns, which included the appearance (to say the least) of a conflict of interest. The journal eventually published our paper, but only after insisting that we make an unusually large number of revisions. Sometimes it seems that medicine is neither an art nor a science but a battlefield!

Well-informed orthopaedic surgeons now believe that titanium alloys should not be used on the articulating surface of the total joint implant because of its sensitivity to scratches. Many still choose to use femoral stems made of titanium alloy. Unfortunately, the inventory of titanium alloy ball-and-socket articulating joints seems to have been quite large. These obsolete implants are marketed and sold in underdeveloped countries. After all, medicine is medicine and business is business. Whenever the two conflict, it seems that business interests always emerge victorious.

As the new millennium begins, titanium continues to be the metal of choice for use in noncemented hip implants. (Charnley's original system used an innovative cement to attach the cup portion of the prosthesis to the pelvis.) The noncemented prostheses were originally developed in the belief that gradual deterioration of the cement could cause the implant to loosen and become extremely painful. I and others believe that noncemented prostheses might eventually create a significantly higher incidence of complications than the Charnley prosthesis, such as deterioration of the bone around the implant, because of metallic debris arising from the soft nature of the metallic implant. I have already stopped using titanium implants and suspect that others, too, will return to stainless steel alloys. We can always hope, of course, that some refinements in the design and manufacture of titanium hip joint prostheses will prove me wrong. The refinements will probably consist in hardening of the alloy without compromising its other good qualities.

Toward the end of my stay at Charnley's Hip Center, I traveled to Bern, Switzerland, to meet with Maurice Muller, Europe's leading expert on fracture surgery. Unfortunately, I found Muller rather aloof and not easily approached. Questions similar to those that had led to dynamic discussions with Sir John Charnley proved beneath the interest of Herr Professor Dr. Muller. In frustration, I cut short my visit to Bern, and returned to England for the remainder of my unofficial sabbatical. I eventually acquired great respect for Dr. Muller. Like Charnley, he is a great thinker, a brilliant innovator, and a remarkably skillful surgeon. I kept in touch with both of them over the years and developed what I think was a good personal relationship. My allegiance to Charnley, however, was based on deep affection and a strong commitment to similar philosophical ideals. My admiration for Muller, while quite different, was equally intense.

My own philosophy on nonsurgical treatment of fractures clashed directly with Muller's philosophy of a totally rigid surgical approach. My ideas about the role of the biological environment on fracture repair are also totally opposite to Muller's. We have been waging our debate for more than a quarter of a century. In the 1971 volume of the *Encyclopedia Britannica*, the chapter on "Fractures" mentioned our opposing philosophies and rhetorically asked which will best withstand the test of time.

I have not wavered in my premise that motion between fracture fragments is good for healing. Our clinical and laboratory experiences have given me sufficient information to justify my stubborn commitment to the concept. Muller based his theory on the premise that rigid immobilization of fractures provided the ideal environment. He later modified his ideas. Recently, the Arbeitsgemeinschaft für Osteosynthesefragen (AO), an organization that he founded and that steadfastly espoused and perpetuated his principles, modified their teachings and began to recommend limited motion between fractured fragments as the ideal environment for healing.

At a recent meeting of the Orthopedic Trauma Association in Vancouver, Canada, Stefan Perrin, the Swiss scientist who for nearly thirty years was the main spokesperson for the AO, preceded me at the podium. He was to talk about the biomechanics of fracture healing under surgical conditions and I was to discuss the effects of an environment where immobilization does not take place. During his presentation, he stated that there had been a major change in his philosophy, and that he now he felt that some motion at the fracture was beneficial. For thirty years, we had loudly argued about our differences. It was good to hear him acknowledge his error, but disappointing that even then, he did not acknowledge the relevance of our work.

In all fairness, I must admit that functional bracing never gained the popularity and acceptance of Muller's theories, as advocated by the AO throughout the 1960s, 1970s, and 1980s. I believe, however, that my theories might eventually find much more widespread acceptance. The popularity of the AO approach to fracture care is closely tied to the popularity of surgery over less aggressive treatment with functional bracing. Surgery may carry more risk than less aggressive treatment, but it also carries more glamour. It also produces more income for the physician. This in no way implies that I believe the nonsurgical treatment of fractures is always superior to the surgical one. Quite the contrary, for a very large percentage of fractures, surgery is the treatment of choice.

The heavily marketed AO system taught orthopaedic surgeons how to reunite broken pieces of bone with no shortening and no deformity in most instances. If the AO did not bother to point out that routine attempts to obtain perfect anatomical restoration were not always necessary, that surgery is almost always more expensive, and that surgery carried some inevitable risks, we can understand their reluctance. The AO system was perfectly sound from a mechanical viewpoint. Only physicians who concern themselves with the physiology of healing recognized its many flaws. In spite of the flaws, the AO system remained attractive to the surgeons, and surgery remained the treatment of choice for many patients. That is why the AO system prevailed for nearly three decades.

I must also point out that virtually all insurance plans, including Medicare and Medicaid, provide higher payment for surgical than for nonsurgical treatments. It would be wrong for me to say that all orthopaedists advocate surgical treatment simply for financial reasons. I firmly believe that the vast majority of my colleagues treat patients according to their best medical judgment. It would be equally wrong, however, to ignore the enormous economic temptation to adopt surgical treatment. There are those who overuse surgical treatments simply because in that manner they increase their income.

Ironically, often the strongest impetus for unnecessary surgery often comes from the patients themselves. Quite frequently, one hears the argument that patients demand surgical treatment because they believe it to be the best treatment and the one most likely to restore them quickly to their preinjury status. Consequently, fewer and fewer orthopaedic surgeons even offer their patients nonsurgical options. Many orthopaedic residents no longer know enough about the biological fracture healing process to understand the advantages of nonsurgical fracture care.

During a recent trip to Germany, where I was invited to participate in a major meeting dealing with fractures of the tibia, I met a young orthopaedist who was just completing his training. He told me that every fracture patient admitted to his hospital underwent surgery. I was reluctant to accept such a blanket statement and made further inquiries. It turned out that he was right. The hospital had virtually abandoned nonsurgical treatment.

After completing my prepared comments that afternoon, I added comments questioning the wisdom of making surgery the treatment for all fractures. I reminded my audience of the added risks, of the evidence that many fractures did well when treated by nonsurgical means, and of the economic advantages of nonsurgical treatment. I even suggested that the financial burdens resulting from such an approach would eventually result in restrictions imposed on the surgeons.

Two of the most prominent traumatologists in the country then discussed my paper and my comments. Both explained that there was nothing the surgeons could do about the current trend since their patients all demanded surgery. In my rebuttal, I suggested that it was their responsibility to convince their patients to accept the most appropriate treatment. I also suggested that their patients' bias toward surgery most likely reflected their own attitudes rather than the reverse.

I argued that, perhaps unwittingly, we often failed to inform patients that surgery always carries the risk of complications; that surgical treatments typically require a second surgery for the removal of implants used to stabilize the fracture; that the broken bone, when treated surgically requires a longer period of time to heal. My German audience received my comments politely. I left the conference, virtually certain that I had not convinced even one of them to change any aspect of their fracture management protocols.

In attempting to understand the current trends and practices, it is important to realize that surgical implant manufacturers have convinced the orthopaedic community that surgery is the superior treatment. While surgery is often the treatment of choice, it is not always the best treatment. For example, a broken femur (the thigh bone) usually requires surgery, but a broken humerus (the upper arm bone) typically heals quickly and soundly when treated with a functional cast.

After many years of documenting our experience treating fractures with functional braces, Loren L. Latta, Ph.D., and I wrote a book about our observations and conclusions. Dr. Latta was a young man, fresh out of college, when I recruited him to be the first engineer to join the faculty of the department of orthopaedics at the University of Miami in the early 1970s. We became very close friends and have worked together ever since. He has been extremely influential in most of the research we have conducted in fracture healing. Springer Verlag, a German publisher of medical works, accepted our manuscript. We knew that Springer Verlag also published many books for AO, the organization that most rigidly defended the widest possible use of orthopaedic surgery, but we naively did not anticipate a conflict of interest.

Springer Verlag did a magnificent job and produced a beautifully illustrated volume. Shortly after its release, we lectured at a meeting of the AO in Switzerland, and noticed that our book, along with AO publications, was displayed at a Springer Verlag booth. On the second day of the meeting, I noticed that all copies of our book had disappeared. I was delighted by this remarkable phenomenon, which I thought indicated that the book had sold out. Upon further inquiry, however, I discovered that a different kind of sellout had occurred. Someone from the AO had requested the removal of the book from the display, and the publisher had acquiesced.

The book was later translated into Spanish, German, Japanese, and Portuguese. The Chinese pirated it and published it in an abbreviated version. The German-published books never sold in large numbers. I once apologized to the president of Springer Verlag for convincing them to publish an elaborate book that never became a financial success. He responded by telling me that he never expected the book to be a best-seller. Before I had a change to ask why he had chosen to publish it, he added, "Your book will be a classic." I never really understood his remark, but it made me feel much better about the poor sales record. We recently issued a second edition of the book.

It is much less elaborate, with far fewer illustrations, and once again, will never be a "classic."

When I returned from England, I immersed myself completely and exclusively in total hip surgery. In accordance with Mr. Charnley's protocols, I have tried to follow all of my patients as carefully as possible. By the time I left Miami to go to California in 1978, eight years after my return from England, I had already performed over one thousand total hip replacements. From California, I wrote a letter to every patient every year and asked for information about the condition of their hips. I also requested them to send me a recent X ray. Because the overwhelming majority of my patients cooperated, I have built an excellent data bank of follow-up information.

I continued the same practice during my stint in Scotland in 1994 and upon my return to Miami. While my patients continued to cooperate, some orthopaedic surgeons proved less willing to help. They accepted my patients for follow-up work but refused to send me their evaluations or their X rays. I suppose that it just shows one more way in which medicine continues to transform itself from a profession to just another business.

In 1976 I was elected president of the Hip Society and held that position for two years. I attempted to make some meaningful changes but succeeded only in a small way. I was able, however, to get approval for a modified bylaws, which increased the number of members of the society creating opportunities for younger orthopaedists to join the ranks. I also established an educational subcommittee; presided over the first open meeting of the society to be held during the annual meeting of the Academy of Orthopedics; and promoted the creation of several awards for contributions to the field, made by young orthopaedic surgeons.

The project to which I more seriously committed my time was the establishment of a Total Hip Joint Registry. I felt very strongly at the time that a national registry was not only feasible but most beneficial. The society had less than thirty members, and the number of different total hip prostheses on the market probably did not exceed half a dozen. It was impossible for me to successfully deal with powerful egos, which felt threatened by such a development. They were concerned that their "unique" systems of individual recording of data (often identified with their own names) would be eclipsed by the national registry.

Twenty years later the American Academy of Orthopaedics has embarked on the development of a hip registry. I should have received the news of such a move with enthusiasm, had it not been for my awareness that times had changed. The number of implants on the market has gone from the earlier half a dozen prostheses to over three hundred. More importantly, the role that industry plays in the development and promulgation of products is of a different nature. Today industry controls the field, designs and makes modifications without consultation with orthopaedic surgeons, and engages in fierce internecine competition between companies producing implants. The industry, I am certain, will do its best to prevent the creation of the registry, since it will be perceived as a loss of control.

I officially stated my position by writing a letter to the editor of the academy's bulletin. In that letter I raised the rhetorical question of the number of prostheses (among the three hundred on the market) that will be included in the registry. Obviously all of them will not be included for logistical reasons. Which ones will be chosen, and how will the choosing process take place? How will the registry determine which of the many industrial concerns fabricating prostheses will be given a place in the registry? How will it discriminate against some of them? Since industrial concerns produce new implants on a frequent basis in order to "beat" the competition, will every new implant enter the registry? How will it handle the issue of the few orthopaedists who have their own manufacturing companies, or those influential surgeons who have their own prostheses and receive handsome royalties from manufacturing companies?

The academy has used the example given by the Swedish Hip Registry to promote a similar system in the United States. I have questioned the wisdom of such an analogy based on the fact that Sweden is a small, disciplined, and homogeneous country. Quite different from ours.

I trust my views will prevail and that the plans to get the registry going will be postponed until the issue has been more carefully studied. Jumping into such an expensive and encompassing undertaking at this time is likely to become a future embarrassment.

chapter 23.
to the top
of the academic ladder

"Fame is proof that people are gullible."
—Ralph Waldo Emerson

The search for a chairman of the department of orthopaedics and rehabilitation at the University of Miami had begun before I left for England. The administration completed its search while I was still abroad. I was delighted to learn of my selection. I assumed the newly created chair on January 1, 1971, a little more than eighteen years after I had arrived in the United States to begin my internship.

On the day that I took over the new post, there was a regular meeting of the Miami Orthopedic Society. That morning, the *Miami Herald* and local TV stations carried the news that a local orthopaedist had performed surgery to treat the broken ribs of a player with the Miami Dolphins football team. Ribs heal themselves remarkably well. All orthopaedists agree that treating such an injury with surgery is inappropriate and unnecessary. During the course of the business section of the society's meeting, I took the floor and asked the group to appoint a task force to investigate the situation. I suggested that we might have to consider taking some kind of action against our fellow member who performed the surgery.

I had anticipated that my suggestion would be supported by all present. It was obvious to everyone that the surgery was presumably unnecessary. My motion was seconded, but the discussion moved quickly from questions of high principles to concerns about less exalted matters. A senior member of the society urged the members not to support my motion. He noted that the proposed investigation could result in a retaliatory lawsuit from the surgeon in question. He reminded the society that on a previous occasion, the same surgeon had successfully sued another orthopaedist whose accusations had led to his dismissal from the American College of Surgeons (ACS). In that case, the surgeon had won not only his lawsuit against his accuser but also reinstatement in ACS. The speaker admonished the members of the Miami Orthopedic Society not to support my motion lest we encounter a similar fate. I tried to argue that ignoring such surgery threatened our own high ethical standards. We had the responsibility to stand up and be counted. Remarkably, the audience silenced me with boos, and the president declared my motion out of order. Only then did I realize that I had started my new position with the university by making powerful and influential enemies in the community.

Only later did I learn that when the dean announced my appointment to head the new department, a group of leading orthopaedists had gone to his office to inform him of their strong opposition to me. They threatened that if he followed through with my appointment, they would resign from the voluntary faculty. Happily, the dean remained steadfast. He told them that he supported my appointment and that no change would be made.

None of them followed through on their threat to resign. Furthermore, I do not recall a single time during my seven-year tenure in Miami as chief of the department when another major confrontation with the voluntary faculty took place. Some continued to oppose me. Several made it extremely obvious that they wished I had never been born, or, failing that, had never come to Florida.

As chairman, I did my best to persuade medical students, residents, and faculty alike of the importance of rehabilitation in the everyday life of the orthopaedist. I established formal rotation through the rehabilitation service for all residents. Many of them dreaded that rotation. While serving in rehabilitation, they were denied opportunities to participate in surgery and compelled to spend most of their time dealing with chronically disabled patients. Working constantly with amputees, victims of stroke and head injuries, spinal cord injuries, and similarly disabled patients can be extremely depressing and frustrating. It can also be the most rewarding and important part of a physician's education.

I have often stated that orthopaedic residents who spend time dealing with chronically disabled patients become better doctors and, more importantly, better people. Dealing with patients who have suffered such devastating conditions is a humbling experience. It exposes surgeons to a side of medicine that is typically hidden from them in their daily routines.

The ability to make such vital changes proved to be one of many exciting opportunities that opened to me when I assumed the department chairmanship at Miami. Over the next eight years, I would oversee a vital, growing program. We were able to recruit several young, intelligent people who brought great enthusiasm to our program and great satisfaction to me personally.

Within a few years, we built our department into one of the most visible, powerful, and profitable components of the medical school. We were conducting research, presenting graduate and postgraduate educational seminars, and providing top-quality medical care. The leading peer-reviewed journals all regularly published articles by faculty of the department of orthopaedics and rehabilitation. We frequently served as visiting professors in many institutions and at conferences around the world.

Those pleasant memories prevail whenever I think about my years leading the program at Miami. I also, however, learned a great deal about the unpleasant facets of academic administration—activities and decision making that typically remain hidden from faculty who do not carry top-level responsibilities. These problems oftentimes consumed a disproportionate part of my time and energy. Over my years as a faculty member, I had come to admire the senior administrators. As a department chairman, I learned far too much about their human frailties. Erasmus of Rotterdam, were he alive today, would have successfully written a sequella to his famous *The Praise of Folly*.

I watched the dean of the medical school, a doctor and a man I had admired, became involved in what seemed to be a never-ending spiral of compromises and special arrangements with special interests. On one occasion, I was drawn into an extended battle between the medical school admissions committee, the dean, and the president of the university. At its heart was the preferential admission of the dean's son-in-law. Before we were done, it had degenerated into a full-scale battle over faculty and administrative prerogatives that threatened the reputation of the entire university.

As I recall, William Harrington, chairman of the department of medicine and a man of impeccable integrity, refused to back down and order the committee to admit the dean's son-in-law. As you might expect, the entire admissions committee stood with him. In response, the dean threatened to dissolve the committee and have the administration assume responsibility for admissions. Harrington, in turn, demanded an investigation by the office of the president of the university.

The "investigation" became a meeting of the department heads, the president of the university, and other university officials. Instead of discussing the issue at hand, the president began to praise the accomplishments of the dean of the medical school. He gave special praise to his skill in building several departments. Now, with three decades of additional administrative experience, I know that I should simply have remained quiet. I can only tell you that at the time I was younger, more naive, and more idealistic. I said to the group, "I thought that we assembled here today to discuss the issue concerning the dean threatening to dismiss the admission committee, allegedly because of their refusal to admit one of his relatives, not to discuss the dean's other accomplishments."

My remarks embarrassed some members of the group, but not enough to make them debate the issue in earnest. Obviously, the upper echelon had already made up their minds that they were not going to take any punitive action against the dean. He kept his job and soon he began to retaliate against anyone who had dared questioned his actions. Because of my comments, I found myself among his targets.

The seven chairmen who had opposed him became known throughout the university as the "dirty seven." One by one, we felt the ire of the dean in different degrees. He eventually forced many of them to resign. Others simply had to endure his criticism. At first, the dean did not pressure me directly. Our department had become one of the medical school's leading sources of revenue and prestige. In retrospect, my departure could have dislocated that important unit and caused substantial embarrassment to the school. That did not prevent the dean from making my life as an academic administrator much less comfortable.

At one meeting, which I did not attend, the dean announced that he was going to transfer rehabilitation from the department of orthopedics and rehabilitation to the department of neurosurgery. I could not believe my ears. It had been at my request that my department had been given the name "orthopaedics and rehabilitation," and at my insistence that the two programs had been combined in my department. We had been the first medical school in the United States to make that connection; several other prestigious universities had followed our example. Our leadership was a source of pride not only to me but to the faculty and the school as well.

I immediately wrote to the dean to express my profound unhappiness with such a plan and requested an appointment with him. At our meeting, he denied having made such a comment. He then told me of his strong support for me and of his satisfaction with the way I had built the department. He added, however, that I should not have written the letter and insisted that if in the future I had any important matters to discuss with him, I should do it verbally and not in writing.

A few weeks later, I was told that another meeting had taken place, and that the dean had again discussed the issue of rehabilitation. At this meeting, he requested confidentiality and then "clarified" the "confusion" caused by his earlier comments. This time, he told the group that he was considering moving the spinal cord injury program to the department of neurosurgery, and leaving the rest of rehabilitation as part of orthopaedics.

Again, I immediately put my strong objections in writing. This time, I did not bother to request an appointment. As I expected, I received a call to report to the dean's office as soon as he had read my letter. He angrily reminded me that he had made himself very clear just a few weeks earlier. Delicate matters, such the one I was discussing, were to be addressed to him in person, not in writing. Playing stupid, I replied that I was not skilled at debating issues in person, and felt more comfortable doing it in writing. I said that I had found that by writing things out, I was able to avoid the need to "clarify" any resulting "confusion." He proceeded again to deny the charges and pleaded with me not to believe rumors. We retained all the components of the rehabilitation program.

I chose, instead, not to believe the dean. He had recruited a new chairman of neurosurgery, and I was certain that the intentions voiced at administrative meetings had been planned in order to fulfill promises made to his leading candidate.

My relationship with the dean remained cordial, formal, and somewhat tense. A year later, I again found myself caught up in a confrontation. This time, the dispute involved Dr. Robert Zeppa, the chief of general surgery, who was insisting that orthopaedic residents continue to rotate through his department, as they had done when the orthopaedics program had been a part of his department.

In order to maintain good relations, I had acquiesced when I first assumed leadership of orthopaedics, but had specified that I was only willing to continue the arrangement for the next two years. When I realized the impact of our required rotation through rehabilitation, however, I informed the chief of surgery that as of the following July, orthopaedic residents would no longer rotate through general surgery. I gave him the reasons for my decision in writing.

We had a stormy confrontation over the issue, at which we both held our ground. Then the CEO of the hospital called the dean of the medical school and the two of us to meet with him and resolve the issue.

The dean proceeded to inform me that he had thought over the issue carefully. He had concluded that he had to support the department of surgery. I would have to rotate our residents through the general surgery service. Having said that, he passed a document to the CEO, who signed it and gave it to the chief of surgery. He, too, signed it with great ceremony, and passed the document to me. I read it, and found it a brief statement in which I, as chairman of orthopaedics and rehabilitation, agreed to begin the rotation of orthopaedics residents through general surgery beginning the following month. Their show had really been quite impressive.

I returned the document, unsigned, to the dean. I told the assembled group that I did not accept their decision and was quite willing to take the matter to the next level of the university administration. The dean exploded. He accused me of insubordination and asked me if I was aware of the fact that I served as chairman of the department at his whim. He had the authority, without any consultation with any higher authority, to remove me from the chair. I quietly responded that I had always been aware of his authority but that I was also aware of my responsibility to my students. On that note, the meeting ended.

I fully expected to receive my letter of termination as chairman the next day. That letter never arrived, and the orthopaedic residents never again rotated through general surgery. My relationship with the dean remained unchanged, but my relationship with the chief of surgery never recovered. He died, still a young man, several years after I left for California. He was an outstanding surgeon who was totally committed to his patients and to high academic standards. Dr. Zeppa succeeded in establishing a wonderful first-class trauma center at Jackson Memorial. I still regret that we were not able to work together more closely.

I suspect that it was inevitable that I would encounter obstacles in the development and running of a department within a medical school. However, those obstacles and the unhappy hours they required did not lessen the enjoyment the job generated. Throughout my stay at Miami, I found the establishment of new programs and the recruitment of new faculty and residents to be extremely stimulating. And while Miami did not have the magnificent research facilities that I would find at USC, our research activities proved enormously gratifying.

I was able to surround myself with a superb group of orthopaedists who were sincerely committed to excellence. They were equally dedicated as teachers and physicians. Most were also remarkably "good people," intellectually honest, warm, and devoted to their school and their colleagues. It was a wonderful era. Our salaries were comfortable. Our facilities were not luxurious; our "perks" were not particularly impressive, but we lived in a supportive and rewarding community. Most importantly, we were part of a medical environment where practicing good medicine and doing the best possible job as a teacher was "the name of the game."

Times have changed dramatically over the past few years. The commercialization of medicine, as I indicated earlier, began with the establishment of Medicare. The change transformed medical schools from drains on university resources into income-generating profit centers. The clinical faculty, once subsidized, became self-supporting. That was a mixed blessing. Faculties increased in number, but most faculty members devoted less time to academic pursuits and more time to their remunerative private practices.

This change pitted teaching physicians in competition with full-time community-based physicians. As the academicians devoted less time to teaching and more time to fee-generating activities, private-practice physicians became increasingly resentful. They argued that the "teachers" were neither teaching nor conducting research but were only taking unfair advantage of the aura of university affiliation.

Largely, this is even truer today. Large numbers of "full-time" faculty members in medical schools do virtually no teaching and never lecture to a medical school class. The students, interns, and residents provide primary care for indigent patients. In some schools the "teaching faculty" treats insured patients and avails itself of whatever assistance it may require from the students.

This trend has already done great harm and will continue to cause more problems. While it is true that medical students, residents, and faculty need to be exposed to the private practice of medicine, much is lost when the teachers do not participate in the care of the indigent. Medicine requires humility and empathy—qualities that cannot be learned from a textbook or by simply participating in caring for the educated and the better-off members of our society.

Catering to the educational needs of residents and seeing them grow during their training years is, by far, the most gratifying part of academic medicine. I know that many other academicians have enjoyed the job as much as I did. Many of them become heroes to their students. Frequently, one sees alumni groups created to perpetuate their names and to honor them during their later years. I must admit, however, that no such groups have ever been formed to honor me, even though I served for twenty consecutive years as chief of residency programs, one of which was the largest in the United States. I suspect that I may have expected too much from my students. I never tolerated mediocrity in any form. I always demanded excellence and discipline. My reward came from watching their success as they reached important positions throughout the orthopaedic community.

I love to question virtually everything, particularly my actions and behavior. I recognize the many flaws in my character with little difficulty, so I occasionally wonder about my contributions as a teacher and administrator. I occasionally wish that I had been more tolerant of others and had treated others with greater consideration. I often wish that I had given more time to my family. None of that self-evaluation, however, alters my satisfaction with my overall conduct over the years.

I have always had the greatest confidence in destiny. I am proud of the success that I have achieved in my personal and professional life. Many of my accomplishments vastly exceeded my goals. Those accomplishments, however, meant little more than opportunities to accomplish still more by doing a good job in influential positions.

I suspect that some may have accused me of having worked hard to achieve the chairmanship of the departments of orthopaedics at Miami and USC, and the presidencies of the Hip Society and the American Academy of Orthopedic Surgeons. Those charges, if they actually have taken place, are false. I have participated in the scientific program of the American Academy of Orthopedic Surgeons for forty consecutive years. It is quite a record and I am proud of it. Never once, however, did I try to influence the program committee to have me involved. I accepted the fact that as long I was submitting worthy material I would be included in the program.

I also served on some committees of the academy for long periods of time and in various capacities. I admit that I occasionally resented the success of others when I watched them attain high office even though I felt my contributions were more significant. I was angered when the chairmanship of a committee on which I had long served went to others with less seniority and fewer accomplishments. As for the presidency of the academy, I always assumed that it was beyond my reach.

When Newton McCollough III became president my first reaction was of great excitement and happiness. For more than thirty-five years, Newt had been my closest friend and most loyal colleague. He had been my student, associate, and for a number of years, my co-chairman of the department of orthopaedics and rehabilitation at the University of Miami. When I moved to California, I tried unsuccessfully to entice him to join me in Los Angeles. When the academy announced his nomination to the presidency, I felt a momentary envy of which I have always been ashamed. Our friendship, however, proved strong enough to carry us through the moment. I totally supported his efforts during his year in office. Two years later, when I became president, he, in turn, became my strongest supporter.

chapter 24.
criticized by the master

"You have the mind of a gynecologist."
—Sir John Charnley

My success as a hip replacement surgeon was greater than I had ever imagined. A remarkable chain of events had led, like an inviolable destiny, to that end. From my first exposure to orthopaedics as a student in Bogota, the structure and diseases of the hip had always fascinated me. My residency in the county hospital in Columbia, South Carolina, had led to my work with Austin Moore, the foremost hip surgeon in the United States and the pioneer of partial hip replacement. Most recently, my three months in England at John Charnley's Hip Center had increased my knowledge exponentially and further refined my surgical skills.

The honor of performing the first total hip replacement in Florida went to Dr. Mike Leinbach, in Saint Petersburg. I was the second Florida-based surgeon to perform the procedure. That gave me a head start. Within a short time, I was carrying out a large number of surgical replacements. As I gained experience with Charnley's procedure, I began making efforts to improve on what I (and others) perceived as deficiencies in Charnley's original technique and prosthesis.

My efforts to improve on Charnley's system eventually produced mixed results. In some aspects, I was able to contribute slightly to simplifying the procedure. Most of my modifications, however, eventually proved not to have been solid contributions. At the time, I believed that our device would be the world's first to comprise titanium as a weight-bearing surface in a total joint implant. Later, I learned that Dr. Pierre Boutin, in France, had already begun to implant hip prostheses made of a titanium alloy. My version of the Charnley implant, however, was the first to use titanium for both the ball and the stem components. I later visited Dr. Boutin at his home in Pau. We shared our common interest and experiences with our respective prostheses.

After what I thought was adequate research, our titanium alloy hip prosthesis went into production, and I began using it extensively. Our initial results proved encouraging. We seemed to be experiencing fewer stress failures, and I began to believe that we had made a major improvement on the Charnley implant. Even at the end of our sixth year of implanting our titanium alloy prosthesis, it appeared that the new prosthesis was better. A year later, however, we began to see more negative indicators. A year after that, the titanium implant demonstrated radiological changes suggestive of possible future failures.

During the early years of my enthusiasm with the modifications I had made in the implant, as well as with the surgical technique, I wrote to Mr. Charnley, informing him of the changes and of my partial deviation from his overall philosophy. I told him that I was no longer using his stiff stainless steel prosthesis and had chosen the more elastic titanium; that I was not producing a fracture of the tip of the bone during the surgery as he had recommended; and that rather than approaching the hip joint from the side, as he did, I was making an incision on the buttock and reaching the joint "from behind." I wanted him to learn of my ideas and experiences from me directly and requested his comments and advice.

His reply was most interesting and somewhat unexpected. He stated that he appreciated my sharing of views with him and he added that my "youth" was the reason for my wanting to make changes to his well-proven approach. The tone of the letter then changed rapidly; it became obvious that he was angry with me. He added that he had concluded that I had changed his surgical approach only because I had "never learned to do his operation correctly." He concluded by saying that I "had missed my calling and had chosen the wrong surgical specialty." He felt that if I was approaching the hip from behind rather than from the front it was because I had the "mentality of a gynecologist."*

I saved his letter. A couple of years later, while my relationship with Mr. Charnley was still rather cold, I presented a paper at the

---

*Letter to the author from Mr. John Charnley, 1976.

meeting of the International Hip Society in Bern, Switzerland. Mr. Charnley was also attending the meeting. I was reporting on my experiences with the titanium prosthesis for the first time in front of the group. I began my talk by flashing a slide dedicating the presentation to Mr. Charnley, and entitling my talk "A Gynecologist's Experience with Total Hip Arthroplasty." I told the story behind my title, and Mr. Charnley joined the audience and me in the general laughter. Happily, our relationship returned to its previously friendly level. We remained close friends, and until his death I continued to benefit from Mr. Charnley's friendship and advice.

A few years later, Mr. Charnley's widow told me that he had shown her the letter before he mailed it. She assured him that the letter was merited, and urged him to go ahead and send it. She said that he had always held me in high esteem.

When I was president of the Hip Society in 1976 and 1977, I again invited Mr. Charnley to come to the United States to present his philosophy of hip surgery in person. This time he not only accepted the invitation but also actually came to the United States. He had realized that his words needed to be heard. American surgeons also realized that they needed to learn from the great man in person. I had the opportunity to introduce him to the audience of more than 800 orthopaedists by stating, "Mr. Charnley needs no introduction. The height of his accomplishments is only surpassed by his impeccable integrity." The entire audience stood as one and gave him a long and enthusiastic round of applause.

During that visit to Miami, I invited Mr. Charnley to serve as visiting lecturer at the university. To my great pleasure, he agreed. It was a great honor for us.

At the end of a magnificent presentation on the subject of hip replacement, I asked him if he felt comfortable predicting the future of research on arthritis in general. He responded, with his rather sharp, high-pitched voice and classical English accent that "one day, probably in the near future, there will be a cure for rheumatoid arthritis but that never, never will osteoarthritis be prevented or cured without surgery." Ten years later, when he again visited us in Los Angeles, I asked him the same question. His answer was the same. He believed that osteoarthritis had been in the genes of humans since the beginning of time and that to try to offset that generic fact was impossible.

He could not have anticipated that a few years later, molecular biologists would be openly claiming that they expected to identify and manipulate the genes that produce osteoarthritis. That has not happened yet. Mr. Charnley's prediction remains intact. He was right so many times, about so many things, that I would not be surprised if he again proves the rest of us to be mistaken.

On one occasion during my first visit to Charnley's Hip Center in England, he discussed his views on evolution. He told me that after he retired from practice he would write a book refuting Darwin's theory of evolution. Charnley had no quarrel with the philosophical basis of Darwin's theories. He simply believed that life had not existed on Earth long enough for evolution to have progressed so far. The true source of biodiversity, he felt, must lie elsewhere. He believed that creationism, therefore, should be regarded as equally valid on a theoretical level. He found the overwhelming support of Darwin by the scientific community to be scientifically insupportable.

A few years later, I reminded him of his plans for his retirement. He responded that his remaining days would probably be occupied with other matters. Unfortunately, Mr. Charnley never got around to correcting Darwin. I am sure that his work would have been fascinating, innovative, and convincing. But he never found time to write the book. He continued to practice surgery until his last day.

By the end of 1977, I, too, found that I was experiencing a shortage of time to handle important activities. I was performing an average of six total hip surgeries a week. Although I was enjoying both the surgery itself and my success as a surgeon, I was becoming dissatisfied with my lifestyle. I had gone into academic medicine because I wanted to teach and to conduct research. Doing so much surgery required me to sacrifice other, more important areas.

During the late 1970s, I received several offers to become the chief of joint replacement surgery in other hospitals throughout the greater Miami area. Mount Sinai Hospital, in Miami Beach, offered to give me an entire building within the medical complex for establishing an Arthritis and Joint Replacement Institute. That concept had long been a dream of mine. I found the offer extremely tempting. I received a similar offer from the Cedars and Lebanon Hospital, which was (and is) situated adjacent to the medical school. A patient of mine, a wealthy woman, offered me one million dollars just for research. These offers held out the temptation to continue building on my surgical practice and conduct advanced research while making a great deal of money. I could not do that as a full-time member of the faculty at the medical school.

Then I received an offer to chair the newly created department of orthopaedics at the University of Southern California. This time I could not resist. The California offer changed my life and my academic career.

chapter 25.
to california:
chasing the rainbow

"Life is a nightmare from which I am trying to awake."
—James Joyce

After twenty years at the University of Miami, first as a resident in training, then as a member of the faculty, and finally as department chair, I moved to California chasing the rainbow. I had achieved both academic and professional success beyond reasonable or even irrational expectations. I had become chairman of a large, successful department. Our department was second only to ophthalmology in the generation of revenues from the private practice component. I was the single largest revenue-producing faculty member in the entire medical school and, of course, in the university.

Our continuing education program had earned national recognition both for my university and for me. My research on functional bracing of fractures had gained international attention. I had become involved in the development of a private practice plan for the University of Miami Medical School faculty, and, like many other professors, had built a successful practice for myself. Increasing numbers of patients anxiously waited for their turn on my operating table; my schedule stretched a full year ahead. The day I left Miami in March of 1978, there were well over one hundred patients remaining on my surgical waiting list.

At Jackson Memorial, I had taken over the abandoned third floor of the Colored Hospital for use as our first orthopaedic rehabilitation ward. The building was termite-ridden and lacked air conditioning. The "lighting fixtures" consisted of a few bare bulbs hanging from wires. That facility remained hazardous to the health and welfare of staff and patients alike for several years. Even when we expanded into space intended for other departments, the facilities remained minimal, at best. When I left Miami, we were just dedicating a new, state-of-the-art rehabilitation center with good facilities for patients and staff. It included the latest rehabilitation equipment, conformable offices, and airy, well-ventilated, cheerful rooms in which patients could recover their dignity as well as their mobility.

Why should I, under such circumstances, leave Miami? Dissatisfaction and ambition are strange creatures that know no rest. They gnaw at the soul. In my own case, I discovered that I wanted more from my career in academic medicine than success and popularity as a surgeon. I had long known that teaching and conducting research were my true raison d'être, and my favorite activities. Surgery had become only a means to an end. Administrative power had become little more than a way to prevent other administrators from interfering with my life, professional goals, and career. But my busy schedule was forcing me to neglect other, more important areas of life.

I remember one night when my family went through a terrifying personal experience. It was a Sunday, and, in a rare exception to my usual patterns, I was at home that afternoon. Gus Jr. had left the house that morning to go fishing with some of friends. We expected him to be back before dark. By 9:00 that evening he had not returned. We called the police at midnight, but they could only tell us that he had not been involved in a traffic accident. That was small comfort, since it was the thought of an accident at sea, not on the highways, that we feared.

Barbara and I huddled by the phone. We tried to keep the other children from worrying. As I recall, they even went to school the next day, unaware that anything out of the ordinary was going on. I, of course, cancelled my scheduled surgery and rounds.

At about noon on Monday, we finally learned that another boat had located the boys, adrift in the ocean between Florida and Bimini. Instead of a brief fishing trip, they had decided to go adventuring! The engine of their boat had broken down, possibly because none of them really knew much about operating it. They did not have a radio onboard. Their boat was totally adrift, floating north in the Gulf Stream, when they were found.

I suppose that the youngsters were never in any real danger. The seas were calm that week. The weather was clear. There were no storms and little wind. The boys had stayed well within heavily traveled sea-lanes. Throughout their ordeal, they had always assumed that someone would spot them sooner or later. They had not even run out of food.

Neither Barbara nor I knew any of that, of course. Visions of shipwrecks filled our imaginations as we huddled close to the phone and contemplated the worst. Both of us tried to reassure the other, but both of us feared the nightmare of losing our son. It became a most painful and humbling night. It also made me aware of the extent to which I had neglected my family. It made me want to spend less time in surgery, in my office, or at the hospital. I wanted to devote myself to research, to teaching, and to my wife and children. With the return of Gus Jr. to dry land, I soon lost sight of that promise to myself, but it never receded far from my consciousness. While I did not cut back my activities, I was constantly seeking ways to restructure my life in a more meaningful way.

There were other difficulties as well. The University of Miami Medical School had not, at the time, mastered the art of obtaining grants for research. This shortage of funds continuously strangled my department's research activities. These financial shortfalls severely limited our productivity, especially compared to other well-known medical schools. We also did not have the financial resources needed to hire additional faculty, which, inevitably, further limited the academic potential of the department. We would never be able to recruit the distinguished faculty needed to further improve our national reputation.

On a trip to Edinburgh, where I attended a combined meeting of the English-speaking orthopaedic associations, a well-known hand surgeon from Los Angeles approached me and told me that the University of Southern California Medical School had just created an orthopaedics department. He told me that they were seeking to recruit the most distinguished faculty in the nation. He asked whether I might be interested in joining this great new adventure. He also indicated that the Orthopaedic Hospital of Los Angeles, one of hospitals affiliated with the university, had received an endowment of thirteen million dollars for research.

His suggestion fell on fertile ground. A few years earlier, Dr. Paul Harvey, USC's chief of the division of orthopaedics, had invited me to be his visiting professor at their first alumni day. I had enjoyed the experience and held an extremely high opinion of Dr. Harvey, who had spent several days as a visiting professor with us in Miami. I had also seen him in action at meetings of the American Academy of Orthopaedic Surgeons Committee on Injuries, which I chaired for several years. I knew he was a demanding, outspoken administrator. He and members of his faculty had published several articles in the *Journal of Bone and Joint Surgery*. I also knew that he had developed a good program at USC. On several occasions I had mentioned to others that USC was going to be a major force in trauma care and would set the pace for the rest of the country.

When I returned to the United States, I received a call from the dean of the USC School of Medicine inviting me to visit the institution and be interviewed for the chairmanship of the new department. My first question to him concerned Paul Harvey, since I had surmised that after sixteen years as chief of the division he would be the logical candidate to hold the chair in the newly created department. Without any hesitation, he told me that Dr. Harvey would not chair the new department. That decision had already been made. I agreed to visit USC the following month.

Upon my arrival to Los Angeles, I told the dean that the first person I wanted to meet was Paul Harvey. Our meeting was cordial, as I had anticipated, since Paul is a charming, socially skilled, gracious person. I said that I admired his accomplishments, assured him that I had no desire to interfere with his career, and told him about the dean's statement that he was not being considered for the chairmanship position. He responded that he was keenly aware of the school's decision and that he had accepted it. He indicated that he had made too many enemies in the community. He regretted that state of affairs, but had to recognize that many powerful people within the university and the community were also opposed to his advancement.

I started my tour of USC's facilities at Los Angeles County (LAC) Hospital, where I discovered an institution that would have been more at home in some developing country than in a great U.S. city. It appeared that the operating rooms had not been improved since the hospital had opened, some seventy years earlier. It reminded me of Jackson Memorial.

In addition to Paul Harvey, there were only two orthopaedists on the full-time faculty at the LAC-USC Medical Center. One more orthopaedist, the famed Jacqueline Perry, was at Rancho Los Amigos Hospital, a rehabilitation hospital affiliated with the university.

The division lacked sufficient support personnel. At Miami, we had recruited approximately forty physical and occupational therapists to cover the department. LAC-USC Medical Center had virtually no rehabilitation coverage for orthopaedics. Overall, I calculated that one and a half therapists provided rehabilitation therapy support to a service with more patients than we had in Miami.

The orthopaedic outpatient clinic, where approximately two hundred patients were seen every day, had no physical therapist on staff or even on call. A mere handful of physical therapists covered the entire institution, which featured more than one thousand beds. For all practical purposes, that meant that LAC-USC provided no rehabilitation at the hospital.

I gathered that the same sad state of affairs prevailed for other departments. Happily, I discovered that the pediatric orthopaedic surgeons operated in another building within the complex. I soon realized, however, that the physical facilities were equally as appalling in the pediatric center as they were in the main building.

The failings of the USC program extended well beyond the physical environment. Too few faculty members supervised too many interns and residents. That left the students and other trainees frequently unsupervised. The three attending orthopaedists on the full-time faculty rotated through the services. They moved from one operating room to the next to oversee surgery in process and to respond when the residents found themselves in serious difficulties. For all intents and purposes, the residents were running their own residency program. I am sure that they found that situation most gratifying to their young egos, but it was dreadful both for the patients and for the long-term development of the doctors in training.

I quickly learned that most of the voluntary faculty had stopped attending hospital functions because of the poor conditions that prevailed throughout, and because of "difficulties dealing with Dr. Harvey." I should have recognized that bright red flag that was waving right in front of my face. After several visits to USC, I had no doubt that Harvey was committed to his work. I had no doubts about his loyalty to the institution to which he had dedicated his life. I realized that the source of any problems must lie elsewhere.

Five hospitals throughout the Los Angeles region were affiliated with the USC Medical School. It did not take me long to recognize that relationships between them were acrimonious. Mutual animosity reigned supreme. I should have recognized that they could be united only by their perception of a common outside enemy (such as a new department head) but I ignored this red flag, as well.

The Orthopaedic Hospital, to which the large research endowment had been made, turned out to be a small institution located a few miles away from the medical school and the County Hospital. I met there with the trustees of the hospital whom, I was told, were "very powerful and influential" members of the community. The chairman of the board was Robert Dockson, chairman of the board of the California Federal Bank and former chairman of the department of economics at the University of Southern California. I found him a most knowledgeable, dedicated, and charismatic individual. By the end of the meeting, I was telling myself that with the support of people like Dockson, I could make the USC department of orthopaedics the best in the United States. In retrospect, my arrogance and pride must have had led me to that conclusion, because I had never seen an academic program so deficient in so many ways.

My conversations with the dean, the vice president for medical affairs, and the trustees at Orthopaedic Hospital all led me to believe that I had their full support. I outlined many of the changes that I had in mind. Everyone in authority agreed that the changes that I was suggesting were, indeed, necessary. What is more, they assured me that the changes could be accomplished relatively easily.

I knew that I would need the full cooperation of all senior administrators if I were to have any hope of correcting the problems at County Hospital and harmonizing the relationship between USC Medical School and its hospital affiliates. The senior administrators convinced me that they all sincerely desired to see matters improve and would support my efforts. I fully believed that they were sincere in the commitment to support the chairman of the new department. I felt comfortable with the challenge. I knew that I had been able to build a respectable orthopaedics and rehabilitation department from scratch at Miami. I assumed that I would be able to build a world-class department from the existing materials in Los Angeles.

I would have many powerful tools with which to work. To begin with, the research money at Orthopaedic Hospital was to be placed in the hands of the new department chairman, who would unify and finalize plans to occupy, staff, and organize the research program there. The university had already taken several important steps along those lines. The hospital had already provided space and financial support to a distinguished group of scientists. They had already begun construction of new laboratories.

During my written and personal communications with the dean, he had made it clear that as chairman of the new department I had the authority to select and appoint the chiefs of orthopaedics at the five affiliated institutions.

During the initial negotiations, the university administration also strongly supported my intention to build a private practice plan, which the university until that time lacked. I had been deeply involved at the University of Miami in the development of our successful private practice plan. I knew from my experience in Miami that a strong private practice plan strengthened the university and could dramatically increase its influence within the community.

I had no desire to develop a private practice in total hip surgery as large as the one I had built in Miami. I had little interest in rebuilding the predicament I had encountered in Miami. In Los Angeles, I wanted to have the time to be more involved in education and research. I also wanted more personal time to devote to my wife and children.

I also knew the Los Angeles county area was already saturated with orthopaedic surgeons. Despite that saturation, I told myself that I would have no difficulty in building a referral practice in hip surgery, since I had an international reputation as a hip surgeon. At that time, I was president of the Hip Society. I anticipated that local Los Angeles area orthopaedists would refer many cases to me, since the continuing education courses I had presented in Miami had always drawn a large number of students from the West Coast.

John Wilson, a distinguished Los Angeles orthopaedist who had previously served as president of the American Academy of Orthopaedic Surgeons was one of the people who had a major influence in my moving to USC. He was a trustee of the university and one its most influential leaders. His efforts to recruit me seemed enthusiastic and sincere. Those efforts included many promises that his office would refer numerous patients to help me develop a thriving private practice as quickly as possible. John died about twelve years after I moved to California. During that entire time, neither he nor his office referred a single patient to me.

Shortly after John's death, however, I received a call from one of his associates. He told me that one of his patients, Dorothy Chandler, wanted me to see her in consultation. She was a prominent member of Los Angeles society, and one of the most generous supporters of music and the fine arts in the region. She had sustained a fracture of the femur, and was considering surgery. I offered to visit her at their hospital before the end of the day. Her doctor told me over the phone that such a visit was not necessary. He would bring the X rays to my office. I replied that I could not consult without personally examining the patient, and assured him that I would visit his patient within the next few hours.

Twenty minutes later, he appeared in my office carrying her X rays. I assume he must have been afraid that the Mrs. Chandler might ask me to be her surgeon. I decided not to make a major production out of the situation, and made my recommendation based on the radiographs. The incident confirmed my belief that neither Dr. Wilson nor any of his associates had ever intended to refer patients to me. That promise had been one more false commitment.

I decided to accept the position at USC in spite of the enormous obstacles I had been able to identify during the three visits I made to the university. I was highly impressed with the people I had met. I fully believed that they would work with me to transform USC into the nation's leading center of orthopaedic excellence. I had a lot to learn about the differences between image and reality.

When I announced that I would be leaving Florida for Southern California, Henry King Stanford, the president of the University of Miami, visited me to ask if there was anything he could do to keep me in Miami. I was so infatuated with the picture of USC, however, that I could only say that I appreciated his words but that my mind was firmly made up. The Sarmiento family was moving to California, where I would become the first professor and chairman of the department of orthopaedics at USC.

I had no written contract. I totally trusted those who were to play a major role in my future and in the future of the department. In turn, I asked colleagues throughout the nation to trust me, and to help me identify the best possible candidates for the chief positions at USC's affiliated hospitals. I met with these candidates in Miami, and shared with them the grandiose plans I had for the new challenge. Three outstanding orthopaedists agreed to join our Los Angeles crusade. One of them was slated to become chief at the LAC-USC hospital, the second would assume the leadership of Orthopaedic Hospital, and the third would take charge at Rancho Los Amigos.

Although I was tempted to purchase a home as soon as we came into town, we elected, instead, to rent an apartment until we became more familiar with the community. My family was thrilled with the move. We were all excited by the new prospects. It was a wonderful time in our lives. None of us had the slightest anticipation of the way our world would be turned upside down in an instant. Even as we were completing preparations for the start of our new life, we learned that Barbara had breast cancer.

This was Barbara's second encounter with cancer. Ten years earlier, her doctors had discovered a malignancy in her uterus. Now, after ten years of freedom from disease, she again faced surgery. We postponed the move as long as possible, but we finally ran out of time. I moved to Los Angeles, alone, anticipating that she would join me a few weeks later. During a follow-up visit to her surgeon, however, he discovered that the cancer was also present in the other breast. Within a few days, she was back in surgery. Happily, she recovered quickly. She and Gregory, our younger son, soon joined me in our new home.

We lived on the seventeenth floor of the Bunker Hill Towers, a building located close to the Orthopaedic Hospital and the medical school. A few months after the move, I took a trip to South America to visit my mother. One morning, while reading the local newspaper, I saw a photograph of a burning high-rise apartment building in Los Angeles. I still remember the slowly expanding horror with which I recognized the building as my own residence, the place where my wife and youngest child should have been at exactly that moment. I tried to reach them by telephone, but there was no answer. I immediately called my secretary. Within a few minutes, she confirmed that my building had caught fire the night before. She also confirmed that the family was safe and staying at a downtown hotel.

Barbara later told me about that terrible night. The fire started well after midnight. She thinks that the noise of people running down the hall woke her up. She woke up Gregory. When she opened the apartment door, however, smoke had already filled the hallway. I am still amazed by the calm and wisdom she exhibited under the stress and terror. She did not panic and run. Instead, she placed wet towels at the bottom of the door and waited for the fire department to put the fire out or rescue her. Fortunately, the fire had started two floors below ours. The fire department had put it out before it spread. But three people died that night.

A few days after I returned from Colombia, while I was home by myself, the fire alarm went off. The occupants of the building panicked and I was no exception. Barefooted, wearing only my underwear and carrying my pants in my hands, I ran down seventeen flights of stairs, possibly setting a new world record for my speed. Only when I reached the outside did I pause to put on my pants. I was not the only resident who chose to finish dressing outside that night. Happily, this time, there had been no fire after all. It was just a false alarm.

chapter 26.
an unexpected shock

"Not as bad as it sounds."
    —Mark Twain (on the music of Richard Wagner)

Filled with enthusiasm and anticipation for the new challenge, I assumed the chair of the orthopaedics department at the University of Southern California on March 1, 1978. Ann Karg, my administrative assistant in Miami who had been my "right hand" for many years; my secretary, Dorothy Preston; and Dick Tarr, a young and extremely promising bioengineer, came to Los Angeles with me. Dick later left us to pursue a successful career in industry. Loren Latta, the bioengineer who had assisted me with investigation in fracture healing and with the development of fracture bracing and total hip replacement had also made plans to move to California. However, at the last minute his wife persuaded him to stay in Miami. His decision devastated me for a while. We have remained very good friends and to date we continue to cooperate in a variety of research projects.

I chose to locate the seat of the new department headquarters at the Orthopaedic Hospital. I felt that it was most important for me to solidify my relationship with that institution. I planned to use Orthopaedic Hospital as my model institution and make it an example to the other affiliates.

Just a few days after I arrived I addressed the medical staff at Orthopedic Hospital. Several members of the board of trustees also chose to attend the meeting, which offered me my first opportunity to share my ideas and plans for the hospital and the university's new department of orthopaedics. I had looked forward to the occasion for weeks, and planned my remarks carefully. I knew that it was extremely important to present a positive image, so I spoke with genuine enthusiasm about the bright future that I envisioned.

I identified the areas where I intended to concentrate my efforts and told them that the administration had assured me of its full support. Working together, I said, we were going to make Orthopedic Hospital the envy of the world, the Mayo Clinic of the West. They applauded enthusiastically, and I heard them talking to each other with genuine animation as I left the room. I was sure that I had said exactly the right things and at the right time. It was my last moment of undiluted enthusiasm and pleasure in California.

Robert Dockson, the chairman of the board, left the auditorium with me. As we stepped into the beautifully bright and clear Los Angeles sunshine, he casually remarked, "Gus, you made a few guys nervous." Unfortunately, I did not pay much attention to the meaning of his words and interpreted them as a compliment. I did not yet know that I was standing on one side of a giant communication gap. I still fully believed that I had rallied the staff behind me. The truth made itself visible within a few days when it became obvious that I had done nothing but brace the staff for conflict.

I had never fully understood the true state of affairs of USC orthopaedics. The medical school had five affiliated hospitals, but none of them were *closely* affiliated. The five hospitals all saw themselves as fully independent institutions. Throughout my early career, I had witnessed the weakness of nonacademic teaching hospitals. I had always sought to embrace academia. I had made my own academic values and standards clear to the USC officers and administrators throughout our negotiations.

Where I had assumed that the medical staff would share the support pledged by the Orthopaedic Hospital trustees, the opposite turned out to be true. They prized their independence and feared entanglement with USC. They preferred to judge themselves and their interns and residents by their own standards. They viewed me not as a teacher but as a competitor. Where I had intended to create an encompassing alliance, I was seen as having declared war. The good news was that I had united my faculty. The bad news was that I had brought them together in battle against me. I was about to undergo advanced on-the-job training in academic politics, California style.

BETRAYAL

Within days, I realized that the many promises for support made during negotiations had not withstood this first test. During my first meeting with the dean, I learned that Rancho Los Amigos Hospital had appointed a new medical director. They had promised that I would have authority to select the new chief; the dean had "approved" my candidate; my candidate had agreed to accept the position. The dean squirmed a bit and insisted that I did not need to worry. He told me that "political problems" beyond his control had crept into the situation. Before long, I would learn that "political problems" always interfered with proper decision making at Orthopedic Hospital and throughout USC.

I soon learned that the dean did not himself have the authority to hire and fire chiefs at the affiliated hospitals. In fact, under the existing structure, he had no authority even to comment on candidates for positions of chief of the various services at Rancho Los Amigos or any of the other hospitals affiliated within USC. He certainly had no authority to promise, as he had, that I would have such power. But he did have the authority to order me to call my designated candidates and withdraw my offers of employment.

The trustees at Orthopaedic Hospital did authorize me to interview Newton McCollough III, whom I had recommended for the post of medical director, and whom I hoped to appoint as vice-chairman of my orthopaedics department at USC. Newton came to Los Angeles, but after a rather short visit, declined my invitation. I may have failed to notice that there was something "rotten" in the state of USC, but Newton's instincts proved more reliable. He went back to Miami where he was appointed to succeed me as chairman.

Affairs at Orthopedic Hospital continued to deteriorate. The trustees soon learned of the medical staff's opposition to my leadership. They quickly took every opportunity to assure me of their unwavering support. I later learned that they had moved equally quickly to form alliances with various staff members. Despite such opposition and maneuvering, I continued my efforts to institute needed changes.

The medical staff at Orthopaedic Hospital was composed of a small group of active surgeons whose standards were good but whose interest in working with the university was guarded if not outright negative. They preferred to maintain the hospital's autonomy and their authority within the hospital administration. They were proud of the independence of their residency program. They did not realize that by distancing the residency program from the university they lost a great deal of respect and prestige. In fact, throughout the country, accrediting boards were targeting independent residency programs, encouraging their elimination, and merging them with programs staffed and managed by strong medical schools. The surgeons at Orthopaedic Hospital sought to maintain the *image* of medical school affiliation and the *reality* of independence.

The day after my first address to the medical staff, one of the surgeons came to my office to tell me that I did not need to worry about finding an "outsider" to run my proposed program in sports medicine. He strongly felt that he was the best person for the job. He told me that he had completed a year of special training in the field and assured me that he was committed to see his area excel.

I expressed my pleasure in meeting him and asked for a copy of his resume. He had never written a scientific paper, never given any lectures at major national meetings, never carried out any investigative research. It was the resume of a practicing surgeon, not the documentation of an academic life and a scholarly career. Yet, he felt that he was not only an outstanding academician but also fully qualified for administrative responsibility. I would soon discover that the majority of the medical staff members fell into the same category.

Had I been born with more common sense, greater political skills, and the ability to read tea leaves, I might have acted quite differently in my overall relationship with the medical staff at the various affiliated hospitals. With 20/20 hindsight, I can see that I should have moved much more slowly. Tradition and job security were deeply rooted in the minds of those who had grown up with these institutions. They saw change as threat. They pictured themselves being replaced by the outsider and his imported cronies. I can understand that viewed from their perspective they had no choice but to oppose every change that I sought to implement.

During my negotiations with the dean and trustees of Orthopaedic Hospital, I was assured that I could merge the two residency programs into one, which would be known as the University of Southern California Affiliated Hospitals Residency Program. When I took over at USC, I immediately initiated conversations with the Board of Orthopaedics and prepared the necessary paperwork. When I sent the documents to the hospital trustees, however, they informed me that they had changed their minds and had decided to retain the autonomy of their residency program.

I was appalled by such an action and strongly protested their decision, which in my opinion represented a flagrant breach of contract. The dean of the medical school refused to involve himself. I was left to fend for myself. My first reaction was to resign. I was beginning to realize that the situation was beyond my ability to maintain control. I finally sensed that I would have to fight, alone, for every change. Neither the medical staffs nor the university administration would stand by my side. If I really wanted to transform USC into a world-class orthopaedics school, I would have to do so over a lot of dead bodies, possibly including my own.

Instead, I chose to call for help. I contacted the advisory group to the American Board of Orthopaedics and requested that they visit Los Angeles and assess the awkward situation in which I had been placed. The advisory group assigned to task to Dr. Ed Henderson, the chief of orthopaedics at the Mayo Clinic and past president of the American Academy of Orthopedic Surgeons.

Dr. Henderson arrived in Los Angeles a few weeks later and spent several days reviewing the program. His verdict made it clear that if the Orthopaedic Hospital did not merge with the LAC-USC program, the American Board of Orthopaedics would probably be forced to disapprove its residency program entirely. The review forced Orthopaedic Hospital to merge its residency program over the objections of the medical staff. The medical staff, in turn, never forgave me. Indeed, their retaliation was awesome and, as intended, extremely embarrassing. Worse yet, it had a terrible result on the life and career of an innocent bystander.

From the start, I had planned to establish a strong group of full-time academician-practitioners based at the hospital. As headquarters for this group practice, I selected a floor of Orthopaedic Hospital where my future associates and I could temporarily see our private patients. I anticipated that we would eventually move into a specially designed new building.

As I began to see the few private patients who sought my services, the medical staff provided minimal support. Possibly consequently, I became overanxious to recruit at least one associate. I identified a young man from upstate New York who had approached me seeking a job. He had completed a pediatric fellowship in addition to his orthopaedic residency. His references were a bit weak, but I decided to hire him anyway. (In retrospect, I know that I should have brought a full team of associates with me from Miami. Moving to Los Angeles without bringing my own support team proved to be a major error.)

The young man began to work a few days later, and his ordeal began the day he arrived. In the opinion of the medical staff, he could not do anything right. They followed every step he made and found fault with everything he did or said. His youth and inexperience would have made it difficult to function under the best circumstances. The concerted opposition by the medical staff made it virtually impossible for him to succeed. The medical staff filed daily reports on him with the quality of care committee.

A few weeks later I was called to meet with the dean and the chairman of the board of trustees of Orthopedic Hospital. According to the official agenda, we were meeting to discuss several issues concerning the relationship between the two institutions. The chairman of the board had his own agenda. Without any warning, he informed the dean, in my presence, that "they" were terminating the young man's contract the following week. The dean pretended to be taken by surprise. (I learned the next day from a member of the administration that the dean had known about the issue prior to the meeting; he had discussed it with other trustees in advance.)

I protested the way in which the matter was being handled. I reminded the two "leaders" that the young man had received an academic appointment from the university. It seemed to me that he could not be dismissed without appropriate notice and due process. They agreed to grant the young man the rights to which he was entitled. I did not pursue the issue any further. I knew that he had no future at Orthopaedic Hospital. He later accused me of betraying him.

The hospital then withdrew from my control the area where I was seeing patients. The trustees called a special meeting to discuss the issue of my seeing private patients on hospital grounds. The physicians accused me of "unfair competition" with the medical staff. The trustees agreed, and literally evicted me from the premises. They also promised that they would find and provide better quarters as soon as possible.

An older member of the medical staff offered me space in his office to see my few private patients. I gladly accepted the invitation and settled into his small office suite across the street from the hospital. His wife served as his secretary, receptionist, nurse and X ray technician. I stayed there for nearly a year before two other young orthopaedists and I rented space in a downtown Los Angeles building, a mile away from the hospital. It was not an ideal or convenient location, but it was the best we could do under the circumstances.

As time went on, I began to discover that Orthopaedic Hospital had been hiding other, more serious problems. The trustees had led me to believe that it was a viable institution and did not face any problems in regards to occupancy, growth, or similar business matters. They repeatedly spoke of the continued success of the Hospital Foundation and the large number of donations that continued to pour in. These gifts to the Hospital Foundation should have ensured the success of the research program—the main reason for my having sought a close association with Orthopaedic Hospital in the first place.

Orthopaedic Hospital had been a first-class hospital some years earlier, but by 1978, the hospital was experiencing serious difficulties. The number of patients being admitted had decreased rapidly over the last few years; several of the physicians who most heavily used Orthopedic Hospital had moved their practices to other institutions in the community. The hospital no longer treated sufficient clinical material to sustain a residency training program.

I reached that conclusion after analyzing the surgery schedules for 1975–1978. I then asked the hospital CEO to provide me information on a number of areas, but he made no effort to accommodate my wishes. After repeated failed attempts to get information from him I decided to obtain it on my own. My administrative staff befriended lower-echelon employees, who provided us with the information I needed. When I read it, I was appalled. I was looking at a dying hospital.

I then organized the data and prepared myself to discuss it with the trustees at one of their monthly meetings. I began my presentation by paraphrasing John Dean, former President Nixon's attorney, who first brought the Watergate cover-up to the attention of the president with the phrase "There is a cancer on the White House." I told the trustees that there was a "cancer in the Orthopaedic Hospital. It needs radical surgery if it is to survive."

I flashed a series of slides with bar graphs illustrating the critical yearly decline in admissions, surgery, and academic productivity. At one time one of the older trustees interrupted me and accused me of exaggerating. He said that I was "letting my Latin blood boil" prematurely. I chose to ignore the ethnic slur and responded professionally: "I am sure that you, as a businessman, would be deeply concerned if the comptroller of your firm were to show you data as dismal as the data I have shown you today."

The president of the board then instructed the secretary to stop taking notes. He was taking the meeting into executive session. He did not want any records to be kept. He excused me from the room. As I left, I suggested that the board members consider making me a member of the executive committee.

It turned out that the trustees were keenly aware of the declining situation of the hospital. They were deeply embarrassed not only by the facts of the impending hospital failure but also by the fact that I had confronted them with the data. They feared not just the collapse of the hospital but the possibility that their well-kept secret could become public.

Within a few days, they invited me to attend another of their meetings. They welcomed me to the executive committee, and informed me that they had hired a consulting firm, which would review the hospital's economic health. For the first time since my arrival in Los Angeles, I felt enthusiastic about my decision to join USC.

Richard Casparis, from San Francisco, headed the review group. We met privately and at a number of meetings with an appointed task force. Everyone, including me, found Casparis to be knowledgable, articulate, and a sound thinker. He took much longer than I had expected before he was ready to report. He concluded his report to the trustees by suggesting that they either follow a rigorous set of demanding recommendations, or put the hospital up for sale.

The Casparis plan coincided, almost to the letter, with the recommendations I had presented to the trustees when I first arrived in Los Angeles. Among the most important issues was the establishment of "centers of excellence" in arthritis and joint replacement surgery, sports medicine, spine surgery, and others. This was the first time that I heard the term "centers of excellence." I greatly admired the concept, which cleanly and clearly expressed my own passion. I felt it to be extremely important to identify our programs in this forceful manner. I was also delighted to hear Casparis urge the trustees to support the recruitment of nationally known orthopaedists to head those centers of excellence.

The trustees accepted the consultant's recommendations with enthusiasm and immediately started planning to implement them. They dismissed the CEO of Orthopaedic Hospital, a man who had been in that position for a number of years but who had become the spokesman for the group that most vocally opposed my efforts.

I, in turn, began to outline the organization of the various centers of excellence and to plan their implementation. Sadly, before long, the trustees began to lose their enthusiasm. By the time I had completed my planning and had outlined the final moves required of the board, the trustees began to balk and find excuses.

Most critically, the board sought to assure itself of continued authority in staffing the centers of excellence. Many of the trustees probably had close friends on the staff or were intimidated by their threats to move to other hospitals. Each sought to make sure that they maintained their authority. I began to suspect that again, I would be denied the ability to raise the standards at Orthopaedic Hospital.

Probably, again from the benefit of 20/20 hindsight, I should just have gone along with them. The board members sought only to protect one or two people. I was fighting for an entire academic program. One member of the medical staff in particular continued to cause disproportionate contention.

Upon my arrival to Orthopaedic Hospital, I offered every orthopaedist on the medical staff a clinical academic position in the university. All of them accepted, except for the one man who was now causing problems. I repeatedly attempted to bring him into my camp, not only because he was politically important in the institution but also because he was a good teacher.

One night I invited him out to dinner and we had a friendly conversation. At one point, I begged him to work with me. "When I get old and find myself rocking in a chair somewhere in Florida," I said, "I am going to enjoy reminiscing about the many things I tried to do. I can see you rocking in a chair somewhere in Texas, but you can only remember the things you were against."

His opposition was based on emotion rather than practical experience or common sense. He believed that the university should not be involved in the affairs of "his" hospital. He was not willing to compromise. As I look back, I find that I now admire his loyalty to his principles more that I resent his opposition. I still regret that I was unable to persuade him to see things differently. He was bright, dedicated, and highly professional. If he had chosen to work with me, we could have accomplished some great things together. I cannot say that I never held a grudge against him. I can, however, say that I knew when to let it go. When I became president of the American Academy of Orthopedic Surgeons, I appointed him to an important committee. I know he enjoyed working with the academy.

Twenty years after my initial conflicts with the medical staff, Orthopaedic Hospital is still experiencing the same difficulties and still struggling to survive. However, it continues to receive great financial support from the community. That continued support still makes it possible for the hospital to keep its doors open. In its present location, however, and with its independent status, I am certain that its days are limited.

(As I neared completion of work on this manuscript, Orthopedic Hospital announced that it would close. It plans to construct a new facility on the grounds of Santa Monica Hospital, an institution affiliated with UCLA. I am told that the leaders of Orthopedic Hospital have signed a contract that will ensure its full autonomy.)

To me, the reorganization of the fledgling Orthopedic Hospital research program was of equal importance to the recommendations made by Casparis. When the hospital trustees moved to begin implementing the Casparis report, they also authorized me to recruit a nationally distinguished full-time director of the research program. I appointed a search committee, which identified and recruited James Reswick, Ph.D., the only individual in the United States who was a member of both the National Academy of Medicine and the National Academy of Engineering.

We knew that as director of research, Reswick would be able to unite the activities and personnel of the five affiliated hospitals under one umbrella. His appointment convinced me that our research program would soon become one of the strongest in the country and among the most influential in the world.

Again, however, our vision of world-class excellence would be frustrated by the paranoia of Orthopaedic Hospital and the medical staff's desperate commitment to mediocrity. Again, the medical staff's fear of lost autonomy and inability to meet global standards of excellence carried the day. They convinced the hospital trustees that the university was about to "steal" the research program, Orthopaedic Hospital's crown jewel.

I discovered the medical staff's concerns and activities only by accident. While in the process of preparing a report on a totally different topic, I found myself in need of an earlier document prepared by the board of trustees. I had misplaced my own copy, and requested that the executive secretary of the board send over another. She graciously and quickly complied with my request. She had not noticed, however, that a paper clip had accidentally picked up a page from another document—the minutes from a recent board committee meeting. In the middle of the page, I found the notation, "We must watch out for Sarmiento. He is very strong and wants to move this institution too close to USC."

The other shoe fell a few days later when, without any explanation, the Orthopedic Hospital trustees appointed Dr. June Marshall as "director of research *for the hospital*." When I objected to this peculiar appointment and even more peculiar title, I was told that Dr. Reswick, my appointee, could continue to be "director of research *for the department*." Dr. Marshall would represent Orthopedic Hospital, since the program was located on its grounds, and would have final authority over all financial decisions. Dr. Reswick resigned a few weeks later and moved to Washington, D.C., where he became an influential medical research administrator.

Dr. Marshall, an anatomist who had served at both the university and the hospital, was well liked at Orthopaedic Hospital and at the university. She suffered from severe rheumatoid arthritis and was barely able to walk. In her later years, she became wheelchair-ridden. She was strong-minded and managed to intimidate just about anyone who crossed her path. Everyone who knew her admired her determination and commitment to work.

My relationship with Dr. Marshall remained friendly. I felt that she shared my commitment to unifying the USC research activities and we worked well together. I fully supported her efforts to produce and maintain a coordinated research program. Nonetheless, she was neither an orthopaedist nor an engineer. She brought no experience in medicine. She never fully comprehended the philosophy and theory of orthopaedics, or the needs of its practitioners and patients. She tried to acquire that appropriate knowledge and learned a great deal, but never truly succeeded. Consequently, while the USC orthopaedic research center became the best equipped and most up to date in the world, she could not have succeeded in making it a global center of excellence.

Dr. Marshall died a few years later, and I again took over the direction of the research laboratories. I made some major changes and within a relatively short time, the program blossomed. Three investigators received major grant awards from the National Institutes of Health before I left the university and moved to Scotland in 1994.

chapter 27.
rethinking my roots

"Si la llevo en la sangre,
si la siento subir por el tejido de mis venas
como un indio desnudo por las lianas
bajo el embrujo de la luna llena."

["I have it in my blood.
I feel it rise through the lumen of my veins
like a naked Indian ascending the vines
under the bewitchment of a new moon."]

Colombian Poem

Remarkably, one of the most emotionally rewarding and stimulating events of my life interrupted the continuous combat of those early years in California. Without warning of any kind, I received a letter from my native land, informing me that the president of Colombia had chosen to honor me with the *Cruz de Boyaca,* one of the country's highest civilian medals.

I had never anticipated such a great honor. Accompanied by my wife and three children, I went to Bogota for the presentation. To my great amazement and greater delight, several family members and old friends had come together for the ceremony. My mother was there, along with my brother Hector, who had returned from Italy, and my uncle Rafael, the bishop. Bill Vargas, the orthopaedic surgeon who had persuaded me to intern in the United States, also joined us for the great day. I was overcome with emotion even before the beginning of the formal ceremonies.

As the president's representative placed the medal around my neck, I realized that the audience expected me to make a few remarks. For many years in the United States, I had dreaded speaking before large audiences. I had always assumed that my difficulty came from my lack of comfort with the English language. Now I faced an audience of old friends from my native country. For the first time, I would be able to speak in my native language.

I wanted to speak with the heartfelt eloquence that the moment deserved. Instead, overcome by the enormity of the honor and a sudden feeling of unworthiness, I choked.

I found that I could not utter even a few of the most obvious phrases. I tried to say that I was surprised by this great honor from my country, but the words would not come. I tried to say that my accomplishments were small, that it was difficult for me to see why they merited such attention. Instead, I found myself apologizing for having betrayed my land and my people. I told my family, friends, and assembled dignitaries that I was sorry that I had given my talents to a foreign country that did not need my services. I said I regretted my failure to return to my native land, where my knowledge, talent, and abilities were more urgently needed.

A North American internship can be extraordinarily valuable to a young physician. The lure of staying and practicing in the United States is obvious. Those who, like me, choose to practice in North America do a great disservice to our native countries. We deprive them of the services that we could have given to them after training abroad. This concern had never bothered me before the day that I received the *Cruz de Boyaca*. Ever since that day, I have felt a nagging guilt about having contributed to the brain drain that has accelerated the decline of my country.

In the days following that emotionally explosive ceremony, I finally began to recognize the importance of my background and upbringing. I suddenly realized that despite my academic interest in Western culture, I had never appreciated the strength of my roots in Colombia. For the first time, I realized that those roots were just as strong as the roots of a giant redwood that had withstood the winds of centuries. Like the trunk of that big tree, I had been totally unaware of the nourishment that I had drawn from my native soil and from the generations that had preceded me. Years later, I read the words of political scientist Walter Lippmann: "What can be taken along is at best no more than the tree which is above the ground. The roots remain in the soil where they first grew."

Ever since my emigration from Colombia, I had minimized my ties with the country of my birth. I wanted to become a North American. I believed that I had to think, act, behave, and speak like a North

American. I learned the English language and did everything possible to eradicate my Latin American accent. In the process, I came close to losing the things that my country had given and meant to me: the cultural and religious environment in which I grew to maturity; the values and ethical principles that guided my conduct just as they had guided my parents and ancestors. Though nationalism has been called "the curse of mankind," it is, in my opinion, more likely to succeed than the now popular idea of globalism. Samual Huntington's recent book, *The Clash of Civilizations*, has reinforced that belief.

I never taught Barbara or any of our children to speak or read Spanish. I had occasionally regretted that omission as a weakness in their education. Now, I found it an inexcusable lapse. I also regretted my failure to teach my children more about the history, culture, and people of my native land. I wished that they could have an opportunity to know and love the country and culture that had nurtured me and made me the person that I am. How foolish it was for me to pretend I had no need to stay in contact with my native country and culture; how blind to believe that my past was irrelevant, that only the future had substance.

Unfortunately, I neglected many other aspects of my relationship with my children as well as our common heritage. I love them dearly and care about them in the most profound way. But I also told myself that the quality of my relationship with them was more important than the quantity of time that I found to share with them. I have learned that such a distinction is ludicrous. I now recognize (and remind my own children) that quality and quantity of time are equally important. I urge them to spend as much time as possible with their own children. I tell them that all of their shared time is quality time.

The immigration experience of today is vastly different from that of the great Atlantic migration of earlier years, and different even from my own experience in 1952. At one time, not all that many years ago, the decision to emigrate was permanent. In the days before air travel, immigrants rarely had opportunities to return to their native countries for visits. Today's immigrants travel back and forth almost routinely. Not long ago, immigrants had to learn to speak English or face economic failure. Today, many immigrants believe that it is neither necessary nor desirable to abandon their native tongue. Only their children learn to speak English, and even that does not necessarily happen. Today, many children born in the United States remain illiterate in English. Today, the American-born children of immigrants are often caught between two worlds. Their language and culture comes from neither world. It sometimes seems to be a unique creation of the back-street neighborhoods of Miami and the barrios of Los Angeles or other cities.

It is wrong, however, to criticize those who continue to see merit in preserving their native culture. Pride in one's country and traditions are not a crime. I have learned the hard way that it is important to pass the values of past generations on to one's children. Immigrants must learn, however, that they can maintain tradition, even while being infused with the culture of the adopted country.

When I returned to Miami after a twenty-year absence from the city, I was amazed by the changes that had taken place. A huge number of Latin American immigrants, particularly Cubans, had transformed Miami into a gateway city that is as much Latino as it is North American. In many ways, Miami has become a truly cosmopolitan city. Industry, commerce, and the arts have flourished. In other ways, however, the change has not been healthy. The deliberate effort to make Miami a Latin city troubles me. Such a move invites conflict and resentment. The spectrum of Quebec, a city divided against itself by language and heritage, hovers today over Miami.

My wife does not speak Spanish. She resents the fact that in most stores, the clerks at merchandise stores address everyone routinely not in English but in Spanish. The same is true in many restaurants, including those that feature North American menus. Many English-speaking people, both recent arrivals and those who have lived in Miami for most of their lives, resent the demotion of English to second-language status. They expect to feel more at home in a city that has been part of their country since its inception.

Foreigners visiting any country where its citizens speak a language they do not understand always fear the problems that come from not being able to communicate with the others. When I first came to the United States I experienced that fear. In Miami the problem has taken a different shape. English-speaking people who cannot communicate in Spanish are experiencing the problem. This sounds like an exaggeration, and to some extent it is. However, I have witnessed at the hospital a number of times, English-speaking people struggling to communicate with nurses, nurses' aides, and other paramedical personnel. The same is true in restaurants and other public facilities. The problem is magnified when communication is carried out over the telephone.

In my office, we have over twenty secretaries; all of them are Latin Americans, and the overwhelming majority of them are Cubans. The CEO of the hospital is Cuban, as are the people responsible for recruiting clerical staff—who prefer to hire other Cubans. Many of our patients are not Spanish-speaking people. Ideally, our office staff would be truly bilingual. All of them are fluent in English. However, when it comes to the written language, problems ensue. Many of them do a wonderful job dealing with patients either face to face or over the telephone, but cannot type letters in English. On the other hand, although they communicate among themselves exclusively in Spanish, the letters they type in Spanish are often very deficient.

Similarly related problems threaten the efficiency of the hospital wards and operating rooms. Technicians assisting us with surgery often do not understand English. Communicating with them while wearing modern surgical helmets becomes almost impossible and enormously frustrating.

An associate was assisting me in surgery one day. He became extremely irritated with a young technician who did not speak English and could not follow instructions. The technician allowed too much blood to accumulate over the wound, making surgery difficult. My associate kept trying to tell him to maintain constant suction. The technician did not understand his repeated instructions. Finally, my associate lost his temper and began waving the medical equipment around and shouting instructions mixed with obscenities. I can laugh about the incident today, but the situation had become quite dangerous. Worse still, the same scene is repeated today, far too often, in far too many operating rooms.

The operating room incident reminded me of something that had happened many years before when I was delivering a lecture during the annual meeting of the Academy of Orthopaedics in Dallas. For some reason, the projectionist had a difficult time synchronizing the slides being displayed simultaneously on two screens. I became extremely frustrated with the continuing problem. I leaned away from the lectern to speak privately with the moderator, who was seated next to me on the dais. In a stage whisper, I said to him, "What a stupid son of a bitch that guy is!" The audience burst into laughter.

I had forgotten that I was wearing a microphone attached to my chest. I immediately apologized to the projectionist, and later walked to his booth to apologize personally. But the damage was done—not only to the projectionist but also to me.

Miami has become complacent with a strange form of linguistic mediocrity. Many do not seem interested in mastering either language anymore. They are happy to speak Spanish, and satisfied if they can barely get by in English. English speakers seem equally complacent if they can say *"buenas dias," "muchas gracias,"* and *"adios."*

chapter 28.
to the presidency
of the academy

"Ships are safest on the harbor, but they were not built to stay on the harbor."

I never expected to be elected president of the academy. I knew that my Hispanic name, Colombian birth and education, and remaining Spanish accent all militated against such an ambition. I also knew that I had often alienated influential members of the academy by taking unpopular positions. I knew, too, that I had passed my sixtieth birthday, and that presidents were typically chosen to serve during their late forties or early fifties. I had seen younger colleagues move past me in the line for academy executive posts. I had already put to rest any illusions that I may have entertained in the past.

I learned of my nomination less than twenty-four hours before it was to be publicly announced. Even then, I heard of it only because I ran into the chairman of the nominating committee late in the evening before the announcement. We were standing in the hotel lobby, when he said to me: "Gus, would you be interested in being president of the academy?"

A few hours earlier, an orthopaedist whom I had known superficially through the years stopped me in the hall and asked if I had a moment or two to share my views on a matter of current interest. I was not even aware at the time that he was not only a member of the American Board of Certification but also an elected member of the nominating committee. At the time, the controversial issue of requiring practicing orthopaedists to earn recertification periodically topped our agenda. The board favored adopting a recertification requirement. The majority of our members opposed it.

The issue was on everyone's mind. I was not surprised when this colleague asked my views and unhesitatingly responded that I did not think recertification was a good idea. I believed that its supporters had not fully thought through all of the ramifications. I suspected that some members of the board who favored recertification were primarily motivated by a desire to enhance the influence of the Board of Orthopaedics.

Our brief and informal meeting ended when the elevator arrived. Only later did I learn that this colleague was a key member of the nominating committee. To this day, I have no idea what he said during their deliberations, but I suspect that he did not vote against me. We became better acquainted in later years, and I found him a person of high integrity. He eventually became department chairman of one of the most prestigious orthopaedic programs on the West Coast, and has excelled as an academic administrator.

When I became a member of the board, I had no idea how to handle such a responsibility. My experience had been limited to running medical school departments of orthopaedics. In my experience, academic administration had never required the formalities of parliamentary procedures. I had managed departmental debates by relying not on *Roberts' Rules of Order* but on "Sarmiento's Rules," which were simpler, more efficient, and more reliably yielded the desired results. I never saw any need for the formal introduction of motions and amendments or rules about debate. Our discussions were open and informal.

I did not run my orthopaedics departments in arbitrary or dictatorial ways. I believed it to be my responsibility to develop and maintain a strong basic philosophy; every member of the department shared responsibility for the implementation of that philosophy. We often argued and quarreled over specific details. I won many debates but also yielded on many occasions when faced with logical or concerted opposition. My faculty and I enjoyed the camaraderie of our shared mission. As I reminisce about my style of management, I regret not that I was too dictatorial but that on too many occasions I failed to act with sufficient authority to cut short or excise some threat or negative influence.

The board of directors of the American Academy of Orthopaedic Surgeons functioned differently. The board conducted all business in strict accordance with *Roberts' Rules of Order.* Throughout my years of membership, those restrictions and constraints continuously irritated me. I believe that our strict adherence to those rigid, outdated rules stymied constructive discussion and often forced members to vote in the absence of sufficient information. The problem was compounded by the fact that the board met only four or five times a year; at each meeting, we had to clear a lengthy agenda. Further encumbered as we were by the tedious formalities of parliamentary procedure, we didn't always have the opportunity to explore every issue fully.

During my early years on the board, I served as a member at large. Only later did I become part of the presidential chain of succession and a member of the executive committee, which held an additional meeting the night before the full board meeting. As a member at large, I received a copy of the agenda and volumes of supporting material just a few days before the board meeting. Many times, we cast our votes without an opportunity to truly understand the issue, without appreciation of alternatives, and without recognizing the full consequences of our actions.

I attended my first board meeting in Cancun, Mexico, in 1987. I enjoyed the experience, but it left me with a bad taste in my mouth. I could not understand why our meetings should be held at such a great cost. I wondered why we met in a resort, instead of in Chicago, where the academy had its headquarters. I wondered why our wives were invited to attend at academy cost, since the wives had nothing to do with our administrative responsibilities.

I later tempered my initial criticism of the combined business-social format of board meetings, and came to recognize the merit in inviting the wives to attend. I continued to oppose exaggerated social agendas and extravagant locations that required us to travel to remote, expensive, and exclusive sites. In one of my few accomplishments, I succeeded in cutting down the number of social meetings and reduced the expenditures of the organization. In retrospect, I sometimes wonder if this financial conservatism may have cost me the support of some members on other, more critical issues.

Prior to my elevation to the presidency of the Academy of Orthopedic Surgeons, I had become increasingly concerned over trends in medicine and particularly in orthopaedics. The evidence at my disposal, however, did not fully support those concerns. Sadly, my entry into the upper echelon of organized orthopaedics only confirmed my many suspicions about impending crises in our medical world.

Promptly, however, I would learn that my beloved academy was becoming more concerned with its pocketbook than with professional ethics. I would learn that throughout the United States and around the world, business interests were transforming U.S. medicine into a medical-industrial complex. I would come to understand that the health care industry expects the members of the medical profession to accept industry's values and ethics, as we abandon ours. Finally, I would have to face (if not accept) my own inability to reverse the trend. A former chairman of the academy's ethics committee told me recently that he had given up convincing the board of directors to allow his group to address in a serious way issues related to ethical concerns dealing with orthopaedic relationships with industry.

Prior to being elected to the board of directors I had strongly felt that the academy had failed to coordinate its educational efforts appropriately. At the time of my last report to the board as chairman of the continuing education committee, I brought this concern to their attention. "The system you now encourage is obsolete. You must develop a method of communication between the major educational areas of the academy," I said. "Having them work in isolation from each other, simply because we must respect sacred cows, is a mistake."

Later that evening, the executive secretary said to me, during the dinner meeting and cocktails, that I had done a good job at expediting my demise as an active participant in the academy. She was wrong. Better days were ahead.

At a meeting of the directors, during my first year as member at large, the board discussed possible involvement in the publication of scientific books. The issue took me by surprise. The executive committee seemed to favor academy involvement in this new endeavor. I disagreed, and pointed out that many reputable publishing firms already supplied the orthopaedic community with the latest information. Many of the subspecialty societies had their own journals. A plethora of throwaway magazines issued by industry inundated the market.

I suggested that instead of adding to the flood, the academy should use its influence to persuade others within its jurisdiction to stem the flow. Was it possible, I asked, that the academy's only motive for entering the publishing field was that publishing was a profitable venture? The academy ignored my challenge and became a successful publisher.

Several years later I learned that the flood of medical publications was greater than I had anticipated. The *British Medical Journal* provided the following information: in 1996 there were approximately thirty thousand medical journals in print worldwide; three thousand new articles are published each day; one thousand new articles are added each day to the online Web site Medline; during a three-year clinical training one million medical publications will be added to Medline.

Food for thought. Was I correct in raising questions about the academy's involvement in the "publication business"?

The board regularly met with the national membership committee to consider new applicants. At one such meeting, the committee recommended that a certain individual be denied membership because he seemed to charge excessive fees and because colleagues in his community felt that he was performing unnecessary surgery. I remarked that the board should support the recommendation of the committee. A distinguished past-president of the academy remarked that we had no business questioning the billing practices of any member of the organization. He added that "there is no clear definition of a high charge. It is a matter of taste." The board overruled its committee and admitted the applicant.

On another occasion, the membership committee recommended that an applicant from Washington, D.C., be denied entrance into the academy. They presented a comprehensive list of reasons, but based the decision primarily on charges of highly questionable ethical practices. One member argued that we were dealing with an influential, well-connected individual who would not hesitate to sue the academy. The board voted to deny membership. The applicant's sponsor then submitted the application for reconsideration, with the same result. After a sustained lobbying effort, however, he won on a third effort. I was horrified by the entire episode, which indelibly demonstrated our inability to maintain clear and well-understood ethical standards.

Over my years on the board, I repeatedly expressed concern over the academy's drift toward becoming little more than a trade union. I frequently said to my colleagues that if we allowed the trend to continue, the academy would suffer the same fate that had so seriously damaged the American Medical Association, which had lost its relevance as an educational organization and became primarily a political body. I felt that the academy had been created and maintained to represent the moral, ethical, and professional concerns of the orthopaedic community. I found myself witnessing a continual increase of "pocketbook" issues. I felt then that the academy, an educational organization par excellence, should not abandon or alter its mission. I watched sadly as board meetings, which in the past had devoted a great deal of time to education and related matters, became the forum for discussions that dealt primarily with economic issues.

Several years after I left office, the academy created a parallel organization with different tax status. Ideally, the nonprofit academy will be able to rededicate itself to its educational mission. The for-profit sister organization will sell merchandise with the academy logo, publish textbooks, and lobby government agencies for changes in Medicare and insurance provisions. I greatly fear, however, that the tail will wag the dog, and the new entity will become the more influential representative of professional orthopaedics.

Another controversial issue that surfaced involved the question of academy endorsement of Certificates of Added Qualifications for hand surgeons who met specific criteria, including a written examination. Although I usually supported academy programs designed to ensure high standards, I objected to this idea. I believed that the certificates would become divisive, discriminatory, and subject to abuse. I stated my belief that many competent and ethical orthopaedists would not want to take the required test. I also noted that there were no criteria designed to prevent unethical individuals from earning these certificates.

I further suggested that rather than concentrating on more costly and time-consuming examinations, the Hand Society should devote its time and efforts to reinforcing the fabric of orthopaedics. I expressed my strong concern that by advocating academy endorsement of their certificates, the Hand Society was helping to accelerate the formation of subspecialties and further fragment our profession.

At the time, the board found itself unable to reach a compromise on this issue. Only now, several years later, do I have the distinct feeling that my views have prevailed. At the time of that divisive discussion, we all believed that once the Hand Society instituted its system, all other subspecialty societies would do likewise. That did not occur. In recent years, I have heard little discussion of Certificates of Additional Competency. To date, no other subspecialty society has tried to implement them.

On one occasion, a group of members raised the issue of public education. They claimed that the public was not sufficiently aware of what orthopaedists do. I thought the plan was ludicrous and fought the new initiative. I believed that everyone in the United States fully understood that orthopaedists were specialized physicians who took care of broken bones, replaced arthritic joints, straightened crooked backs and feet, repaired cut tendons, and cared for the musculoskeletal system in many other ways. In any case, most patients who required the care of an orthopaedist would be referred by an internist or a general practitioner.

I believed that advertising our services was demeaning to the profession and that it would do more harm than good. I reminded the board of the words of Warren Burger, former chief justice of the United States, who remarked at the annual meeting of the American Medical Association, "I would not seek the services of a physician who finds it necessary to advertise his services." The board dismissed my views and authorized $700,000 for public education. The board has added to that initial investment on several occasions. I doubt that these efforts have helped the profession. I have never seen any hard evidence on the subject. I suspect that the project simply gave an opportunity to the assigned academy spokesmen to market their names in their communities.

Toward the end of my tenure on the academy's board of directors, we entertained a proposal that the academy initiate a program of selling shirts, caps, cufflinks, ties, and other merchandise. All of these materials would carry the seal or logo of the American Academy of Orthopaedic Surgery. Again, I argued strenuously against the concept. I said that we did not need the few dollars that such products would generate. I felt that selling our identity would cheapen the organization. One of the other board members noted that in spite of my criticism, I was wearing a coat that had buttons with the academy's emblem on them, as well as a watch and an academy presidential broach, which displayed the academy's seal.

"That is true," I responded, "but I did not buy these items. They were given to me by the academy in recognition for services and accomplishments. I have treasured these gifts as symbols of those honors. If they can be purchased by anyone for a few dollars, however, they will no longer be meaningful to me." The board approved the plan, and many members now proudly display their academy souvenirs.

I spoke vehemently against the establishment of an educational center within the walls of the academy's headquarters, although I had strongly supported the idea at an earlier time. The center was to be a facility where structured courses, particularly those dealing with manual skills, were to be conducted on a frequent basis. I felt it was unwise to embark on a project whose financial success was questionable and that would eventually force the academy into dependency upon the medical industry for its continued operation. A vote was taken with everybody in support of proceeding forward. The only dissenting vote was mine.

A few years after its opening, the center has experienced support from the fellowship. Its success suggests that I may have been mistaken in my predictions. The center continues to have financial difficulties, however, and as I feared, its survival has become more and more dependent on industry support each year. Inevitably, the educational content of the center's activities will reflect industry's viewpoint. We will have given industry one more powerful tool with which to distort our once-proud profession.

As I look back at those years on the board of directors and my year as president of the academy, I regret that I did not better prepare myself for the job. When I first won election to the board, I asked the retiring member whose seat I was taking to brief me on my duties. He responded that they consisted primarily of seconding motions. I did not believe him. I immediately wrote a letter to the president and informed him that I was not going to waste my time. As a member of the board, I fully intended to involve myself in all issues under discussion.

IN RETROSPECT

I now know that I should have planned more carefully and focused more of my energies on the overriding issues—the loss of professionalism, the ominous growth of the orthopaedic/industrial complex, and the collapse of medical ethics. Instead, I let myself be distracted by a myriad of less significant proposals, "being distracted from distraction by distraction," as T. S. Eliot wrote. These distractions prevented me from taking full advantage of my moral authority when I finally rose to become president of the academy.

I should have accomplished much more than I did during my year of academy leadership. Many others who have led the academy have done so with more distinction and more impact. Those who performed most effectively were those who most carefully planned their agendas from the outset. They knew exactly what they wanted to accomplish during their brief tenure. They focused their moral authority on concrete proposals that brought narrowly defined but valuable reform. Consequently, they were able to make the most of their brief time in office.

Unfortunately, the academy's organized agenda unfolded in unanticipated ways. I wanted the academy to take a good look at itself; I wanted it to limit the time devoted to pocket-book issues and concentrate on more important ones. Even though I knew that I could not expect to effect change in just a year or two, I focused my energies on the relaxation of ethical conduct among the fellowship; the potential evil of excessive fragmentation of the profession; and the damage that the growing orthopaedic-industrial complex was inflicting on members. I also worked hard to convince the academy to make a serious commitment to orthopaedic research.

None of those issues were easy to deal with, let alone resolve in such a short time. I ended up concluding that I should be satisfied if I could, at least, provoke a discussion on them and generate an awareness of their importance. In retrospect, I did not succeed to the extent that someone else, better organized, would have.

I recognize that my contribution to the deliberations of the board of directors was primarily that of questioning the propriety of our actions and their potential future adverse repercussions. I was negative perhaps too often and questioned the need or worth of many of the projects the organization was embarked on. To many of the directors I became little more than an annoying gadfly who raised far too many questions. I opposed many resolutions I thought to be inconsequential to the future of the organization; I voted against projects that gave a hint of self-serving motives; I argued against expenditures that I considered trivial and unnecessary; I almost never prevailed.

chapter 29.
a strange experience

"There's a sucker born every minute."
—Attributed to P. T. Barnum

During the stormy days in California, I had an experience quite so far from the ordinary that it defies classification. Even today it seems profound yet absurd, and climactic yet irrelevant. The episode demands retelling, and I have, in fact, retold it often. If it seems surrounded by a Daliesque surrealism, I can assure you that it seemed quite real at the time.

The episode started not with a fire bell in the night but with a telephone call at 5:00 A.M. One of the advantages of a practice in orthopaedic surgery devoted to elective procedures is that we are rarely called out for emergencies. In the many years since I limited my practice to hip replacement surgery, I have rarely been called for a medical emergency. So, when the telephone rang in the middle of the night, Barbara and I both assumed that a personal crisis of some kind had occurred.

Not so. The caller stated he was calling from the Israeli Embassy in Washington, D.C. (where it was 8:00, I quickly realized). He wanted to discuss a medical matter of great importance to his government. An important Israeli scientist had sustained a fractured ankle. It was not healing properly and urgently needed highly skilled attention. Several people had given the caller my name, but he would not give me his. He would say only that his sources had assured him that I was the best man to treat the scientist.

There must be a bit of James Bond in every man. Instead of seeing the absurdity of such a situation, I found it extremely flattering. I also found the predawn call and the mystery of anonymous contacts delightfully exciting. I agreed to see the injured man, set up an appointment, and told the caller how best to reach my office.

The next morning, a man in his late twenties or early thirties walked into my office. He was of slightly dark complexion, with raven-black eyes, curly black hair, and sharply delineated facial features. Usually, I am not a particularly observant man. I am more likely to recognize a patient's X rays than his face. This time, however, I took instant inventory of my visitor's physical features.

He was dressed in a tailored three-piece suit and spoke English not with a Hebrew accent but with a slightly high voice that spoke the pure tones of Oxford and Cambridge. His bearing, language, and self-possession created the strong impression that this was a highly cultured individual, a man of power and privilege. He proceeded to inform me that before bringing into my office the injured scientist, it was important that we discuss the problem in advance. He wanted me to understand the seriousness of the situation. He then apologized for having to take time to inform me who he was and why matters had to be handled in a somewhat unorthodox manner. He assured me that the information he was about to provide would make me understand the importance of total confidentiality.

He informed me that he was a physicist, and that he also held a medical degree. He had earned his medical degree at the age of sixteen from the University of Milan, and his name appears in the *Guinness Book of World Records* as being the youngest graduate from a medical school; he had elected, after his graduation from medical school, to pursue studies that led to his obtaining a doctoral degree in physics. He then opened a large leather portfolio similar to something much like my brother used to carry prints of his architectural drawings. He showed me photographs of his graduation day from medical school and clippings from several major European newspapers, calling him the youngest person ever to graduate from medical school. He showed me congratulatory letters from the pope and from the prime minister of Italy.

He showed me photographs of himself in the company of a number of European and American dignitaries, including Willy Brandt, the mayor of Berlin, and Prince Philip of the United Kingdom. He also had pictures of himself standing with the prime minister of France, Senator Ted Kennedy, President Ronald Reagan, and Secretary of State Alexander Haig. He then reached for a tape recorder, and played a recording of the secretary of state thanking him for a "job well done," and inviting him to visit with him again in the near future.

By this time, I was totally mystified by this elaborate introduction to someone who was not even my patient. But he was not finished. He informed me that his IQ was over 250 points; it was so high that it could not be accurately measured. He had been asked to donate sperm by scientists in the United States who were secretly building a sperm bank in Washington. He also assured me that he had been invited to participate as a consultant to the Nobel Prize Committee in Sweden.

By now, you are probably saying, "What a fruitcake." I can only say that you had to be there to understand the man's impact. "What a remarkable young man," I said to myself.

Only after he had shown me the many photographs in his leather case did he finally began to talk about the patient. He said the injured person was his older brother, "the smarter member of the family," who held an important position in the Israeli scientific community and who was working in an extraordinarily top-secret research project. The project was totally unique. It could well involve enormous consequences not only to the nation of Israel but to the world as a whole. He hinted that it had to do the harnessing of energy from black holes in space.

He reached his smaller briefcase and produced two X rays that showed a two-week-old fracture of the ankle. His scientist brother had allegedly been seen by orthopaedists in Israel, Italy, Switzerland, Germany, the United Kingdom, New York, and Washington, D.C. All the examining physicians, without exception, had indicated that surgery was the only way to deal with that type of fracture; two of the surgeons had indicated that I was probably the only person who could treat him successfully without surgery.

I looked at the X rays and immediately concluded that the fracture required surgical treatment, particularly in view of the fact that two weeks had passed since the original injury. I told him that even if I had been asked to treat the injury when it first occurred, it would have been extremely difficult, if not impossible, to treat it properly by nonsurgical means.

I asked why they were so adamantly opposed to having the fracture treated surgically. He responded that the Israeli government was concerned that the patient, under anesthesia, might reveal important secrets. I replied that the surgery could be carried out under spinal anesthesia. The patient would remain fully awake, and fully in control. There would be no security risk. This answer did not satisfy him. He said that under no circumstances would they permit any type of anesthesia, not even a local one. Then he said that if I agreed to treat his brother, they would not only pay my usual fees but would also provide a check for $1 million for research.

We all know that if something seems too good to be true, it probably is. The offer of a $1 million research grant should have raised a red flag. In truth, had they offered to pay me the $1 million, I might have become suspicious. Their offer of a research grant, however, just made me more curious and involved me even more in this extraordinary family and these mysterious circumstances.

We arranged for an examination of the patient that night. The brother insisted that their visit take place outside of normal hours. They did not want to be seen in public. I agreed to the peculiar (but dramatic) arrangements, and met them in the plaster room at the Orthopaedic Hospital a few hours later. The older scientist resembled his younger brother, though his expression was somewhat sullen. Speaking with a soft, almost satin voice, he agreed with his brother's opposition to any type of anesthesia.

I removed the cast that had been applied two weeks earlier, and found a moderately swollen ankle and foot. After a careful examination, I told myself that it would be impossible to successfully manipulate the displaced bones into place, or to successfully maintain any possible reduction I could achieve. I tried one more time to convince them that a spinal block was a benign procedure and that surgery was the only reasonable way to restore the ankle to reasonable condition. The reiterated their total opposition to any kinds of anesthesia.

The patient was sitting on a high examining table. His leg hung over its side. Again, I took hold of the broken leg to examine it more closely. I told the patient that manipulation, without an anaesthetic, would be painful, and that I would need his cooperation. I told him that it would help if he relaxed as much as possible. A moment later, as quickly as I could, I applied all the force I could summon and twisted his broken ankle into what I thought it would be the position of reduction. I heard the sound of bones moving into position.

The pain must have been excruciating, but the patient made no sound at all. But his face was pale and clammy, and tears ran down his cheeks. I then applied a new cast, as carefully as I could. I wanted to avoid causing my patient any more pain, but I was more concerned to avoid displacing the bony fragments—in the event that I had somehow been successful in relocating them properly. We waited while the cast hardened. A few minutes later, I took X rays of the joint and sent them through the automatic processor.

Much to my surprise, the X rays demonstrated that I had anatomically reduced the fracture. I could hardly believe it. My patient and his brother seemed to take it all much more calmly, and much more as the expected outcome, than I did. I emphasized the high risk of subsequent displacement of the fracture, and suggested the use of a wheelchair for a few days. I even found a wheelchair for them to use while they stayed in Los Angeles. I encouraged the patient to keep his leg elevated on pillows and to avoid activity. We agreed on an appointment for a follow-up visit to the hospital for additional X ray evaluation. They asked me to make a house call at their hotel. I promised I would visit them the next day. Without further comment, they returned to their hotel.

After work the next day I drove to Hollywood and spoke with the younger brother from the hotel lobby. He warned me that I might run into some of their bodyguards when I arrived on the floor. He assured me that they were expecting me, and would cause no difficulty. I did not see anybody. "Perhaps they had been distracted for a few minutes," they suggested.

During the course of two weeks, I visited the patient frequently. Every few nights, they moved to a different hotel. They claimed to be afraid to stay in one place for long. They told me that there was a high risk of being recognized. They greatly feared kidnapping attempts. The government of Israel was deeply concerned by that threat, which was why they had assigned bodyguards. I never saw the bodyguards. I assumed that the Israeli security men were more skilled at concealing themselves that I was at identifying them.

Seven days after the initial encounter, they returned to the X ray department at Orthopedic Hospital. Again, we met in the evening, after the close of regular business. Incredibly, I discovered that the reduction of the fracture had maintained itself. The patient told me that he had avoided all movement. He had just transferred, when necessary, from his bed to the wheelchair. He had not even moved his toes during the week.

One month after the manipulation, we discussed the possibility of their leaving town and returning later for further follow-up and eventual removal of the cast. We made an appointment for them to return in four weeks. They promised that on their way to Los Angeles International Airport, they would return the wheelchair we had lent them the night of their first visit to the hospital.

I never saw them again.

The two men totally disappeared. When I called the telephone number they had left with me, an operator said that it had been disconnected. I then called my old friend William Fielding in New York. He was among the many orthopaedists they had claimed to have consulted. He started laughing immediately, then said, "Those two, they're first class con artists." They had given him the same stories about the graduation from medical school at the age of sixteen, their political connections, and the rest of them. "Don't worry. You'll never see them again," Fielding added.

I asked how he had been able to draw his conclusions so quickly. He just laughed some more. "You don't live in New York for thirty years without learning to pick up the phonies a mile away."

One hour after our conversation, Fielding called me back. He wanted to tell me that his office files on the "scientist" had disappeared. He asked me to look for mine, while he waited at the other end of the line. My files had also vanished.

Three months later, I received a postcard from the younger brother apologizing for their long silence. He wrote that his brother was back to work in Israel and that he had been extremely busy with the Nobel Prize Committee. The postcard carried a Swedish stamp, but there were no cancellation marks, or any other markings to suggest that it had followed regular postal routes. The brother promised that he would return to the United States within the next thirty days. At that time, they would pay my fee, return the borrowed wheelchair, and follow through with the promised $1 million donation.

I never heard from them again.

Over the years, I have enjoyed many laughs about my adventure in the world of international intrigue. The hospital administrator, however, did not find pleasure in the loss of a wheelchair or in the free X rays and plaster casting materials. Sometimes, however, I still think that perhaps there is a brilliant scientist working on a mysterious new source of energy that will save the world.

Fifteen years later I shared this story with a young German physician working in the office of a colleague of mine. He was a very talented person and very knowledgable in computer matters. He asked me for the name of the alleged Israeli physician. I gave it to him.

A few days later my friend handed me thirty pages of Internet information regarding the interesting and "brilliant" physicist/physician. It made my day. I had found out that I was not the only fool who for a while believed the stories fabricated by the professional con artist. According to his former teachers, he had been a mediocre student in his early school days; and had not graduated from the Milan School of Medicine. He did, however, manage to get a medical degree from the University of Perugia, in Italy. According to the records I read, the officers of the University of Perugia had later apologized for the errors they made in granting him a degree without having carefully confirmed his alleged record of outstanding performance.

It appears that some time around the episode in which I was involved, the young man went into the banking business and other business ventures. He convinced wealthy people into financing a venture dealing cryonics, the preservation of bodies by means of freezing techniques. He made millions of dollars serving as president of the company, until he was finally discovered as a fraud and was fired.

He then returned to Israel and ran for public office. He came very close to being elected to the Israeli Parliament, and rumors were spread that he might run for the presidency of the country.

In early 2001, his name surfaced again in relation to the broadly announced plans by a group of Italian scientists to clone the first human being. Though the scientists argue that he is not a member of the team, he advertises himself as one of the associates. He sat in the front row during testimony given to the U.S. Congress by alleged experts in the field, giving advice to the those given testimony. Severino Antinori, the Italian gynecologist whose name is associated with plans to pursue human cloning in a vigorous way, at a press conference in Rome, announced that my patient "would be ready to underwrite the cost of the research project."

It appears that the "hero" of my story has not changed very much over the last fifteen years. He still carries with him his leather case containing the photographs of his powerful "friends" and tells the same stories. And he finds suckers everywhere who believe him. Perhaps in some ways he has changed: he has gotten bolder. He has gone as far as claiming that "Roman Catholic Church leaders support human embryo cloning after he suggested that they could replicate

Jesus from DNA fibers extracted from the Shroud of Turin." Not wanting to leave any stone unturned, he has suggested to "Jewish friends that the biblical patriarch Abraham, of monotheistic faith, could be brought for a return engagement with a few scraps of genetic material from bones in the Cave of Machpelah."

I have the distinct feeling that we will hear more about this corrupt Houdini. He may even make the evening news announcing his own cloning. Neither will I be surprised if during the next Summer Olympics in China, his brother, the one with the broken ankle, runs and wins the marathon.

The story reminded me of previous experiences where I had naively allowed myself to be fooled. Only a few months after my father's death, when I was only thirteen years old, a neighbor from down the street asked me if I would be interested in earning a few dollars by completing some simple forms, placing them in envelopes, and taking them to the post office. For several nights I worked on the tedious job and awaited payment. It never happened. The neighbor left town and I never saw him again.

During my second year in medical school, I ran into a fellow whom I had met in grade school years earlier. Our respective parents had been friends. He had not pursued a professional career and was apparently involved in several businesses. One of those businesses, a lamp factory, was located a few blocks from the apartment where I was living. I asked him if he could give me a part-time job, since I was living on the small amount of money my uncle was sending me on a monthly basis.

I worked as many hours as I could squeeze in the afternoons. I not only made many lamps by myself but also supervised the work of his twelve or fifteen employees. After a few weeks, I was an expert lamp maker. I also enjoyed the distraction from my studies, but my friend, the owner of the factory, had not yet paid me. He explained to me that he had encountered a short-term cash flow problem because of the expansion of one of his other businesses. He swore that he would pay me shortly, with extra compensation because of the delay. A few days later, he, too, left town without letting anyone know, and without paying any of his employees. I never saw him again.

During a recent trip to Budapest, I attended a reception for the faculty of the medical congress at a beautiful, old castle. The taxi driver dropped me at the entrance to the park. The castle lay only a short distance away, but I could not read any of the signs and had no idea how to get to it. I walked around for a while, until I found someone who gave me directions.

Not far from the castle, two tall, heavyset men approached me. They showed me badges and informed me that they were members of the Secret Police. They asked for my passport and I promptly accommodated their request. The older of the two men looked at my photograph and carefully looked at my face. In heavily broken English, he indicated that he was satisfied. Then, he asked for my wallet. I instantly became alert to the possibility of robbery and asked the reason for such a request.

"We are investigating a dangerous black market," he said. Reluctantly, I handed him my wallet.

He unfolded it, and removed a few thousand Hungarian florins and about 550 U.S. dollars. He carefully counted the money in front of me. Then he said, "Be careful with the dollars. Don't put them in the wallet the way you have them. Rather, fold them and put them behind the local currency."

He folded the U.S. dollars and showed me what he had done. Then, suggesting that I may not have understood his instructions, he took the dollars out of the wallet again and repeated his actions. I thanked him and left.

Later in the afternoon, on my way to my hotel, I stopped at a newsstand to purchase an U.S. newspaper. When I opened my wallet, I discovered that the U.S. dollars had vanished. The man had stolen my money in broad daylight, while I was carefully watching him.

From Budapest, I flew to meet Maurice Muller in Zurich. He had invited me to ride with him to Davos, in his private limousine. The board of trustees of the AO had invited me to be the keynote speaker at their annual meeting. I told Dr. Muller about the unpleasant episode in Budapest. He convinced me that a layperson couldn't detect the practiced, fast motions of the professional magician. He knew, because he was a magician himself. Then he demonstrated his skills for me.

The next night, in Davos, another magician entertained the group with his tricks. No matter how carefully I tried to follow his moves, he fooled me every time.

chapter 30.
the orthopaedic-industrial complex

"The hottest places in hell are reserved for those who in times of moral crisis preserved their neutrality."
—Dante Alighieri

"We seem incapable of appreciating the degree of spiritual, political and moral degradation that has permeated throughout the West."
—Václav Havel

I first became concerned over the overwhelming influence that the manufacturers of orthopaedic equipment had gained in orthopaedic health care long before I joined the academy board of directors. As I recall, I first publicly expressed my growing concern at a 1978 meeting in New York. At that meeting, I paraphrased President Dwight Eisenhower's comments on the "Military Industrial Complex" with my own reference to the ominous growth of what I called the Orthopaedic Industrial Complex. Others have since sounded a similar theme.

By the time I became an academy board member, the Orthopedic Industrial Complex had become overwhelming. Industry largely contributed to the financial success of the annual meeting of the academy and was subsidizing the costs of an increasingly larger number of continuing education programs. Meetings throughout the nation featured a growing presence of industry, with displays of their products and presentations of hands-on bioskills laboratories—that is, sessions where students have an opportunity to practice surgery in plastic bones.

In return, industry often named the experts who participated in those courses and the orthopaedists who would serve as visiting professors at countless meetings of universities, hospitals, and societies. Industry grants funded and defined activities in progress throughout the country, through subsidized (usually product-oriented) research conducted in departments of orthopaedics. On a global level, the AO, while not officially an industrial venture, had already achieved virtual hegemony over the practice of orthopaedics throughout Western Europe. Few researchers today will risk alienating the hands that feed them. If the tail is not yet wagging the dog, it most certainly is telling the dog when, where, and how to wag. And the dog totally understands that it must never, never bite the hand that feed it.

Many physicians tell me that I exaggerate a perfectly normal situation. I accept the domination of the automobile industry by a handful of manufacturers as normal. What has happened to medicine is not normal. Industry today has changed the essential nature of medicine and redirected its focus. Modern medicine centers not on the patient but on the insurers, hospitals, rehabilitation centers, and industry. Even the language has changed. We are no longer physicians. We have become "health care providers."

Nothing symbolizes this change more graphically than the widespread confusion over the most recognized symbol of medicine. Since ancient times, the medical profession has been symbolized by the staff of Aesculapius, the Greek god of healing. The winged staff of Aesculapius is entwined by a single serpent. Today, we usually see medicine symbolized by the caduceus, a winged staff entwined by *two* serpents. The caduceus with the two serpents, however, was carried not by a healer but by Hermes, the god of commerce and thieves. I have no idea how this change of popular images occurred. I know only that the change in symbols parallels the transformation in reality.

Because orthopaedics depends heavily on technology, it provides a good model for all of medicine. Without the partnership of industry, orthopaedics may have not progressed in a major way over the past four of five decades. The major advances made in the discipline have been made in areas such as fracture fixation, joint replacement, correction of congenital and developmental deformities, and arthroscopic surgery. Modern orthopaedics cannot function without a partnership with industry. We depend on industry for a wide range of technological tools. The changing relationship between industry and medicine, therefore, has had a particularly dramatic effect on orthopaedics.

For industry, orthopaedics offered medicine's most dramatic opportunities. The challenge for industry was to find a way to encourage conservative orthopaedists to change their ways. To meet this challenge, leading executives developed integrated marketing strategies. The global fascination with total joint replacement surgery provided a perfect opening. Industry invited successful orthopaedic surgeons to become involved in the design of new products. They made these high-profile surgeons industry "stakeholders" through royalties and even part ownership of specific products. At one point, it seemed that any orthopaedic surgeon with a busy joint replacement practice was using his own implant, designed by him in concert with leading manufacturers from around the world.

Consequently, more than three hundred different hip prostheses are available on the market today. Most of these new implants are virtually indistinguishable from each other. More tragically, many of the new implants proved inferior or even defective in design. These defective implants are quickly removed from the market in the United States, but industry sometimes continues to sell remaining inventory in developing countries. This practice, which I suspect is widespread, is contrary to the most basic tenets of professionalism.

If industry and medicine shared a common goal, the domination of one by the other would not be a problem. For medicine, the goal has been, above all, to help the patient. The logical and appropriate goal of industry, however, is to maximize shareowner profits. Because patient welfare is only one of many means for industry to achieve its goal, the two philosophies are difficult to reconcile.

Yet, medicine has chosen to ignore the growing power of the industrial philosophy. The problem is that medicine, unaware of potential dangers, has allowed industry to gain far too much control of professional medicine. Whenever industry generously offers financial support for educational activities, medicine happily accepts. As the cost of educational activities has grown, so, too, has medicine's reliance on industry. Industry has developed a subtle and effective stratagem to lull us into a slumber that keeps us from realizing the degree to which we have become subservient to them. The perks and help we receive from industry are distractions to allow it to control our destiny.

During my years at the University of Miami, I ran many continuing education courses. These programs were successful and never required any support from industry. Registration fees funded all course expenditures. My success with such courses led to my appointment to the continuing education committee at the academy, and my eventual selection to chair that committee. Never, during all those years at Miami, did industry ever seek to interfere with the programs or courses.

After I moved to the University of Southern California, I continued my involvement in continuing education. Late in my tenure at USC, I invited hip surgeons from around the world to participate in an international program on hip surgery. I issued announcements of the meeting to several manufacturing companies, and offered them the opportunity to display their products in the hotel exhibit hall. I charged them a fee for that opportunity. We planned to use the income from the sale of display space to defray the expenses incurred by visiting faculty from abroad.

All the manufacturing companies accepted the terms and contracted with us for display space. However, I was struck by the fact that three of the responses added a new dimension. In almost identical language, they asked how many of our speakers they would be entitled to "nominate" in return for underwriting our program. I had organized almost 100 continuing education courses, and had never before encountered such a request. I replied that all speakers had already been selected, that our program was complete, and that industry should not expect to gain control of the faculty in any way. All three of the companies honored their contracts.

I soon learned that this practice had become commonplace, and that my continuing education programs were among the last to learn about it. For the first time, I understood how many educational programs had become so elaborate and so lavish in their accommodations. Industry had been, directly or indirectly, selecting members of the faculty of the courses and paying their expenses. That freed the sponsoring organization to use income from display areas for other purposes. Before long, the program sponsors had become almost totally dependent on industry's support.

A similar phenomenon has produced industry control of education in an even more insidious fashion. For a long time, I had failed to realize how effectively industry had managed to influence visiting lectureships in this country. Only recently have I recognized that a large percentage of visiting speakers have their expenses paid by manufacturing companies. Industry representatives suggest to directors of medical schools' educational programs, as well as officers of medical societies and other organizations, the names of individuals who will be available to lecture at their respective educational meetings. Obviously, industry will subsidize their expenses and provide an honorarium. Typically, the "selected" speakers are the developers or frequent users of products sold by the underwriting company.

It saddens me to see orthopaedic surgeons lower themselves by serving as salespeople for industry. Among them you now see individuals we had held in the highest esteem traveling all over the world advertising industrial products. Since written and unwritten rules require that they identify any commercial ties with the products they discussed, many of them comply with the mandate. However, contrary to initial expectations, such an identification does not seem to militate against their credibility; quite the contrary it appears to enhance it.

These practices provide training institutions with funding for needed educational programs. It becomes a problem when it distorts the educational balance of a program. It becomes a crisis when it transforms an education forum into a marketing presentation. The lines are fuzzy, hard to identify, and easily crossed. Many state orthopaedic societies and similar groups rely heavily on underwriting by industry for their survival.

Our own powerful American Academy of Orthopaedics annual meeting is also heavily subsidized by industry. The academy earns several million dollars by renting display space for commercial exhibits. More than half of the attendees at the annual meeting are sales representatives and other staff of industry. At the moment these lines are being typed, the Academy of Orthopaedics has announced that the attendance to its continuing education courses has decreased significantly. The future financial viability of such an endeavor is in question. Therefore, plans are in the making to join forces with industry and structure a program whereby the two organizations produce educational programs as cosponsors. We do not know the outcome of this plan. I feel, however, that if it comes to fruition it will represent the betrayal of the academy's educational mission, and the equivalent of driving a strong and irremovable nail into its own coffin.

Increasing numbers of orthopaedists from other countries now

attend the academy annual meeting and other educational conferences. Most attend as the guests of industry. It is wonderful that these
people are able to attend the conferences. To qualify for such generosity, however, many of these visitors must first commit themselves
to use implants or other devices manufactured by their sponsors.

The orthopaedic profession has not only built its own trap but has
lined the cage with mink. Today, no orthopaedic society of any kind
could afford to produce a scientific conference, educational symposium, or any other kind of meeting without the support of industry.
For many years, my profession rationalized the process. It reasoned
that orthopaedics suffered no damage and gained many benefits. The
meetings became more appealing and more enjoyable.

Publishers of medical journals find it impossible to produce a
product that does not fill at least half its pages with commercial
advertisements. As the price of those ads increases, so does the
dependency of the publishers on the supporting business organizations. The dependency is not recognized without probing deeper into
the issue. It can be detected when one realizes the reluctance of the
editors to publish any editorials that might be critical of the industrial
body.

Nothing exemplifies better the control industry has gained over
the publishing medical field than a recent experience I had with a
popular orthopaedic magazine. This magazine has gained great popularity and boasts having a circulation larger than all other publications, and it has become the most effective vehicle for industry to keep
the orthopaedic community abreast of its activities. Every page
announces new products, the merging of companies, as well as summaries of presentations that emphasize the success of surgical
implants. These summaries are limited to presentations made at various medical meetings without subjecting them to any semblance of
peer review.

An old friend of mine serves as editor-in-chief of the magazine,
and with him I have discussed several issues dealing with the current
condition of our profession. He regularly writes the editorial and a
number of times has written very provoking and interesting statements.

Recently, I sent to him a "Letter to the Editor" commenting on the
problems that frequently arise in the operating room during the performance of total hip surgery, due to the fact every manufacturing

company makes its implants and instruments different. When a failed implant needs to be replaced with a new one, it is often impossible to tell who manufactured the one to be removed and replaced. This creates pandemonium because in the middle of the surgical procedures the surgeon finds out that the instruments necessary to complete the intervention do not fit the failed implant. Its removal becomes impossible. Other times, when only one segment of the implant needs revision, a failure to appropriately identify prior to surgery the manufacturer of the implant precludes the completion of the procedure. Once the manufacturer is identified by visually examining the prosthesis, the nurse in charge gets on the phone and tries to locate the vendor of the respective company. Sometimes at least one hour passes before the vendor arrives, bringing the needed parts.

I feel this problem is extremely disturbing to the surgeon and may be associated with problems to the patient. Leaving a wound open for a long period of time waiting for the necessary parts to arrive may set the stage for an infection. Furthermore the prolonged anaesthesia time is not at all desirable and free of potential complications. Addressing the issue in writing, I suspected, would generate debate and hopefully a solution to the problem.

The editor agreed with my logic and informed me that he had sent it to the publisher for publication the following month. When my letter failed to appear in the next issue, I contacted the editor, who candidly admitted that the publisher had decided not to publish it. Allegedly, they were afraid to antagonize the manufacturing industry, on whom they depended so heavily.

Undeterred by the bad and unsavory experience I wrote another letter three months later in which I commented on an article written by an industry representative in which she had discussed a presentation I had made at a recent symposium held during the annual meeting of the American Orthopaedic Association. Once again, the editor agreed to publish it. However, my comments never had a chance to meet the printing press. I must assume that the publisher, once again, did not want to offend the generous industry supporters! Enough for Jefferson's inalienable rights, and the viability of the First Amendment to the U.S. Constitution. Industry has gained the power to dictate when such rights are allowed!

Only in my maturity have I recognized what every economist is taught from birth: "There is no such thing as a free lunch." The organized orthopaedic community has accepted industry's offer to pay the piper. We have no right to complain now that industry calls the tune. I can only assume that industry has employed the same strategy and tactics with other branches of medicine, wherever pharmaceutical products, surgical implants, or medical products and supplies of any kind can be marketed and sold.

Today, it is almost impossible to run a continuing education course, offer a visiting professorship, or run a medical conference without the support of industry. We no longer have a partnership. We have a new type of relationship in which medicine has become a tool that functions primarily as a marketing arm of industry. Patient welfare has become little more than a desirable (but not essential) byproduct.

As the past chairman of two of the United States's largest and more influential medical school departments of orthopaedics, I feel comfortable in stating that the education of today's orthopaedists is structured, to a great extent, to satisfy the marketing needs of industry. Today's students have little use for traditional learning and less use for scholarly research. They use "educational systems" provided by industry to learn to use industry's tools.

Daniel Callahan, one of the leading medical ethicists in the modern United States has stated, "There is no necessary correlation between the kind of innovation generated by the market and the kind of technology needed to improve overall health."[*] He is right. Industry provides all the fuel needed to drive the medical marketplace.

On a number of occasions, I have referred to a deeply troubling experience I had with an orthopaedic resident. The young man sat in the back of a classroom where I was lecturing several years ago. While I was giving my lecture on the effects of the environment on bone healing, he was reading a newspaper. I suppose that at first, I was more insulted by his rudeness than troubled by his inattention. When confronted by me, he responded not with embarrassment but with amazing candor. He told me that he was reading the newspaper because he was not interested in knowing how fractures heal, much less about environmental factors on the healing process. He simply wanted to know how to fix fractures.

Only later, after long and sad contemplation about the state of

---

[*]Daniel Callahan, *False Hopes* (New York: Simon and Schuster, 1998), p. x.

medical education, did I recognize what the young intern was actually saying. In effect, he was telling me that he had not learned to be a physician, but had been trained as a technician. He was a new kind of orthopaedist, a product of industry, a cosmetic surgeon of the skeleton.

That experience had a profound impact on my thinking regarding the future of medicine. At first, I thought the young resident was an aberration and that others reasoned differently. After probing further into the matter, I concluded that he was, in effect, speaking on behalf of many of his contemporaries. He had expressed, quite accurately, the ethos of the times.

After all, his education had taken place in an environment that emphasized technique over the biological sciences. The lectures he listened to were, for the most part, related to the technical aspects of treatment modalities. The sight of an X ray depicting a fracture instinctively provoked the question, "What operation does this fracture need?" That question had replaced the traditional inquiry, "What treatment is best for this patient?" The technician's instinct to use the latest tools and implants had replaced the physician's desire to use the most appropriate treatment.

The plethora of "new and improved" products we use in surgery are not, in many instances, the result of research designed to solve a problem. Instead, the research is designed to prove a new device "safe and effective." There is no need to prove that its use promises improved outcomes. Few surgeons today provide the kind of follow-up care that would provide them with data on their success rates. Today's surgeons rely on marketing materials provided by manufacturers and distributors to inform them about the latest devices. Some devices are produced not to improve outcomes but simply to stay one step ahead of the competition.

The next explosion of knowledge in orthopaedics will come from research conducted through genetic engineering and molecular biology. It is likely that the face of the profession will experience the most radical changes. Early investigations appear promising, however, the clinical application of the new technology has not yet happened. Nonetheless, industry has already begun to market products, the results of those investigations, in a major way, without any evidence of their clinical value.

The president of major industrial concern said to me a number of years ago that by the time his company released a new prosthesis to the public, they had already begun work on the next version. He said that they could not afford to wait for their competitors to come out with a more attractive product. He was concerned only with identifying those surgeons who were the most likely to be good salespeople for his products, with giving them "appropriate" incentives, and with making sure that they had a "state-of-the-art" product to sell.

I reminded him that Dr. John Charnley produced a higher rate of successful outcomes than any contemporary hip replacement surgeon did. He smiled in a way that wordlessly but powerfully expressed his lack of concern with such amusing but totally irrelevant data.

During my year as president of the academy, I chose to address the issue of the giant and still growing Orthopaedic Industrial Complex in a formal, official way. I called for a board of directors' workshop on the subject. I invited representatives from industry to participate in our discussions. We had several frank, animated discussions. In retrospect, I must admit that nothing meaningful took place during those two and a half days. For the most part it resembled a meeting of a mutual admiration society, during which time we heard the usual platitudes: the marvelous relationship between the two parties; the great progress that such a harmonious relationship had wrought to all concerns; and industry's generosity and unselfish support of education and research. Few attendees expressed any concern about developments that, to me, seemed ominous. Perfunctory reports were drafted, which were soon shelved and have long been forgotten. Industry continued its campaign. Its influence has continued to grow.

Physicians in all specialties express widespread frustration with HMOs and managed care organizations. The media frequently cover disputes between primary care providers and HMOs that require staff bureaucrats to review proposed treatment plans. In orthopaedics, the new generation, to a greater extent, rarely recognizes any "choice" of treatment. They simply follow the latest and most fashionable surgical trends, which rely totally on the newest and most expensive equipment that industry can provide. Clearly, the Orthopaedic Industrial Complex has even overpowered the managed care industry.

Comfortable in its position of power and influence, industry has assumed that the ethics of business should become the ethics of the medical profession. Accepting such a change would, no doubt, prove highly profitable to a small medical group. It could also prove expensive, well beyond price, to patients.

Several years ago, a vice president of one of the major medical device manufacturing companies in the United States visited me in my office in Los Angeles. After the usual small talk, he placed a velvet-lined box on my desk. It contained a brand new, shining hip prosthesis. At first, I thought that he was there to tell me the merits of the new implant. I wondered, however, why a senior corporate executive would assume a responsibility usually reserved for field representatives. He answered my unexpressed concern by saying that the new implant was the result of efforts made by his engineers to develop a product that reflected my philosophy of hip surgery. His company was presenting to me the new implant "in recognition of the many contributions I had made to hip surgery over the years." He then added that they wanted to market the implant as the Sarmiento Hip Prosthesis. Without pausing, he reached into his pocket, then handed me a check for $250,000. He also assured me that his company was also prepared to pay a substantial royalty on futures sale of the device.

I had known this gentleman for a number of years, and I had long admired his social and business skills. I would even have described us as "old friends." I asked what had prompted him to believe that I would accept his offer: "What have I done for you or said to you that would lead you to suspect that you could buy me? Why do you think I would be willing to allow my name to be attached to a product that I had nothing to do with developing?" Without another word, he put the check back in his pocket, closed the box, and left my office.

About three months later, I saw a large ad in our main orthopaedic journal illustrating the prosthesis that had allegedly been developed "according to my philosophy." The ad mentioned the intensive research that had gone into its production and promised that it would provide answers to many of the problems had been encountered with other implants. When I asked the distributor who had developed the prosthesis, he gave me the name of a senior professor at a respected medical school in the eastern United States.

The same year, I received a visit from a major distributor of orthopaedic implants in southern California. He was bemoaning the loss of business because of stiffer competition. He was in my office to "make me a deal." Since I was the chairman of the department of orthopaedics at USC, and five different hospitals fell under the USC umbrella, he offered to pay me $200 for every implant he sold to any of those institutions. He assured me that no one would have to be aware of our arrangement.

As in the case of the vice president that visited me the previous month, I had known this man for quite some time. We called each other by first names. I responded after a brief pause, "I am not sure I like the figure of two hundred dollars. Is it negotiable?"

"Of course" was his reply.

"What about two hundred and fifty dollars per implant?"

"It's a deal."

I made the same comments that I had made to his competitor a few weeks earlier. I told him that I was not for sale. His response differed only slightly. Through his embarrassment, he assured me that the deal he had offered me was common practice. "We do it all the time. The other companies do it as well."

I do not pretend to know if these practices are, in fact, widespread. I am sure that many other physicians share my ethical concerns, and that most are ethical, law-abiding people. I hope and suspect that industry has not found us to be so easily corrupted. The fact remains, however, that industry now expects the medical profession to accept industry methods and ethics. That should not be surprising, since they have already seen us sell out in so many other ways.

A few years ago, medical schools and universities paid the expenses of faculty members attending professional conventions and seminars. As the cost of attending these programs rose, most schools had to cut back on their support. Consequently, many surgeons now routinely travel to the annual meeting of AAOS and other conventions as the guests of industry. While I was visiting Europe recently, a professor told me that an implant-manufacturing firm underwrites his trips to the United States to attend such meetings. He added that he pays his gardener and other domestic staff, both at his home and at his summer place on the Mediterranean coast, with money from industry.

Quite recently, the academy, witnessing a decline in the attendance to its continuing education courses, began to discuss the possibility of having industry become a cosponsor of its educational endeavors. I happened to learn of such plans just prior to the annual meeting of the American Orthopaedic Association in Palm Beach, Florida, where I had been invited to participate on a panel dealing with the relationship between industry and medicine. I took advantage of that opportunity by expressing my serious concerns that such a move could generate problems for our profession.

On the same panel was another orthopaedist who had, within the past two weeks, received an endowed chair at his university, a position funded by a manufacturing company of orthopaedic products. The other two panelists were vice presidents of major orthopaedic manufacturing companies.

I said during my presentation that bringing industry as a cosponsor of educational activities would be a "grave mistake; a betrayal of the academy's educational mission; and the equivalent of driving a strong and irremovable nail into its own coffin." The reception to my remarks was enthusiastic. I know, however, that the upper echelon of the academy will pay no attention to my warnings, and will proceed as planned. Economic success must be attained, regardless of the harm that such a move is likely to generate, will be the unspoken response from the organization.

The response from the audience was warm because the medical profession is finally becoming concerned over the dominant role industry plays in the education of the physician and its likely harmful consequences. If anyone doubts the degree of control that industry has in the education of the medical profession, I urge you to take a look at the information presented in the July 2, 2001, issue of *Modern Health Care*, based on a report of a study conducted by Scott-Levin. It states that the pharmaceutical industry offered physicians 314,000 meetings, events, and dinners in 2000, an increase of 11 percent since 1995. The cost of these offerings was a $15 billion-a-year promotion effort.

It is evidence such as this that prompted me to state during my address to the American Orthopaedic Association, "Industry has lulled us into a slumber that has prevented us from realizing the degree to which we have become subservient to them."

chapter 31.
fighting the war
on several fronts

"I detest that man, who hides one thing in the depths of his heart, and speaks forth another."

—Homer

"In war there is no substitute for victory."

—Douglas McArthur

I should probably never have left the University of Miami for the golden but empty promises of southern California. I had started at Miami as a resident. My roots went deep in the community, the university, and the hospital. We had built a dynamic research program, a world-renowned rehabilitation center, and created an internationally respected department of orthopaedics and rehabilitation at both the medical school and at Jackson Memorial Hospital. Our personnel system that enabled faculty members to maintain a private practice was being imitated throughout the country. Our continuing education had won national recognition and earned me a respected post with the American Academy of Orthopaedic Surgeons. I had achieved remarkable success well beyond reasonable dreams or expectations. More importantly, my family and I were happy.

California and USC held the promise of substantial professional and intellectual rewards. The lure that had proven irresistible, however, had been the opportunity to lead the research program at Orthopedic Hospital, which offered the opportunity of a stellar research program that included world-class laboratories and top-quality support staff. In theory, it should have provided an ideal situation.

Our research faculty and facilities at Miami had grown up together. Many of us had worked side-by-side for years. We were experienced collaborators who shared our goals and vision. At Orthopedic Hospital I encountered a totally different situation and instant opposition. Despite the efforts of the hospital staff, I continued working to impose my vision and world-class standards on the clinical and research program. I continued to believe that I would eventually convince others to follow me. I fully expected the hospital programs to become models for the international orthopaedic community.

Instead, I became increasingly aware that the divided research program at Orthopedic Hospital was actually causing it to lose ground. Projects and sections continued to function independently, with no concept of common goals. One section director privately patented and sold a product emerging from hospital laboratories. In the absence of strong administrative management, the hospital was unable to document his work and enforce its policies. One researcher insisted on continuing an investigation that had been in process for more than a decade without results. The National Institutes of Health continued to fund the project for a second decade before it was finally abandoned. Other researchers worked on projects that had little to do with the musculoskeletal system, the presumed mission of the laboratory.

My attempts to rein in these practices accomplished little more than to increase resentment. Complaints were voiced to the dean of the medical school I was just another academic administrator who did not appreciate the fact that intellectual vitality required total academic independence. I did not understand the value of pure research. I was just a hip surgeon, not a research scientist.

In my defense, I would point out that throughout my academic career, I had always been a strong believer in scholarly and scientific research. At the University of Miami, my faculty and I had begun our research in the most primitive possible laboratories, using salvaged automobile tools. When I left Miami, the facilities included moderately advanced technology and the staff provided highly skilled research support. During my twenty years as a department chairman, seven at Miami and thirteen at USC, my faculties maintained an uninterrupted record of reporting on research at the annual meetings of the academy. I, personally, have appeared on its scientific program for forty consecutive years. I believed my record of support for research could not be denied.

The researchers at Orthopedic Hospital obviously disagreed. At the annual meeting of the American Academy of Orthopedic Surgeons and the Orthopedic Research Society in Atlanta, I had a rude awakening. When I opened the printed program, I discovered, for the first time, that members of our department were presenting a paper dealing with the effects of weightlessness on fracture healing. The researchers had informed me neither that they had applied to participate in the congress nor that their application had been accepted. The individual presenting the scientific paper was a physician's assistant who served as the animal keeper in our laboratories; the coinvestigator was June Marshall, an anatomist who served as the director of the Orthopedic Hospital research laboratory.

The possible effects of weightlessness on fracture healing had long fascinated me. I had initiated the study a few years earlier and had continuously funded the project through the laboratories' budget. I had sent the animal keeper and others to visit the offices of NASA as well as the Toronto research laboratory of Robert Salter, who had done some fascinating work on the effects of continuous motion on cartilage repair in experimental animals. The project staff's failure to keep me informed insulted and depressed me profoundly. I also found their choice of the animal keeper as senior project representative questionable in the extreme.

The episode forced me to recognize that I had totally lost control of the research program at Orthopedic Hospital. Upon my return to Los Angeles, I decided to resign from the position I held at the hospital and from the hospital board of trustees. I would retain only my responsibility for my ongoing laboratory research in biomechanics. I had obtained funding for those projects from sources outside the hospital. I felt certain that I would be able to continue them without interference.

At the next board meeting, I announced my resignation and expressed my appreciation for the "support they had extended me over the years." I told them that I had concluded that it was no longer in the best interest of the hospital for me to continue my strong identification with its day-to-day activities. In the future, I would devote my time to serving the medical school. I assured them that I still intended to admit my private patients to the hospital.

The trustees accepted my resignation with traditional words of gratitude and good wishes. We all knew, however, that my resignation weakened the professional reputation of the hospital and its competitive ability to win research grants. I also knew that several of the trustees would regard my resignation as a personal insult. Having the chairman of a major department at the university resign from their board was not something they would take lightly.

A few days later, the dean of the medical school announced that he had invited Dr. Kay Clawson, the chancellor at the University of Kansas, to visit Los Angeles to assess the situation and make recommendations. Clawson was a distinguished orthopaedist who had previously served as chairman of the department of orthopaedics at the University of Washington in Seattle. We had met a few times in the past but were not close friends.

I met with Clawson for about an hour, as he began his professional review. He spent the rest of the time meeting with other people from a list prepared by the dean. Later that evening, he called me at home and suggested that we meet for breakfast the following morning.

During breakfast, Clawson advised me to resign. "Gus, this is one battle you cannot possibly win. You took on powerful people who want to get rid of you since you do not fit into their agenda. There is no way for you to win over the combined power of the trustees of Orthopaedic Hospital, Bob Kerlan and Herb Stark. I suggest that you resign, today, before the dean fires you. He is not going to back you up."

When we parted, I headed toward the office to prepare my letter of resignation. His argument was compelling and seemed wise. I planned to deliver my resignation in person at the end of the day, and placed it in my pocket.

At the last minute, I chose to postpone my trip to the dean until the next day. That night, increasingly angry and bitter, I rehashed the events of the last few years, as well as my previous experiences at the University of Miami. I asked myself whether I had created my own problems and misread the signs before me. I concluded that while I had made mistakes, there was no reason for the university to dismiss me from the department chair.

I thought about my relationship with the two men whom Clawson had specifically mentioned that morning—Bob Kerlan and Herb Stark. Kerlan was a former alumnus of the Los Angeles County residency program. When I had assumed the chair at USC, Kerlan was already well known in sports medicine circles. During a courtesy call shortly after my arrival, he showed me the huge physical therapy area in his office and made me aware of the fact that he and his associates were the physicians for the Los Angeles Lakers and other professional teams and athletes. He pointed out that Dr. Harvey had rotated the LAC-USC orthopaedics residents through his office on a casual basis. I assured him that I would look into the matter of making the rotations compulsory, and subsequently acted accordingly.

After our first meeting, I did not see Kerlan again for a long time. A few years later, my attempts to establish a division of sports medicine within USCs orthopaedics department again brought us together. We disagreed on several questions about the new division, including its leadership. My plans for the new division stalled.

When we revived plans for a sports medicine division, I recruited James Tibone to lead the new program. Tibone had recently completed his residency training in one of the local residency programs and had spent a year as a fellow. At first, we had almost no patients. The only clinical material available to him were indigent patients at the county hospital. The residents and staff joked that I instructed everyone to refer to Dr. Tibone all patients coming to the emergency room reporting trauma sustained from attacks with baseball bats—the closest thing we had to a "sports" injury.

Tibone soon built a successful practice. As our department grew, I began planning to approach the athletic department at the university and convince them that we were capable of assuming responsibility for the USC teams and athletes. Those plans fell by the wayside when Kerlan successfully recruited Tibone to join his practice.

So, I was not surprised to learn that Kerlan was among those who were most anxious to see me leave USC. Neither was I surprised to learn that Herbert Stark was also among the opposition, even though he had originally encouraged me to come to Los Angeles. In fact, one of my first actions when arriving at USC had been to reappoint Stark as chief of the division of hand surgery. I had also recommended a clinical professorship for Stark and for his associates. He had assured me of his full support and commitment to the program.

Unfortunately, Stark did not respond to the responsibilities that he had agreed to assume. He rotated his associates through the county hospital clinics and covered the operating room activities in a casual manner. He did not appear interested in increasing the academic standing of the department. After five years, I informed him that I intended to appoint a full-time division chief for hand surgery.

Stark agreed, at first, but our battles over selecting a division chief attracted cross-country attention. A candidate from a prestigious institution in New York retold the story of his "interview" with Stark, and I received several calls from disturbed but curious colleagues. Stark had said to him that if he were foolish enough to accept my offer, he would make it impossible for the candidate to develop a referral practice; furthermore, he would never allow him to become a member the Hand Society.

Stark had served as secretary for the American Academy of Orthopedic Surgeons and had assumed that he would eventually be elected to its presidency. He reacted badly when that honor was not given to him, and died a few years later.

Stark was a complex individual. As he indulged in actions indicative of lack of integrity, he officially preached from the pulpit of the local church the Christian tenets of humility and charity. Was he Stevenson's Dr. Jekyll and Mr. Hyde? A reincarnated Sinclair Lewis's Elmer Gantry? A Tartuffe from the pages of Moliere's classic? Or simply a Manichean expression of good and evil dualism?

I was not surprised to learn of Stark's opposition to my continued service as department chair. I had to accept, however, the fact that Kerlan and Stark, in combination with the trustees of Orthopedic Hospital, would probably prove too much for me.

To this day, I still do not know why I decided not to resign. When I met with the dean the next day, I told him that I had prepared a letter of resignation but had changed my mind. I reminded him that the department had been successful under my leadership, despite his lack of support. I had inherited a second-class program and transformed it into one that was earning recognition in academic circles throughout the country. I threatened to take my case to the university senate as well as to the American Association of University Professors. That was the end of our meeting. I did not hear again from him regarding the issue at hand. Within a few weeks, he left the medical school and the vice president for medical affairs took his place.

The new dean, a former professor and chairman of neurology at USC, soon informed me that Dr. Clawson's review of my department had not been sufficiently thorough, and that he was going to conduct another. I pleaded with him to postpone the review until the dust had settled from Clawson's visit. I pointed out that we would soon be recruiting the next group of residents. News of another departmental review, I argued, would jeopardize our ability to recruit the best applicants. It was all to no avail. He did, however, offer me one choice. He could either conduct the review himself, or select a panel of outsiders to do it. I told him that I wanted to avoid further publicity, and would trust his judgment. I asked only to be informed of changes and given an opportunity to defend myself.

The dean must have met with many people. The residents requested a meeting with him and supported me in strong terms. They even sent a letter to the dean with a copy to the president of the university. All sixty-five residents signed the letter, which stated in the most complimentary terms that my performance as chairman had been excellent. That letter made it possible for me to continue my fight. It would become one of my most cherished memories of my years at USC.

Several weeks later, I was called to the dean's office. He showed me two piles of letters and indicated that the ones on the right were in my support and the ones on the left against me. Before proceeding any further, I asked him if I was going to have the opportunity to answer to the charges against me. He replied that he had elected not to inform me of the charges or the names of the accusers. He had decided to rule in my favor, and in the interest of a smoother future, had decided to keep all materials confidential.

I returned to work hoping to patch up the damage that inevitably had been done. I never did learn any specific information about the charges or about who had opposed my continued leadership. I took strength, however, from this renewed evidence that the university knew that I was doing a good job, and that nothing was going to stop me from making our program one of the best in the country.

chapter 32.
understanding the opposition

"These are the times that try men's souls."

—Thomas Paine

"Al'ouest rien d neuveau"
("All is quiet on the western front")

—A. M. Remark

The events at Orthopaedic Hospital and the hurdles placed in my path by USC administrators ran in tandem with challenges at the Los Angeles County-University of Southern California (LAC-USC) Medical Center. There, too, I encountered unanticipated administrative difficulties. Again, I discovered a well-entrenched home team that simply did not want things to change.

When I had accepted the position as chair of the USC department of orthopaedics and head of orthopaedics LAC-USC Medical Center, I assumed that I would be responsible for the overall education program at the medical school and its leading affiliated hospital. The university and hospital reinforced my expectations shortly after we arrived, when we discussed the merging of the two previously independent residency programs. I soon learned, however, that my assumption was not shared by everyone.

The former chief of orthopaedics at LAC-USC Medical Center had other ideas. He claimed that my appointment as chief of the newly expanded department gave me jurisdiction only over the education of the medical students. He insisted that his seniority at the hospital meant he would remain in charge of the residency education program. In spite of my repeated requests, the dean of the medical school refused to intervene in this delicate situation and clear up the lines of authority and responsibility.

Consequently, I found myself faced with a totally unanticipated administrative nightmare. While I was trying to put the fire out at Orthopaedic Hospital, Paul Harvey's opposition at LAC-USC became increasingly entrenched. He boycotted every change I tried to institute and openly instructed the residents to ignore my recommendations or instructions. It soon escalated beyond an annoying situation and became an intolerable one. Assisting him in his relentless efforts to make my life miserable, he had the support of his underling, an insecure man with the viciousness of the Shakespearian Iago, who masterminded Othello's tragedy.

Our dispute came to a head with a series of meetings and a memorandum in which I threatened to resign from the university. Faced with that threat, the dean finally intervened and supported my position.

In recognition of the former chief's many professional accomplishments, I extended a series of olive branches. I invited him and his wife to join Barbara and me for dinner. He at first accepted, but then declined. I asked him to take over the pediatric orthopaedics division where he could function semi-independently. I reminded him that I had spoken with him when I had first been approached about the position at USC. I had agreed to consider the position only after he had assured me that he knew that he would not be considered for the chairmanship. He himself had told me that he had "too many enemies" long before I became a candidate for the position. He refused to listen.

Fortunately, by the time our disagreements came to a head, I had built a strong base of support within the department. I had successfully lured a few extremely capable young orthopaedists to join the full-time faculty of the department. While their salaries were only marginally competitive, I had given them opportunities to develop their own private practices. I had also involved the hospital's voluntary faculty more actively in the formal teaching program.

My greatest support came from the residents. The brutality of the LAC-USC orthopaedic residency had earned a national reputation. Residents were expected to handle thirty-six-hour shifts. Their patient load far exceeded national norms. Their rotations were difficult, demanding, and complex.

I did not see any value in such a physically and emotionally demanding environment. I came to understand it only after my predecessor and I participated, as part of a group of orthopaedists from the United States, in a series of lecture programs in Belgium and England. I welcomed the opportunity. Unfortunately, the camaraderie that existed during the trip proved to be a mirage. The trip did, however, give me an opportunity to learn more about him and the values that underlay his residency regimen.

At various seminars, each of us presented papers dealing with projects that we had completed or were in progress. I talked primarily about fracture care, discussed my experiences, and presented statistical data. His papers dealt with complications. He displayed a large number of slides showing infected fractures and patients with the kind of grotesque results that one sees only rarely in the developed world. He accompanied this depressing slide show with a humorous and lively narrative. At every session, he was clearly the star of the show.

During the discussion periods that followed our presentations, attendees usually asked him why the complication rate at his institution was so high. He told them that the reason was simple: "My hospital is dirty and my patients are also dirty." His enthusiasm reflected xenophobia and a rare type of a deep-seated scatological obsession. LAC-USC Medical Center provides care to indigent residents. Many of them are African American or of Hispanic origin. Virtually all patients at LAC-USC are poor people from poor families. This was the first time that I had heard anyone speak about them in such stark, antagonistic terms.

As I watched his presentations to our European audiences, I realized that Harvey seemed proud of this depressing state of affairs. He had become a warrior. He approached public health care with the joy of battle. He shared that attitude with many of the residents who trained under him. He trained them to handle battlefield conditions. Most of them took great pleasure and pride in their "wartime" experiences. Many of his former residents still enjoy reminiscing about the "incredible" problems they had to deal with and the fascinating complications they encountered. Medical students throughout the United States had already heard about the primitive working conditions at LAC-USC and the superhuman demands that the institution placed on its residents. Many of the students who applied to LAC-USC were people who relished that kind of challenge.

LAC-USC Medical Center graduated twelve residents every year; we typically received approximately five hundred applications to fill the twelve first-year positions. While I kept my own role in the admissions process small, I have always found it fascinating. Just how does one choose twelve people from a pool of 500 qualified applicants? What should we look for? How do we identify the people who will make the best physicians? What do our choices say about us?

In Miami, the faculty had consisted for several years of the chief, Wallace Miller, and me. Usually, only Dr. Miller interviewed applicants. I remember one occasion, however, when he was out of town and asked me to handle the interview. When he returned, his first question about the applicant was, "Is he tall?" I could not help but smile when I responded that from my perspective, almost everybody was tall. I realized, for the first time, that most of our residents had been substantially taller than me. I must admit that I was somewhat startled to realize the reason for that happenstance.

Interviewers who use more subjective criteria often found that the admission process could be extremely frustrating. Most of the 500 applicants were graduates of good medical schools; we usually assumed that they were well qualified to begin their residency. When we asked questions designed to reveal their medical knowledge, we only confirmed that assumption. Other approaches only revealed that most candidates were well-coached in interview techniques. I later learned that many of them took special classes to prepare for the admissions interview. They prepared in other ways, as well. I saw many applicants wearing well-tailored suits at those interviews, but I never saw any of those suits again. Our residents typically dressed extremely casually, but I never interviewed an applicant in blue jeans.

At USC, I often challenged the applicants to tell us why in their opinion we should select them in preference to other applicants. They typically answered with a well-rehearsed "because I am dedicated to my career and I am a hard-working person." I also frequently asked them to describe their special strengths. Again, the answers rarely varied. When asked to describe their weaknesses, they seldom provided candid responses. I recall only one notable exception. When I asked one young lady to enumerate her strengths, she responded that she did not think she had many and described herself as a "run of the mill" average student. I was both startled and somewhat impressed with her reply. I then asked to describe any possible deficits that she had been able to identify. Her answer: "I have many weaknesses; I lack the assurance and self-confidence that others seem to have; maybe I am just not as smart as others."

By the end of the interview, I found myself hoping that the other committee members would also vote for her. Unfortunately, I was the only one who was impressed with her candor and honesty. I hope that some other program accepted her. She would have made a good orthopaedist. If she chose another specialty instead, I am equally certain that today she is doing well and practicing good medicine.

As I look back at my experiences with our selection process, I believe it needs much improvement. We first looked at the medical school from which the applicants graduate. Then, we checked whether or not they had graduated high in the class, and if they belonged to important academic fraternities. We gave a high priority to those whose curriculum vitae demonstrated a strong commitment to research. We automatically lowered the evaluation for anyone who graduated from a foreign medical school, and did not even consider applicants whose names also happened to be too "foreign."

We were wrong to select residents the way we did. Many who apparently had the "right" qualifications lacked maturity, compassion, understanding, and good judgment. We should have sought to judge applicants by their future potential—not just by academic accomplishments. It is foolish to deny opportunities to future physicians because of outdated prejudices. We have a responsibility to provide opportunities to those who have the passion and ability to make the most of themselves. Those who have enjoyed many advantages from birth and who have repeatedly demonstrated their ability to score well on examinations may make great applicants. They do not always make good physicians.

I particularly remember one applicant with an especially strong background in research. He had involved himself in basic research throughout his entire four years in medical school, and had published several papers in refereed journals. His professors provided the strongest possible recommendations. All agreed that the young man was a diamond in the rough, and that he would one day be a leader in medical research. We knew that every residency program would recruit this student, who seemed destined for future stardom.

We were delighted when he chose our program, and he quickly demonstrated his remarkable intellectual abilities. He even scored in the top percentile in the national in-training examinations. Curiously, however, his evaluations on other aspects of his work, including empathy for patients and peer leadership, were just average for his group. We found it more troubling, however, that as he progressed through the residency, he did not seem interested in resuming his research.

At the beginning of his fourth year of the five-year program, I approached him about the fact that he had not yet begun any research. I reminded him that the main reason for our having selected him was his strong research background. He explained that while he had been involved in research during his medical student days, he had never enjoyed the experience. Then he nonchalantly added, "I only did research because I knew that it would help me enter a good residency program. The truth is, I never want to see the inside of another laboratory for as long as I live."

I now know that many applicants for residency programs do exactly the same thing. In fact, I can hardly blame them. They have accurately identified a systemic weakness and have acted accordingly. I can only hope that they are equally successful when they become practicing physicians.

We all assume that the most successful students will make the best doctors. In fact, there is no evidence to support that view. The skills that make a good doctor have little to do with the skills required by medical schools. I suspect that many of our contemporary problems in medicine—especially the loss of professionalism and exaggerated concern with financial profit—are rooted in the values of medical school and residency program admissions committees. Those committees should pay less attention to grades and more attention to character.

A member of the board of trustees at one of our affiliated hospitals called me one day to request special consideration for one applicant to our residency program. He told me that the young man's father was a wealthy and influential man in the community. The father would probably donate a great deal of money to our research laboratory if we accepted his son. I invited the young man to meet with me so that I could justify adding his name to the list of personal interviews scheduled by the screening committee.

I found the applicant to be a deeply troubled young man. Our interview extended well past the half-hour I had originally planned. The more we talked, the more I wondered why he chose a career in medicine, and how he had completed medical school. I carefully explained the nature of orthopaedics to him. I told him about the responsibilities he would face as an orthopaedist. Finally, and somewhat reluctantly, I encouraged him to select a different specialty. I suspect that he accepted my advice. I know that I never again heard from him. I also never again heard from the trustee.

There were times during my years as department chairman when I had to make unpleasant decisions. Rightly or wrongly, I made them. On one occasion, I dismissed a resident as he began his last year in training. He had transferred to us from a prestigious residency training program on the East Coast and had come to Los Angeles with strong letters of recommendation. Such strong references, unfortunately, are not always what they seem. Sometime, they represent little more than a program's desire to rid itself of a problem without risking a lawsuit. Many program directors seem to be afraid to write objective, critical letters. I am so surprised to receive a critical letter that when I receive one, I usually try to find out what is *really* going on. Such letters always represent a deep-seated conflict that may well have been invisible to the student. Sometimes the fault lies with the student. Just as often, the professor writing the recommendation is more at fault.

This particular student came from an influential, highly respected family. But from the start of his work with us at USC, his clinical performance was, at best, questionable. During his first-year reviews, we assumed that he was experiencing problems due to the difficulty of transitioning from a small program to a large one with extremely busy clinics. Newly arrived residents often found life at LAC-USC hard to handle. After a year or two, however, they usually proved themselves up to the challenge.

Shortly after the beginning of this student's last year of residency, he rotated through my service and I had an opportunity to observe him closely. It did not take long for me to realize that the young man was a fine and ethical individual and that he possessed an adequate knowledge of orthopaedics. I was also forced to recognize, however, that he seemed incapable of functioning under stress. He panicked when he found himself in situations that required him to make quick, critical decisions.

I met with him personally and tried to better understand him and, if possible, correct his deficiencies. Both of his parents were physicians. Most of his family was deeply involved with medicine, some in industry, some in other health care professions. After several lengthy conversations, I surmised that the young man had chosen a career in medicine under a great deal of pressure from his family. With a great deal of reluctance, I concluded that he could never overcome his inability to make decisions and his tendency to panic under stress. We could not allow him to complete his training as an orthopaedist. Finally, I told him that we could not allow him to continue. Using as much decency, sympathy, and courtesy as possible, I explained to him the reasons for my decision.

He was devastated and broke into tears. When he was finally able to talk, the first thing he said was, "What am I going to tell my mom?" I promised that I would help him choose another medical career—a different specialty or some other health care profession where he could take full advantage of his extensive talents and the experiences and knowledge that he had accumulated over the years. Over the next few weeks, I wrote several letters of recommendation for him, and arranged several interviews.

A few weeks later, I saw him in the back of the auditorium where we held our weekly "grand rounds." At he end of the meeting, he joined me at the front of the room. He was carrying a box under his arm. He said that it was a present for me. For a fraction of a second, I feared that it might contain an explosive device that would detonate as soon as I opened it.

I asked him what I had done to justify the gift.

"Doctor Sarmiento, your firing me from my residency was a painful and difficult thing for me to take. I know that it was also difficult for you. I realized that you had no choice. Your letters and calls were very helpful. I have been accepted for residency training in pathology. Thank you for helping me."

I received his remarks with mixed emotions. At the time, I was still torturing myself with the thought that I should have given him the opportunity to complete his training. His rapid adjustment to the situation and his obvious relief, however, convinced me that I had taken the correct action. I was also sure that he would make a good pathologist.

On a few other occasions, I also had the unpleasant duty of firing residents from the program because of their abuse of drugs or alcohol. We always provided appropriate opportunities for rehabilitation. We even readmitted two students after they completed full rehabilitation programs. Both failed again. They were sick people. It would have been immoral and illegal for us to allow them to graduate and practice medicine. A third student recovered fully from his addiction. To my knowledge, he has remained clean and enjoys a successful practice.

I am especially pleased with my memories of one senior resident who was in the process of finding a job in the Los Angels area. One morning, after my weekly Sunday "pass-on rounds," he stopped me as I was leaving the room:

> Doctor Sarmiento, you have done me a great favor. My wife and I were entertained the other night by a group of prestigious orthopaedists in the community. They took us out to dinner, and offered me a position in their office with exceptionally generous financial incentives.
>
> As we were leaving the restaurant, the senior member of the group said to me, with a big grin on his face, "Son, now that you will be working with us, I want you to remember one thing at all times. In life there is only one thing more important than money, and that is more money." I notified them yesterday that I had decided not to accept their offer. I made that decision partly because I remembered the many times that you have spoken about the importance of being ethical in our personal and professional lives. You helped convince me that making money is not the name of the game.

That young man made my day. I suspect that my speeches were just one of many valuable influences on his life, ethics, values, and philosophy. I am sure that he had a strong family and many wonderful teachers. I take great pleasure, however, in the fact that he felt I had played a part in his choice. I need no other reward.

At around the same time that this graduate refused to follow the path to more gold, we learned that our residents' scores on the previous year's in-training examinations had plummeted from the eighty-fifth percentile to something in the mid-forties. As you would imagine, the report badly bruised my ego. I had taken great personal pride in the earlier escalation of those scores. I did not want to be known as the leader of a program whose residents scored so poorly. I was not alone in my concern. The report caused consternation throughout the department. We immediately formed a committee to find out what had happened and what we had to do to correct it.

We quickly discovered that a small group of just three residents had earned extremely low scores. Their extremely poor performance had brought down the average for the entire department. Among the three was a young lady whose grades were in the third percentile.

Before the examinations, this young lady had been performing well and had been earning typical mid-range reviews. After the examinations, I began reviewing her work with a much more critical eye. I began to regard her as a poor student who was making my entire program look bad. I dreaded the inevitable time when she would rotate through my service, and I would have to work with her on a daily basis.

Much to my amazement, she did a superb job at taking care of my patients. She proved herself warm and sympathetic to their needs. She made patient care her top priority. She also proved to be knowledgeable. Her clinical abilities simply did not correlate with her examination results.

The day she completed her rotation in my service, I called her into my office. I told her that I had not looked forward to her rotation through my service, because of her dreadful performance on the in-training examinations. Then I assured her that my experience with her had been extremely positive. I congratulated her for her work with us, and assured her that she would most surely become a good orthopaedist. I have lost touch with her, but I am sure that she has been successful in her chosen career. I can only hope that she never has to take another examination.

chapter 33.
the changing face of research

"The fear of being wrong is a disease."

—Walter Lippmann

I was pleasantly surprised several years ago when the National Institutes of Health (NIH) invited me to join one of their grant proposal evaluation panels. Perhaps I had always assumed that such groups consisted of people with more lofty qualifications than mine. As you know, I had never been trained as a disciplined researcher. My involvement had always been more pragmatic and more administrative. I could only guess that the NIH invitation originated with someone who appreciated my commitment to research. I had also recently received the Kappa Delta and the Nicholas Andry awards. I received those highly coveted research awards for work that I had conducted with Loren Latta, who brought to our study the necessary support from the basic sciences.

At the NIH meeting in Washington, I reported my evaluations of seven investigative proposals and listened to the discussion concerning those and other grant applications. One proposal dealt with the shuffling gait of the elderly. It requested nearly $1 million to underwrite a proposed three-year project. I questioned the proposal's value to society or to science, but was quickly told that I was not capable of appreciating "true research." The panel approved the proposal. I can only assume that the proposal had substantial "scientific" merit. I can assure you that it had no clinical merit whatsoever. That was my first warning of the growing chasm between clinical and basic science research.

In subsequent years, I have spent much more time reviewing a broader picture of funded research. I have learned that much funded research, when viewed from a strictly clinical perspective, seems unworthy of attention or support. By the same token, many clinically worthwhile research projects are routinely denied funding. The scientific community's system for evaluating research proposals appears to be almost as capricious as our residency admissions processes at USC.

When I had occasion to present congressional testimony on behalf of orthopaedic research, I became even more aware that our nation's organized research effort may be based more on political concerns than on scientific considerations. The near monopoly of a self-selected scientific elite produces a remarkable waste of financial resources. I once discussed this issue with a good friend of mine from Harvard. He accused me of being resentful of the large share of research funding that his university received. (He did not know that my own laboratories had three studies in the pipeline that would soon receive substantial funding from NIH.)

My criticism did not stem from jealousy but from extended observations and discussions with orthopaedic researchers around the world. We have created a circular system whereby scientists affiliated with elite institutions approve funding for proposals initiated by their peers and colleagues. Researchers who are not part of this inner circle must find funding elsewhere. Most turn to industry, which is often happy to provide the needed support. Industry's support for research usually relates to product-oriented investigations. A better system for reviewing proposals would probably produce both better science and better medicine. It would also weaken the Medical-Industrial Complex.

During my tenure as president of the American Academy of Orthopaedic Surgeons, and at my instigation, the board of directors approved the establishment of a research center at the academy's headquarters. I had high hopes that such a center would increase the influence of orthopaedic researchers and increase the popularity of research in the orthopaedic community. I also hoped that it would provide a home base for long-term outcome-based study of surgical procedures. During my administration, the academy hired staff for the center and initiated work on the outcomes study. As soon as my year in office ended, however, the board lost interest in the center and soon eliminated its priority funding status.

At the time, the academy had shifted its priorities and begun devoting more of its resources to its own more profitable ventures. I should also have realized that the academy traditionally pays close attention to the pet proposals of newly elected presidents, but loses interest in those projects as the end of the presidential terms approach. Continuity is not one of the academy's strong suits.

During my tenure as president, I participated in a workshop in Washington that sought to identify new ways to increase support for musculoskeletal research. A group of approximately thirty investigators gathered for the meeting. I was particularly impressed by the remarks of an orthopaedic scientist from Philadelphia who spoke about his concern that far too few orthopaedists seemed interested in research. He commented that if the group assembled in Washington that day were to travel home in the same plane, and if the plane crashed, orthopaedic research in the United States would die along with them. He was right. There were only about thirty people in the room, but our small group included almost all of the orthopaedists in the country who were deeply involved in research. He then displayed data demonstrating the extent to which scientists in other disciplines had taken over most ongoing research involving the musculoskeletal system.

In my own comments, I berated the group for their failure to recognize the inevitability of change. I told them that professional orthopaedics had already abandoned research. As a profession, we no longer had the capacity to preside over investigations in the basic sciences. Our residency programs were no longer educating scientists but training technicians. I argued that while we were no longer qualified to lead research teams, we should maintain our interest in participating as members of research teams. I argued that we should modify our mission. Henceforth, we should seek to ensure that research conducted by the highly trained research scientists remained clinically relevant.

On the last day of he meeting I had to make some final comments. I proceeded to concoct a story. I had a nightmare the previous evening in which a group of old men living in a nursing home had assembled to discuss problems they were individually experiencing, such as loss of memory of recent events, fatigue, failure to zip their flies, and many other concerns. They had appointed subcommittees to discuss the various problems and had scheduled future meetings in anticipation of finding solutions. Then, I told the group, I was awakened by the sound of the alarm clock. This morning when I walked into the meeting room I realized that the faces of the old men in the nursing home were the faces of my colleagues. Then I added, "Like the senior citizens in my dream, you are looking for solutions to problems which no one can provide."

Some in the group reacted violently. They accused me of surrendering and betraying our cause. They accused me of selling out to other disciplines. I wish I could agree with them now, but several years later, I am even more convinced that my views were correct.

We orthopaedists continue to admire and advocate research, but we no longer educate our young orthopaedists in ways that equip them for research careers. Unless a radical change takes place in orthopaedic education, the number of orthopaedic surgeons qualified to preside over basic research studies will soon decline to zero.

Scientists from other disciplines are continuing to improve their qualifications to conduct research. They will have to carry our torch. Unless they and the academic orthopaedic community recognize this change, however, and find ways to work together, it is unlikely that either group will produce scientifically valid results that yield clinical benefits on questions of medical importance.

The urgent need for clinically based, scientifically valid orthopaedic research will increase dramatically as our society ages. We are already witnessing a dramatic increase in the incidence of age-related, degenerative musculoskeletal disease. These diseases do not seem interesting to politically influential people. There are no high-visibility associations campaigning to find a cure. There is no euphonic acronym for age-related, degenerative musculoskeletal disease. We do not even have our own ribbon color. But as America ages, most of our celebrities, politicians, newsmakers, and opinion leaders will most assuredly experience these diseases firsthand. For the moment, however, our leaders seem to hope that if we ignore age-related degenerative diseases of the musculoskeletal system, they will just go away.

We can conduct vitally necessary research only if orthopaedists and research scientists learn to work together. We must convince National Institutes of Health and other funding agencies that only such cooperative studies are worthy of public support. I understand that research scientists will have to lead the way. The academic orthopaedist community must accept that new reality. They must identify ways to work with talented, skillful researchers to achieve clinically relevant results.

chapter 34.
enjoying the teaching experience

"For not many men, the proverb saith,
Can love a friend who fortune prospereth
Unenvying; and about the envious brain
Cold poison clings and doubles all the pain
Life brings him. His own woundings he must nurse,
And feels another's gladness like a curse."

—Aeschylus

Despite the constant battles that marred every aspect of my tenure as chief of orthopaedics at USC, I always enjoyed my work and almost all of the people I met and with whom I worked. In addition to my administrative responsibilities, teaching, and research, I had my own private patients. As I had done in Miami, I confined my practice to treating arthritic conditions of the hip in adults. Though my practice never grew as large as it had been in Miami, I continually maintained a steady flow of patients.

In Los Angeles, I limited my surgical practice to an average of two hip replacements each week. That pace proved sufficient for me to meet the demands of my patients, satisfy my own need to continue work as a surgeon, and to provide me with a good income. When I moved to California, I continued the follow-up practices I had established in Miami. I continued my annual request that they visit their orthopaedist for follow-up X rays, and provided them with a questionnaire. I also usually included a brief personal note.

This continued contact with patients has been gratifying in many respects. I have found that maintaining personal contact with my patients has dramatically increased my pleasure and professional satisfaction. It has also enabled me to document accurately the successes and failures of the operation. I have also developed a fascinating data bank with information on thousands of patients.

Every response brought its own unique view of my patients and their lives. One elderly patient whom I had followed for over twenty years wrote, "Doctor Sarmiento, I appreciate your interest in my condition for all these years. However, I do not want to hear from you again, as I am afraid that one day you might tell me that I need another operation. I am too old to go through surgery again and, furthermore, you are not around to do it."

Another elderly lady informed me that she could not afford the expense of an X ray every year. I called her and asked how much it would cost to have one done at her nearest hospital. She told me that it was around fifty dollars, and I mailed her a check for that amount. A few days later, I received a collect call from her. She thanked me for the check, but told me that she did not have enough money to pay for the taxi ride to the hospital and back. I mailed her the cab fare. A few days later I received the X rays.

Usually, my patients visit a local orthopaedic surgeon to have their hips evaluated and X rays taken. The doctor typically mails the films to me. Over the years, the overwhelming majority of doctors accommodated my wishes and mailed me a copy of their office dictation as well as the X ray films. Even when I moved to California, my patients and their doctors in Florida continued to comply with my requests. Only a few refused. Most cited the inconvenience of mailing the films or the costs involved.

During my years in California, I also enjoyed my contact with residents and fellows, and my work in the outpatient clinics at the county hospital. I met with the residents every Sunday morning from 7:00 to 9:30 or 10:00. The residents included those who had been on duty since the previous morning and the new group who were just starting their shift. We called that meeting "pass-on rounds." The departing group would "pass on" information concerning newly admitted patients as well as the patients whom they had operated on during their shift.

Usually the residents who had been on duty for the past twenty-four hours were not in the best physical or emotional condition. They were not fully able to concentrate on my teaching. I nevertheless found this contact with young people to be enjoyable and rewarding. I converted every clinical problem they had encountered into a teaching experience. I also used the time to share my ideas about medicine, values, ethics, and the changing times. I still miss those wonderful Sunday mornings.

Similar pass-on rounds were held every morning. A different attending surgeon presided over them each day. I attended those other pass-on rounds with as much frequency as I could. I found that I often benefited from what others had to say and from their teachings.

Every Wednesday morning I covered an outpatient clinic totally devoted to patients with fractures treated with functional braces, the braces that I had developed in Miami many years earlier. We typically saw about sixty patients each week. I made it my practice to be certain that the responsible resident presented every patient to me. It also gave me an opportunity to continue learning about fracture care, and to teach the residents about the subject. For reasons I do not fully understand, I have always found working in public clinics with poor patients to be uniquely rewarding. That clinic in California became one of the highlights of my career.

The condition of those clinics was primitive to say the least. Patients reported early in the morning and waited in line for a long time—often until the late afternoon—before they were seen. Many had to take two or three buses to reach the hospital, usually without help from anyone. Californians often speak of their compassion and their deep concern for their fellow man. In my experience, Los Angeles limits its compassion to those who can afford to pay for it.

On several occasions, distinguished visitors joined me at these outpatient clinics. Most were horrified by the conditions but amazed by our ability to help our patients. Maurice Muller, the distinguished Swiss surgeon, was especially shocked by our surroundings. Muller himself worked in a most sophisticated and refined environment. He could not believe what he was seeing in California, the golden heart of the wealthiest nation in the world. On the other hand, I know that he was extremely impressed with our clinical results.

It is hard to believe that such a deplorable situation exists in the United States. When I arrived in Los Angeles, I committed myself to do something about the medieval state of the facilities and the totally inadequate staffing. I intended to do everything possible and whatever was necessary to see that at least the orthopaedic program would become more humane and effective. My efforts proved to be an exercise in futility. Those in a position to help could not or would not make the effort. They routinely excused their inaction because of the lack of financial support. They were right. The institution's budget did not provide sufficient funds to implement the necessary changes

When I tackled that problem, I discovered an impenetrable wall of professional bureaucrats backed up by a second barrier composed of professional politicians. Behind them stood the wealthy taxpayers of Los Angeles County, an extraordinary group of powerful, influential, and wealthy lawyers, physicians, entertainers, industrialists, and financiers. I recognize, however, that to a great extent the health care situation in Los Angeles had become worse as a result of recent federal and state mandates that penalized southern California in a major and disproportional way.

I had encountered the same situation in Miami in the 1960s. The conditions at Jackson Memorial had been as bad as those at LAC-USC. In Miami, however, the community responded dramatically and effectively to the challenge. A local group of wealthy philanthropists decided that it was time for a change. They established a trust that took over the administration and management of Jackson Memorial and converted it into a modern institution. (Southern California also has many philanthropists. They do many good works. They help the California condor, save whales, and rescue retired circus elephants and lions. They just are not particularly interested in poor people.)

Even after its total renovation, Miami's Jackson Memorial Hospital remained the place where the indigent received medical care. They filled the emergency wards and the outpatient clinics. In southern California, wealthy community leaders built themselves their own hospitals so they would not have to encounter public patients. In Miami, Jackson Memorial became a facility where public patients and well-insured private patients alike all came for surgery and medical treatment.

During my days at Jackson Memorial, I performed hip replacement surgery on many private patients from throughout the United States and abroad. They included trustees of the University of Miami and leaders of the local and state community. Today, Jackson Memorial Hospital still ranks among the best medical centers in the United States. The hospital is again becoming an institution that primarily serves indigent patients. Many private patients now seek and receive care at other nearby facilities. But Jackson Memorial remains a clean, well-staffed, up-to-date facility.

In the meantime, LAC-USC Medical Center in Los Angeles remains the crowded and underdeveloped hospital it has been for the past seventy or eighty years. Its leaders remain unwilling or unable to make it a respectable institution. Instead, the USC trustees chose to form a partnership with a for-profit medical corporation to build a university hospital that would attract well-paying private, international, and insured patients.

During my earliest days in Los Angeles, I once insisted that the medical director and the CEO of the hospital join me on a visit to the orthopaedic wards and the outpatient facilities. They claimed to be horrified by what they saw, expressed deep concern over the situation, and promised to act. I was new to southern California. I did not yet recognize the typically meaningless bureaucratic jargon. I now suspect that the two of them went back to their offices and enjoyed a hearty laugh about the political naïveté of their new chief of orthopaedics.

At my first meeting of the operating room committee, I spoke about the urgent need to cut waiting times for fracture patients. I placed most of the blame on lack of supervision, an insufficient number of operating rooms, and lack of personnel. The operating room supervisor took my remarks as a personal affront. She wrote a lengthy letter to the administration in which she stated that I perceived her as being incompetent. The medical director immediately sent me a copy of the letter and demanded my response. I sent a brief note to the complaining nurse supervisor, in which I complimented her for being "so perceptive."

The medical director called me to his office and demanded that I apologize to the "injured supervisor." I refused. He then told me that the incident would be recorded on my personal file. I did not consider this to be an overpowering threat. The experience taught me a great deal about the USC bureaucracy.

Throughout my tenure at USC, the hospital, university, and county government in Los Angeles remained unconcerned about the deplorable conditions at their own public hospital. I routinely fought to improve working conditions for the interns and residents, to increase staffing, to add beds, or at the least to set aside one operating room for patients with open fractures who were waiting for surgery.

On one occasion, I thought that I had finally won the battle. In the midst of a particularly grave crisis, the hospital CEO announced that one operating room was to be assigned "exclusively for orthopaedics, and to be functional twenty-four hours per day, seven days a week." We rejoiced at the news of this long-awaited development. Our celebration proved to be premature. We were able to keep the room for our exclusive use for little more than twenty-four hours. The next day, we were told that there were not enough nurses on duty, and other departments would use the room while we waited. The day after that, we were told that most of the hospital's anesthesiologists were attending an important conference. Those remaining in the hospital were swamped with more urgent cases. We got the message. The residents later took to referring to the administration's promise as "the twenty four hour solution," a parody of the title of a best-selling novel featuring Sherlock Holmes.

During all my years in Miami, I encountered only one malpractice suit. The hospital and insurance company stood behind me. After lengthy preparation for litigation, the suit was dismissed. In Los Angeles my first and only experience with malpractice law began with a subpoena. A former county prisoner had sustained a fracture of his wrist. That wrist was now badly deformed, and the former prisoner regarded this bad clinical result as the result of malpractice. The plaintiff's attorney called me to the stand and raised many embarrassing questions. I found myself explaining that what appeared on the surface to be substandard practice was actually routine procedure at LAC. I explained that the hospital did not have sufficient personnel to transport X rays of the two hundred patients seen daily in the orthopaedic clinic, but that all of our clinicians did the best they could, working without ready access to the X rays.

The jury found the hospital guilty of malpractice. At first, I was extremely angry. The clinic staff had done everything possible under the circumstances to provide good care. Only later did I accept that "the circumstances" did not provide an adequate defense. In fact, what we had done to the patient could legitimately be considered malpractice. The jury's verdict was correct and just. Unfortunately, it was directed toward the wrong people. The hospital and hospital staff moved mountains to accomplish miracles every day. They simply did not have the resources to move thousands of X rays. They chose to use their limited resources in other, more critical ways. The malpractice award should, more justly, have been directed against the voters and board of supervisors of Los Angeles County.

In fact, LAC-USC Medical Center faces a staggering level of medical malpractice claims. A large number of attorneys, many working full time for the city, review the chronic avalanche of malpractice suits. In most instances, the city settles out of court. These suits, many of them fully justified, drain millions of dollars from the county economy. I believe that the county could save a great deal of money by diverting the budget allocations that support this legal staff and finance the malpractice settlements to renovating and adequately staffing LAC-USC hospital. The taxpayers should demand an accounting and better use of their tax money. Instead, the politicians and administrators seem to prefer allowing the injurious and expensive chaos to perpetuate itself.

chapter 35.
life gets more complicated

"The game ain't over till it's over."

—Yogi Berra

"When I first wrote it, only God and I knew what It meant. Today, only God knows."

—Georg Wilhelm Friedrich Hegel

"Only crime and the criminal, it is true, confront the perplexity of radical evil; but only the hypocrite is really rotten to the core."

—H. Arendt

While USC was developing plans to build the new University Hospital, the administration appointed a new dean of the medical school. Most of my colleagues and I greeted the news with pleasure. The new man had once been an administrator at LAC-USC Medical Center. He was intimately familiar with our problems. He would be returning to Los Angeles from the University of Massachusetts, where he had been serving as vice-chancellor of the medical school. He appeared to offer an ideal combination of intelligence, experience, pragmatism, and values.

The new dean visited our research laboratory and held meetings with the entire full-time department faculty. He repeatedly congratulated us for doing an outstanding job. He listened to the complaints about the precarious situation at the county hospital and expressed a great deal of enthusiasm about the success of our private practice program.

During the ensuing months, as the medical school became more deeply involved in planning the construction of University Hospital, he repeatedly used orthopaedics as his model of a successful and well-managed department and private practice. I took great pleasure and pride in his attention and comments. My spirits and expectations soared to new heights, far beyond anything I had experienced since the day before I had started work at USC.

Planning for the new University Hospital also seemed to be progressing beautifully. After lengthy discussion, the university contracted with National Medical Enterprises (NME) to build and manage the new institution. University Hospital would be a for-profit facility. It would be located just a few blocks away from the medical school campus and the LAC-USC Medical Center. My only concern stemmed from the philosophy of the basic agreement. NME would provide the necessary funding for construction. The medical school would have "adequate representation" but not a majority vote on the University Hospital board of directors. I wondered if this would open the door for possible future conflicts between "good business" and "good medicine."

My concerns seem to have been accurate. NME was found guilty of a number of fraudulent activities in some of its institutions. NME merged eventually with TENET, another major for-profit chain of hospitals. At the time this book is being written, TENET is confronting litigation regarding possible fraudulent dealings of several physicians.

I met frequently with NME executives to discuss my department's obligations, plans, and dreams. They appeared to be supportive, and I developed a constructive relationship with the person responsible for working out and implementing the University Hospital master plan. He admired the private practice plans that I had learned in Miami and instituted at USC. He believed that we would be able to build a smooth, efficient partnership between my department at the university and the new hospital.

Throughout the discussions concerning the new hospital, we continued to insist that the department of orthopaedics would maintain its strong presence at Orthopaedic Hospital. I suggested that the orthopaedics faculty should admit patients to both Orthopedic and University Hospitals. I also recommended that we transfer the seat of the department to the new hospital.

I soon learned that the dean was not happy with all of our proposed arrangements with NME. His leading concerns involved questions of funding the new faculty who had not yet established private practices but would be needed to cover the full range of the new hospital's activities. Orthopaedists who participated in USC's private practice program paid a percentage of the practice incomes to the university and the department to cover use of facilities and their share of administrative overhead. The dean insisted that our existing faculty would have to increase this payment in order to subsidize the creation of new programs.

We then learned that the dean was offering enormous salaries to recruit faculty for other departments from other medical schools. He was essentially demanding that the current orthopaedics faculty accept a lower income in order to subsidize the high salaries he wanted to pay other departments. As you can imagine, the orthopaedics faculty found this arrangement unacceptable. We met with the dean on several occasions, but my faculty found little satisfaction in his responses. I then met with the dean and told him that if he did not assuage their concerns, we could face an exodus of our most valuable and most productive faculty members—especially those who were producing the most income for the university.

The level of tension between the dean and the orthopaedics faculty continued to escalate. As tensions increased, my faculty hired an attorney and brought him to their next meeting. The dean expressed his objections to their "adversarial attitude" but did nothing to soften his stand. A few weeks later, two key department members resigned. Other resignations soon followed.

Faced with this new reality, the dean responded with unusual speed. Instead of restructuring his proposal, he attacked the department. He announced that in light of the imminent opening of the new hospital, he wanted to review all USC medical school departments. He would start with a full-scale outside review of orthopaedics.

I found this decision personally insulting and professionally embarrassing. I might have been more distressed except that just a few weeks earlier, I had been elected second vice president of the American Academy of Orthopaedic Surgeons. In two years, I would become president of the academy, my specialty's largest and most prestigious professional society. My own university was about to subject me to my third review in less than five years at the same time that the American Academy of Orthopaedic Surgeons had selected me to lead its national operations.

The dean wanted a blue-ribbon panel of the nation's most respected academic orthopaedists to conduct the review. He selected Dr. Philip Wilson, professor and chief of orthopaedics at Cornell University's Medical School and director of the Hospital for Special

Surgery in New York; Dr. Clement Sledge, who held a comparable position at Harvard and directed the Brigham and Women's Hospital in Boston; Dr. Reginald Cooper, the professor and chief of orthopaedics at the University of Iowa; and Dr. James Urbaniak, professor and chairman of orthopaedics at Duke University.

It would be impossible to identify a more respected, more influential, or more powerful group of orthopaedists. The review committee came to Los Angeles and spent three days looking at the program. They met with faculty, students, and staff at the medical school and at all of the affiliated hospitals. My predecessor had his chance at performing his criticism of me in front of a distinguished audience. The reviewers also met with me. I gave them a summary of the status of the department. It included a statement of our accomplishments as well as a description of the difficulties that we were encountering. In our brief but cordial meeting, the committee gave me no hint of their inclination or probable findings.

Wilson, Sledge, Cooper, and Urbaniak submitted their unanimous evaluation to the dean a few days later, but the dean did not provide a copy for the department. Instead, he met privately with other senior administrators. He released the review to the department only when faced with repeated requests from the entire orthopaedic faculty.

In their report, the reviewers spoke in extremely flattering terms about the progress that the orthopaedics department at USC had made under my chairmanship. They identified the remarkable increase in the size of the faculty and improvements in the residency program. They also complimented our successful private practice plan, and stated that they were appalled by the minimal support that the department had received from the medical school and from the university as a whole.

In the wake of the review, the relationship between university administration, NME, and me entered an era of smooth sailing. After years of continuous struggles and constant battles, it seemed that my last few years before mandatory retirement would be friction-free and productive. I found that prospect especially pleasing because of the approach of my year as president of the academy. That year, I knew, would require extensive travel. The affairs of the academy would require much of my time and attention. Under the best of circumstances, it would be difficult to manage my medical school department and the relationships with the five affiliated hospitals while leading the academy.

My vision of calm seas vanished when the dean told me that Bob Kerlan, the local sports medicine man, had just offered to endow a chair in sports medicine. Kerlan and I had never enjoyed each other's company. Our enmity stretched back almost to my arrival in Los Angeles. Despite my objections to his businesslike philosophy and approach to medicine, I regularly rotated orthopaedics residents through his practice, which had become one of the world's most profitable medical enterprises. Ever since my arrival at USC, I had sought to build a sports medicine division within my department. So far, Kerlan had managed to block or derail all of my efforts in that regard. He had also continuously sought my removal from the department chair, and I had managed to defuse those efforts.

We had established a relationship that allowed both of us to function, but only at arm's length. His offer to endow a chair of sports medicine in my department threatened to upset this precarious balance. He knew that his offer of $1 million would bring the dean to his side in any dispute. I felt that it was ethically and philosophically important to maintain as much distance as possible between Kerlan and the medical school.

The details of our escalating dispute would not be so interesting had the stakes not seemed so high to both of us. We squared off not just as personal adversaries but as representatives of two opposing philosophies of medicine. Kerlan viewed me as the spokesperson of an old and out-of-date philosophy that prevented him from marketing himself and practicing medicine according to his own standards and values. I saw him as the personification of the new era of medical business.

As Kerlan anticipated, the dean found his offer of an endowed chair to be almost irresistible. I countered by informing the dean that NME was extremely interested in establishing a division of sports medicine at the new hospital. I pointed out that a division of sports medicine would generate substantial income for the university—far more income, in fact, than would be generated by Kerlan's gift.

The dean then promised to set up a meeting with Kerlan, at which we could work out our differences and work together, in the best interests of Los Angeles, the university, and the University Hospital. I agreed to the meeting, but as I expected, several months passed without it taking place. When I shared my concerns with NME, a senior corporate executive told me to go ahead and develop plans for my own sports medicine division. If the dean chose not to support me, NME would subsidize the division itself.

I then met with the director of the athletic department at USC to discuss my ideas for the new sports medicine division. The university's athletic department would be a golden client for any orthopaedic practice. The high profile position as physician to USC's outstanding "Trojan" athletic teams promised great status within the Los Angeles community and throughout the nation.

When I had tried to form my own sports medicine department several years before, the director of athletics had resisted us. He had expressed his opinion that our full-time orthopaedic faculty lacked sufficient experience in the physiology of athletes. This time, I was better prepared to win his support. I showed him how the new University Hospital division of sports medicine could use the services of the doctor who already treated his athletes. I suggested that NME would be happy to hire an orthopaedist of worldwide reputation in sports medicine to become director of the division. His athletes would have the best of both worlds—top-notch physicians, and brand-new state-of-the art facilities.

Under those circumstances, he said, the USC athletic department would be interested in working with us. He could see that it made a great deal of sense to have USC's athletes treated at a university medical center, especially if they could continue to relate to the doctors he had chosen. I was delighted by his response, and immediately brought the dean up to date on the progress of my negotiations with NME and the USC department of athletics. The dean offered his complete support. With his approval, I recruited Dr. Bill Clancy, the chief of sports medicine at the University of Wisconsin, to become chief of the new sports medicine division at USC University Hospital.

Suddenly, Bob Kerlan, who had not been able to find time to meet with the dean and me in the previous six months, discovered an opening in his calendar. I arrived at the appointed time. Kerlan and the dean were already deep in conversation. Kerlan then told me that he had decided that a million-dollar endowment was not adequate. He had concluded that he would donate $3 million to endow a chair in sports medicine.

I responded that I was delighted with his interest and generosity. I then turned to the dean and offered to initiate a search for someone to fill the new endowed professorship. Kerlan instantly exploded in anger at my remark. It was his $3 million, he said. He would name the recipient. I told him that no university in the world could accept money under those conditions. I would, however, be grateful if he agreed to participate in the search. I told him that he was welcome to serve as a member of the search committee. He responded that my offer was totally ridiculous, and the meeting ended in disarray. We could agree only on a date when we could meet again.

As I left, I requested a private meeting with the dean the next day. At that meeting, the dean pretended that he had been surprised by Kerlan's $3 million proposal. He told me that he was delighted with the progress that I had made, and that everyone concerned in the negotiations was delighted with Clancy's interest in USC. He encouraged me to continue my discussions with Clancy and to do everything possible to convince him to join us in California. He suggested that I leave future negotiations with Kerlan up to him. "Don't worry, Gus. I can handle Bob Kerlan."

Despite his protestations to the contrary, I suddenly felt that I was again losing my chance to establish a sports medicine division in my department. I elected to press the dean to go along with my plans and to convince him that I was moving in the right direction. I began by commenting to the dean that I hoped he had been able to read between the lines and had realized that Kerlan had no plans to endow a chair. Kerlan was simply playing an old game that the two of us had already played out several times before. I told him that Kerlan would do anything necessary to prevent the medical school from developing its own strong sports medicine program.

I pleaded with the dean and urged him in the strongest possible language not to surrender to Kerlan's conditions. If he allowed Kerlan to "buy" a chair and fill it with his own handpicked division chief, we would all be permanently disgraced in academic circles. "USC has been here for a long time and it will be here long after you and I have left this world. I have been in academic medicine for a long time and have maintained the highest possible professional and ethical standards. I have insisted that everyone in the department, including residents and students, do likewise. Allowing Kerlan to make this appointment will irreparably tarnish all of us."

I predicted that once the dean allowed Kerlan to interfere with our plans with NME and force us to break off negotiations with Clancy, the money would disappear. That meeting would prove to have long-term results. I learned the next day just how seriously I had underestimated Bob Kerlan's influence and the buying power of $3 million (at least at USC).

The following afternoon, I learned from the resident who was currently rotating trough Kerlan's office that the university had approved a long-term arrangement. Effective immediately, Kerlan's practice would assume exclusive responsibility for the care of all varsity athletes at USC. I rushed to the dean's office to confront him and to hear him either confirm or deny the rumor. He confirmed it. He said that the "highest levels of the university administration" had met with Kerlan the night before. They had, in fact, approved a contract making Kerlan and his group responsible for all orthopaedic care required by the athletic department. The dean indicated that the issue was extremely delicate and ordered me to support him.

He emphasized the importance of moving ahead, claimed that he agreed with my position but demanded my cooperation. I said that I had lost the battle but did not have to lose my self-respect, even though I did not have the power to undo what he and the senior administration had forged. I continued to express my strong objections. The dean insisted that neither of us had any choice. He repeated that I "had to cooperate" with him and with Kerlan. If I denied them my cooperation, he said, he would have no choice and would be forced to dismiss me from the chairmanship of the department.

It is possible that our meeting was not conducted as a calm academic dialogue. I suspect that both of us began to express our opinions, perhaps, using words that could have been chosen with more deliberation. I responded that I was aware that he had the authority to dismiss me as chairman of the department. I also suggested that if he really believed that he "had no choice," and wished to behave ethically when faced with unacceptable decisions by superior authorities, that he could start with the works of Thoreau and Gandhi in order to learn about the meaning of civil disobedience.

When I left the dean's office, I knew that Kerlan would renew his efforts to have me removed as department chairman, and that he would now, most likely, enjoy the full support of the dean. In anticipation of coming events, I requested an appointment with the provost of the university. At that meeting, I described the recent chain of events and my conversations with the dean. I restated my opposition to "selling a chair." I made clear my willingness to continue to fight the good fight.

The provost protested that he had heard nothing of these events. I responded that according to the dean, the decision had been made by the highest levels of the university administration. I expressed my firm belief that the "highest levels of the university administration" included the office of the provost.

Amazingly, the university did not seek retribution and chose not to dismiss me as department chairman. I suspect that someone looked at the relevant records, noted that I was sixty-four years old, and realized that they could just wait me out. In any case, the storm subsided as quickly as it had begun. NME dropped its plans to fund a division of sports medicine. And I returned to my work, which included increasing commitments to the academy.

I was about to begin my tour of duty as president of the academy and was traveling almost constantly. My agenda for the rest of the year called for my being absent from Los Angeles for a few days every week for the rest of the year. My relationship with the dean had totally collapsed, as had all illusions of support from the "highest levels of the university administration." I realized that if I tried to be chairman of a department in turmoil and, at the same time, preside over a major national organization, I was unlikely to do either job well.

I knew that the university had decided to wait me out. In another ten months, I would reach my sixty-fifth birthday. Tradition called for me to step down as department chair at that age. (I suspected that the "highest levels of the university administration" would be anxious to assist tradition, if necessary.) But after more than a decade of constant battles, I finally understood how the great fighter Roberto Duran must have felt toward the end of his remarkable career. Reluctantly, I decided that it was time to say, "*No mas. No mas.*" I decided not to wait, and chose instead to resign as chairman of the department of orthopaedics at USC. I would continue to serve as a professor in the department, continue to treat patients, and continue my research projects that were still under way in the laboratories at Orthopedic Hospital. I would devote the balance of my time to the affairs of the academy.

Accordingly, I sent my letter of resignation to the dean. To my knowledge, it was the first time in orthopaedic academic history that a sitting department chair chose to resign while serving as president of his discipline's leading professional association. My resignation did not go unnoticed by the academic community or by the "highest levels of university administration." Less than a week later, the dean was relieved of his responsibilities. I have no idea if the two events were related. Rumors had circulated that the dean was on his way out.

Bob Kerlan died five years later. He never endowed a chair at USC.

My decision to free myself of departmental responsibilities before assuming the academy leadership soon proved to have been correct. I quickly discovered that properly discharging all the duties of academy president would be a great deal more demanding that I had anticipated. I traveled often to Chicago, where the academy head-quarters was located. I also attended a large number of meetings held by various councils of the organization, meetings of many of the state orthopaedic societies, and meetings of subspecialty societies. I even traveled to Washington to testify before Congress on issues related to increasing the funding for research on disorders of the muscu-loskeletal system.

I represented the United States at national academy meetings in Christchurch, New Zealand; Bristol, England; Toronto, Canada; and Johannesburg, South Africa. I also spent one week in Israel, lecturing at three medical schools. Altogether, I was away from home more than two hundred days during my presidential year. I could never have undertaken that schedule and represented the academy well, so frequently, or in so many places, if I had continued as department chair at USC.

One of the duties as president of the academy was to place my sig-nature on the diplomas given to the nearly three hundred new members who joined our ranks during the year. The executive secretary of the organization had requested my signature in advance in order to prepare the usual stamp. Several months after the distribution of the certificates, one member asked me why my signature was not on his diploma. He showed it to me. My signature was there, but had been stamped back-wards and upside-down. My handwriting is so bad that no one else had noticed the mistake. The academy promised to issue new certificates, but that never happened. The executive director later suggested that the 1992 academy diplomas would become collectors' items.

When I completed my presidential year with the academy, I returned to my daily activities and devoted more time than ever to the research program at the Orthopedic Hospital. Many of the same people who had once opposed all of my suggestions now welcomed them. We made many changes in the research program. (Those changes eventually proved inadequate to secure the future of the institution. As I complete this manuscript, Orthopaedic Hospital is moving to a new facility on the campus of UCLA, the cross-town rival of USC.)

I continued to attend the Sunday morning pass-on rounds and the fracture clinic for the indigent at the County Hospital. I still had three more years on the board of directors of the academy. I continued traveling to Chicago for board meetings, and accepted many invitations to serve as visiting professor or as a guest speaker.

On a few occasions, I was able to combine the business trips with pleasure. My wife, Barbara, accompanied me on several trips, especially my trips as academy president to represent the United States at meetings of English-speaking organizations. I took Gus Jr. with me to South Africa when I represented the United States at the meeting of that country's orthopaedic organization. We took a few days off to tour the country and enjoy Kruger National Park. I relished the opportunity to be with Gus for a few days.

I took Greg, our younger son who was then about fifteen, with me when I traveled to Australia. The meeting was held in a ski resort, and it was the first time that I had an opportunity to see Greg on skis. Greg and I also spent several days at Heron Island, a magnificent resort on the Great Barrier Reef. Greg and I swam together in the clear waters of the Coral Sea. Those moments in the company of the children are unforgettable. I only wished I had had more of them.

I took our daughter, Janette, then about twenty, to Spain, where I had the opportunity to introduce her to El Prado Museum, observe the magnificent Valley of the Fallen, and spend two days walking around historic Toledo. From Madrid, we flew to Barcelona, where she could appreciate the other side of urban Spain, the land of the proud Catalans. In Barcelona, I shared with her my experiences during my first visit to that ancient city, when I had been the guest of Dr. Joseph Trueta.

Trueta was one of the great stars of modern orthopaedics. A native Catalan and already an outstanding doctor, he fought against the fascists during the Spanish Civil War of the 1930s. During that conflict, Trueta described methods of treatment of war injuries that dramatically improved outcomes. Toward the end of the war, Trueta fled to England, where he eventually became professor and chief of orthopaedics at Oxford University.

During my visit with him, he shared many of his medical and personal experiences in Spain and the United Kingdom. I learned from him about the difficult times he experienced in Oxford and the unfriendly reception he received from the British establishment. The British orthopaedic establishment severely criticized most of his novel ideas concerning the treatment of war injuries, then adopted them during World War II. I still remember the pleasure with which he described the day when Watson-Jones, Trueta's opponent for many years, publicly acknowledged his contributions. A few years later, Trueta came to Miami as my invited visiting professor. We spent several hours discussing medicine as well as philosophy, history, and world affairs. He had a profound impact on my thinking in a number of areas.

chapter 36.
contemplating life in scotland

"Greed is good, greed is great."

Gordon Gecko, in the movie *Wall Street*

In the summer of 1993, as my tenure at USC entered its final phase, I received a call from Dr. Clement Sledge, professor at Harvard and chief of orthopaedics at the Brigham and Women's Hospital in Boston. He was calling to tell me that he had submitted my name as a candidate for the position of chief of orthopaedics at a new hospital located in Clydebank, Scotland, a suburb of Glasgow. Harvard University and several of its affiliated financial institutions were behind the project. They intended to make the hospital "the Mayo Clinic of Europe." The chief of orthopaedics would have an academic position at Glasgow University Medical School, one of the oldest and most prestigious institutions in the Western world. The new chief would be ideally situated to develop a first-class residency program, with research opportunities at both the hospital and the medical school.

My first reaction to Sledge's suggestion was negative: "For God's sake, what makes you think that I would consider moving from sunny California to Scotland?"

Sledge responded in his always friendly, always witty way: "Gus, never turn down a job that has not been offered to you."

I laughed and asked him to tell the new hospital's officials to contact me. Sledge then told me that he was the chairman of the search committee. Two other professors at Harvard and David Hamblen, the professor at Glasgow University, were the other members.

I did not take the offer seriously at first, but the more I learned about it, the more fascinating it became. The £180-million medical center hospital was nearing completion. It would be exclusively devoted to cardiovascular surgery, oncological surgery, and orthopaedic surgery. It would be closely affiliated with Harvard and

Glasgow universities. Patients from Europe and the Middle East would no longer have to travel all the way to the United States to be treated by world-class surgeons. They could, instead, travel by air ambulance to Glasgow, where they and their families would be met by luxury ambulance for the trip to Clydebank. They would be housed in the new five-star hotel, managed by Marriott, next door to the hospital.

The venture was being funded by the Harvard Foundation, leading venture capitalists throughout the United States, and a consortium of European banks. The new corporation, Health Care International, had all the investors it could handle. More investors were waiting in line to provide any additional capital that was needed.

As chief of orthopaedics, I would work alongside the most distinguished surgeons. They would pay whatever salary was needed to attract the best people available to staff the new institution. It all sounded too good to be true. I decided to accept the search committee's invitation to visit the hospital.

Glasgow is the largest city in Scotland. It is an industrial city—a blue-collar working-class city that lacks the charm of Edinburgh, the only other city in Scotland that I had visited. The climate is dreary, at best, most of the year. It can be brutally cold in winter. I arrived in Glasgow in late summer, when the climate is at its best. The day I arrived, clouds filled the sky. The air was chilled and dampened with a heavy mist. Shortly after I left the airport, it started to rain. I reminded myself that I was not looking for a retirement resort, but seeking a challenging new professional opportunity.

That night at dinner, I met several of the key people at the hospital. The medical director, Dr. Larry Hollier, had served as chief of surgery at the Oschner Clinic in New Orleans; he had been chief of vascular surgery at the Mayo Clinic before that. Rose Mary Mackey, the person in charge of marketing for the new hospital, had worked in the marketing department at Michael Debakey's institution in Texas; her husband, Dr. Irving Kroacoff, was the new chief of medical oncology. These were all highly accomplished people who were filled with enthusiasm for the new venture.

As we enjoyed our appetizers, Dr. Hollier told me that the project had started as the dream of two Harvard Medical School physicians, Dr. Raphael Levey and Dr. Angelo Eraklis. They had received initial funding from the Harvard Foundation and the Scottish Development

Agency. Staff at Harvard Management had created the business plan. The city of Glasgow had provided land along the River Clyde, at a site once occupied by famous shipwrights. Glasgow University was looking forward to the arrival of the U.S. surgeons and welcomed the opportunity for affiliation with Harvard University. Dr. Hollier did not tell me that the Harvard team had decided to build in Scotland only after the Irish government had rejected their proposal.

As we enjoyed our soup, Dr. Hollier told me that the government-financed Scottish Development Agency viewed the project as a potential boost to the depressed local economy. The agency anticipated that hundreds, possibly thousands, of local citizens would be employed at the hospital, the hotel, and their support industries. Thousands of wealthy foreigners would be coming for treatment. They would be bringing their families, and spending thousands of pounds in foreign exchange.

Then came the main course. Dr. Hollier told me that the directors of the three departments, as well as the chiefs of the other ancillary medical and surgical departments, were widely recognized professors from various medical schools in the United States. The vice-chairman of radiology at the Massachusetts General Hospital in Boston, Dr. Reggie Green, was already onboard, along with three young radiologists from Harvard, who would be spending two years at the Scottish hospital. The radiologists were just the first of a long list of exchange physicians who would eventually travel between the two institutions. Dr. Gary Lowery, a heart surgeon who had worked closely with Dr. Debaky in Houston, was expected on-site within the next two months.

The plans for the hospital's administrative structure were even more exciting. The hospital was to become the first paperless hospital in the world. Every conceivable aspect of the organization was completely computerized. We would maintain no paper medical records at all. Laboratory reports, anesthesia records, medication orders, and treatment orders would all be electronic. X rays would be available on-demand through the computer, with no need to transport films around the hospital.

Patients throughout Europe and the Middle East were anxiously awaiting completion of the new institution. Extensive market research allegedly conducted in several countries led the administration to anticipate that approximately five thousand patients would be admitted to the hospital by the end of the year. Orthopaedics, "probably the program that had received the most attention," could anticipate performing a thousand joint replacement surgeries. I was told that the first priority of the new chief of orthopaedics would be recruitment of a top-quality, world-class staff. They suggested that I start thinking about whom I would like to hire. I would be able to offer my candidates the prospect of academic appointment at Glasgow University. Money, of course, was no object.

Negotiations were under way to finalize the establishment of residency and fellowship programs in the key three departments. Students from Harvard University, Glasgow University, and other world-class medical colleges would be rotating through the hospital for various periods. All academic programs would be operational within a short time. They were also working on a formal affiliation with Harvard. The plan called for the three department chiefs to hold joint appointments at Glasgow, one of the most prestigious medical schools in Europe, and Harvard, the best medical school in the United States.

By the time we finished dessert, I knew that the next five years of my life would be spent in Glasgow. Everyone at the table shared a remarkable energy and enthusiasm that seemed overwhelmingly contagious. They were all sure that the hospital was a winning proposition that was pure gold—in every sense of the word. In fact, the hospital was offering an extremely generous compensation package. Combined with the low cost of living in Glasgow, Barbara and I would be able to save money for my retirement while living very comfortably.

Staff physicians and surgeons were to be fully salaried employees of the hospital. While there would be no private practices, our salaries would be extremely generous; Dr. Hollier offered me $500,000 plus a generous bonus. The bonuses were to be paid in monthly installments, beginning the day I joined the staff. Dr. Hollier showed me a photograph of an old castle that he had bought, and was in the process of remodeling in order to add the most modern conveniences. Life was to be wonderful in such a picturesque community. It was all too good to be true.

The next day I visited the construction site. As I entered the building, I found myself in a huge lobby that resembled the atrium of a modern Las Vegas or Miami Beach hotel. To the right of the lobby was a five-star hotel that would be operated by the Marriott Corporation. The working spaces of the hospital proved just as impressive. The operating rooms were enormous; so were the laboratories and radiology suites. Evidence of the most modern, cutting-edge technology was everywhere. I could not have imagined or asked for anything better. Health Care International (HCI), the corporation responsible for bringing this dream to life, had clearly committed itself to matching the best people with the best facility in the world.

Jim Wiczai, the CEO of the new hospital, had been CEO of Brigham and Women's Hospital in Boston. As he showed me around the luxurious operating rooms and other facilities, he reinforced many of the things that Dr. Hollier and the others had said to me at the dinner the night before. Wiczai was a strong leader and inspirational recruiter. He was absolutely convinced that HCI would revolutionize international health care delivery. He was certain that the hospital would be inundated by a flood of patients from the moment it opened its doors. In fact, he strongly suggested that if I were to be chosen for the job, I should move to Scotland early in February to start preparing for the March 1994 opening.

While I was talking to Wiczai, Larry Hollier joined us. He told us that he had just that moment completed negotiations with important officials in Egypt. The Egyptian Defense Department had just agreed that HCI would handle all their needs for cardiovascular surgery. The contract between HCI and the Egyptian government would bring one thousand patients a year to Glasgow. It was all beginning!

When I left the hospital, I contracted with a taxi driver to take me on a tour of Clydebank and Glasgow. He talked as he drove me around. I suppose he was telling me all about the city, but I could hardly understand a word he said. I found his heavy Scottish brogue to be almost incomprehensible. That should not have surprised me. I have always had trouble understanding some dialects of English. I had already encountered difficulties with Irish and Welsh accents. Now I was having difficulty with Scottish. Perhaps that is because I was raised speaking Spanish, and English is my second language. Native-born Americans seem to find it easier to tune their ears to those dialects.

The next day provided remarkable relief from the unpleasant climate. Indeed, the remarkably bright sunshine seemed a cheerful omen. I took advantage of it to tour the countryside, which featured pastoral landscapes that seemed almost to be the creations of a talented nineteenth-century postcard artist. I found myself enchanted by the narrow, winding roads and the green, lush grass around the hilly old towns. I was falling in love with Scotland even before the job had been offered to me.

I flew back to the United States, hoping that I would be invited to return for a second interview. Barbara found less cause for optimism in the prospect of our moving to Glasgow. She had never enjoyed living in Los Angeles. On the flight home, I had convinced myself that she would love Scotland. Instead, she found the thought of moving so far from her children to be deeply depressing.

A few weeks later, I was invited to return and the two of us visited Glasgow together. Happily, the weather proved delightful, and she, too, fell in love with the Scottish people and with the countryside. She even began looking around for a house to buy, when (and if) HCI decided to offer me the position. I assured her that I would accept their offer. In fact, by then, my only concern was the possibility that the position might be given to someone else.

HCI offered me the post the next day, and I immediately accepted. My title would be chief of orthopaedics. They agreed with my recommendation to name the new department "orthopaedics and musculoskeletal disorders." I had first envisioned establishing a department with that title at the University of Miami many years earlier. It all seemed to be the perfect capstone for my career.

In accordance with the requests of hospital executives, I immediately began to identify people to bring to Glasgow for personal interviews. Barbara and I also began a serious round of house hunting. We selected a hundred-year-old house about ten miles southwest of Glasgow, near the village of Kilmacolm. The picturesque main street was only three blocks long. It featured one restaurant, a pub, and a few stores. The local barbershop and movie theater were in the next village, just down the road.

An attractive yard with a lovely garden surrounded the three-story half-timbered house, which had more than enough room to accommodate my three-thousand-book library. We had the house fully inspected by a local official, who gave it a glowing report. The price seemed high, but we expected it to be a good investment. We believed that we would be spending the rest of our lives in that house. Our mortgage, however, extended for only five years—the length of my contract with HCI.

Curiously, that contract had not yet arrived. My concern over the incomplete paperwork increased as the end of my contract with USC approached. Mr. Yick, the assistant administrator at HCI, assured me that there were no difficulties. The contract was in process. He would send it as soon as it was completed. "We are so busy taking care of so many last minute things that we are behind finalizing the written contracts," he said. I had no reason to doubt his words. I knew that I was dealing with people of impeccable professionalism and ethics.

Finally, we completed packing our belongings. Everything was ready for shipment to Scotland. In only a few days, I would receive my last paycheck from USC. I had not yet seen a contract from HCI. I was quite angry when I called Scotland and expressed my frustration. Once again, the administrators assured me that there were no problems. My contract would be waiting for me on my new desk in my new office. Reluctantly, I agreed.

Because of the depressed California real estate market, our Glendale home did not sell for several months. We ended up selling it for less than we had paid thirteen years before. I sent a form letter to all of my patients, notifying them of my new address. I also added a brief hand-written note to each. I had done the same thing fifteen years earlier, when I had moved from Miami to USC.

Jim Luck, the CEO at Orthopedic Hospital, hosted a small farewell dinner for us, where we reminisced about my stormy tenure in Los Angeles. He also held a cocktail party in my honor in the hospital dining room.

At the LAC-USC Medical Center, the new chairman hosted a farewell reception in our honor. He compressed every appropriate platitude into a brief speech, and presented me with a small wooden souvenir that he had probably purchased at the hospital's gift shop moments before the presentation. I dropped it in the trash bin as I left. Then I released all of our possessions for shipment to Scotland, and Barbara and I boarded the plane for Glasgow.

chapter 37.
in the land of adam smith

"The grand lesson of History is that nobody learns the lessons of History."
—Georg Wilhelm Friedrich Hegel

"—We were once in love. Do you remember me?
—Ah, I think I remember you.
—What do you rmember?
—I don't remember."

Anonymous

Barbara and I arrived in Glasgow on January 31, 1994. I reported to the hospital the next morning. I had last visited the hospital on a lovely summer day. When I returned, the weather was cold and rainy. The midwinter days at these northern latitudes provide only a few hours of cold sunlight. Unfortunately, the same would prove true of HCI and its Glasgow hospital. In mid-September 1994, commercial investors led by the French bank *Credit Lyonais* and the Dutch bank, ING, refused to lend HCI an additional £15 million. In November, the creditors forced HCI into receivership. By then, I was just another witness to the debacle. I had already read the writing on the wall and resigned.

HCI fell victim to unbelievably bad business planning, gross amateurism in marketing, and self-delusion on a global scale. The collapse of HCI became an international scandal that threatened the government of Scotland. By some estimates, almost £100 million of the original £180 million funding package disappeared mysteriously down the Clyde River. When the dream collapsed, so, too, did high-end visions of the privatization of international health care.

The Scottish newspapers covered the collapse for months, starting in September 1994, when they first realized that all was not going well at the Clydebank institution. With 20/20 hindsight, some reporters and many politicians claimed that the collapse had been inevitable. They pointed out that the economic environment for the international health care industry had changed dramatically since 1979, when Levey and Eraklis had first envisioned a European hospital for wealthy patients in need of advanced surgery. HCI administrators had presented the hospital to me as a guaranteed instant success. I learned only later that the Irish government had rejected their proposal, and that the Scottish Development Agency had only approved it moments before enabling tax legislation would have expired.

By the time HCI finally opened the hospital, many European and Middle Eastern countries had established their own high-quality tertiary-care institutions, and several prestigious U.S. hospitals had already opened European satellite offices. Worst of all, a worldwide recession had cut the ability of patients to pay the hospital's high fees, and or the high charges at the neighboring luxury hotel.

When I returned to Glasgow with Barbara, early in 1994, no one at HCI had recognized or faced up to the changed economic environment. We were all extremely enthusiastic about the venture, convinced that the investors had pledged more than enough capital, and anxious to begin our new lives. I filled my first few days with a bewildering flood of paperwork concerning the purchasing of our house, compliance with government regulations, completing immigration documents, obtaining my work permit, registering with the official civil and medical authorities, opening bank accounts, and purchasing an automobile.

We found a good car at a good price with the help of the secretary to the hospital CEO. She was married to a local police officer. She referred us to a friend who had already assisted other newly arrived physicians in need of transportation. The friend helped us find an excellent vehicle at a real bargain price. The next day, I was once again familiarizing myself with the roundabouts, enjoying the pleasures of learning to drive a car with the steering wheel on the right, on the "wrong side" of the road.

It should have been an exciting time. The hospital would be opening in thirty days. We were all working in temporary quarters on the construction site, watching everything come together in the new hospital and the neighboring hotel. The air was filled with the anticipation of the grand opening of our venture. The first harbingers of doubt, however, began arriving even before the contractors had left the premises. I was especially disturbed to discover that HCI had not yet prepared my contract, and kept offering the same old excuses. Other staff physicians on-site had also chosen to come to Glasgow without written agreements. We were told that in Scotland, a handshake was as good as a written contract. That may well be true for Scots doing business with each other. I would soon discover that it was not necessarily true for Americans doing business in Scotland.

I spent much of my time visiting the medical and engineering schools at Glasgow University, where I discussed my future involvement in educational and research activities. The hospital administration had repeatedly told us of their plans to build a facility adjacent to the hospital, where HCI and major European industrial firms would jointly sponsor advanced research projects. I shared these plans with several of the outstanding scholars on the faculty of the university.

With great pleasure, I renewed my acquaintance with Glasgow University's Professor John Paul, one of the world's true giants in the field of biomechanics. I had first met him many years earlier during one of his visits to the United States. I found the prospect of working side by side with him extremely exciting. I also took advantage of my time to renew my friendship with David Hamblen, the professor of orthopaedics at Glasgow University. I had met David previously, at meetings we had both attended while representing our countries as presidents of our respective orthopaedic organizations.

We discussed my eventual involvement in his department, and, a few days later, he invited me to lecture at one of his weekly departmental meetings. I told David that I was looking forward to my official appointment to his faculty and to his cooperation with us at HCI Hospital. When he did not respond, I became a bit more concerned. The chief of surgery at HCI, however, assured me that negotiations concerning my appointment were well underway, and indicated that issues about my appointment "would be resolved within a short time." A meeting with the dean of the medical school gave me further reassurance.

Ann Karg, my administrative assistant who had been with me since Miami, arrived a few days later. She immediately began helping me plan the organization of the new department and initiated our quest for research funding. Dr. Peter Grigoris also joined us at this time. Grigoris, a Greek national, was a young orthopaedist with outstanding potential as a surgeon and a researcher. Recent changes in United States law had made it impossible for Grigoris to obtain a medical license in the United States. He had received his postgraduate training in the United Kingdom, however. We anticipated that he would encounter no difficulty having his British medical license reinstated in Scotland.

About a month after our arrival in Glasgow, the director of marketing asked Peter and me to meet with her. She was concerned by the lack of activity in Greece, and hoped that the two of us could visit Athens and meet with the people in HCI's satellite office. I was delighted with the prospect of visiting that classical city, and Peter was pleased with the opportunity to visit and show off his "home town." We also had many questions about the Greek patients we were expecting. We knew that HCI anticipated large numbers of patients from Greece, but we did now know how many of them would be seeking orthopaedic care, or what kinds of orthopaedic treatment they were most likely to require. The trip seemed to offer a perfect combination of business and pleasure. We both gladly accepted the opportunity.

I began to prepare for the trip by learning as much as possible about the HCI office in Athens. I soon discovered, however, that HCI Glasgow had little information about HCI's other offices. This made no sense to me. One of HCI's two cofounders, Dr. Angelo Eraklis, had convinced corporate backers that "thousands of patients" from Greece would be coming to Glasgow. Yet no one in Glasgow seemed able to tell me anything about those patients, or about the agencies that would be sending them to us. I became even more concerned when our director of marketing gave me her explanation of the problem: "Frankly, Dr. Sarmiento, we think that the people in the HCI office in Athens do not know anything about orthopaedics. Do you think that you could lend them a book on the subject?"

At that moment, I realized that HCI had no future. I discussed the incident with Ann Karg and shared my concerns with Barbara. I urged Barbara not to make any commitments to begin expensive repairs on our home. (We had just learned that our wonderful house in the country was termite-ridden, and the floor of the second-floor library was beginning to sag under the weight of my books.) Peter and I set off for Athens with less optimism and more foreboding.

The day after our arrival in Athens, Peter and I met with the individual in charge of the Greek operation. He could not (or would not) answer most of our questions. He was still seeking a location for a referral clinic. He understood that the HCI satellite office would have beds and operating rooms. He believed that local surgeons would perform simple operations at the clinic. Only patients who needed major surgery would be sent to Scotland. He did not know where the patients would come from, or how many patients to expect. He did not know if they would be cardiac patients, cancer patients, or orthopaedic patients.

He did tell us that it was difficult to have information in that regard, because the government had established new regulations concerning travel for health care. The new rules mandated that Greek nationals wishing to travel to another country for medical care must first be examined by a panel of local specialists. This panel would determine whether the patient could best be treated locally. He also told us that there were at least seven other offices in Athens representing foreign nations. All were trying to capture medical referrals.

Later in the day, it became obvious to us that Athens had become host to an international feeding frenzy of competition for medical patients. The tidal wave of marketing experts from abroad had totally offended the Greek medical establishment with their unprofessional, unethical campaigns. Some foreign hospitals were reportedly paying local physicians "under the table" for every referral they made overseas. The Greek medical community, understandably, had become deeply troubled by this sudden emergence of foreign competition.

I never fully understood why the international medical community focused so much attention on Greece. It became obvious to me in short order that the orthopaedic community in Athens was capable of handling most of the medical needs of their own countrymen. Apparently, some aspect of Greek law had opened doors to foreign hospitals. Now, however, just as HCI Hospital was finally about to open, the Greek government seemed determined to close the door.

Only once during our meeting with the administration of the Athens office of HCI did we acquire meaningful information. A young physician on the HCI staff produced data suggesting that during the previous year, approximately seventy patients had left Greece seeking medical care in other countries. She did not know the nature of their medical conditions. It really did not matter. HCI Hospital had 240 beds and many operating rooms. Marketing projections had been based on an anticipation of five thousand patients per year. Seventy patients from Greece, even if all of them came to Scotland, would hardly help.

Peter and I spent the rest of the time touring the old city. We visited the Acropolis and I marveled at the sculptures and architectural magnificence of the Parthenon. Peter proved to be a priceless travel companion. Since he already knew of my interest in history and my fascination with the literature and philosophers of ancient Greece, he constantly prodded our guide for more information. Upon looking at the ruins of the old theaters, I visualized the excitement that the native Greek population must have experienced during the performance of the immortal plays of Aeschylus, Sophocles, Euripides, and Aristophanes. When we got through with the tour, I recognized how fortunate I was. One day, I would be too old and too infirm to travel to Greece. I would have regretted missing that trip for the rest of my life. That visit became the bright silver lining surrounding the darkening clouds that were gathering over HCI and the hospital.

We returned home and sought a meeting with the hospital CEO Jim Wiczai, the medical director, and the marketing staff. We were anxious to share our experiences with them and tell them about our profound dissatisfaction with the HCI operations in Athens. We planned to tell them about the apparent scarcity of patients, the competition from other foreign hospitals, and share our concern that the "satellite clinic" was more likely to become a competitor than a source of referrals.

Wiczai first sought to postpone our meeting. When we persisted and finally met with him and his marketing staff they did not seem to be especially startled by our disclosures. Peter and I soon realized that Wiczai and his staff were already familiar with the situation. They also seemed to be determined to ignore the bad news. Wiczai assured me that the situation was well in hand, that the board of directors were fully familiar with developments in Athens, that the hospital had no reason to change any of its expectations.

HCI Hospital officially opened its doors on March 1, 1994. While there were still no calls for my surgical skills, my independent efforts to obtain financial support for my research were progressing smoothly. The European representative of one U.S. industrial corporation indicated strong interest in sponsoring orthopaedic research at HCI. A few weeks later, they officially informed me that they would allocate $1 million for our project. I immediately told the hospital administration about the potential gift, but never told them that we had completed negotiations. I wanted to first convince myself of the viability of the hospital. I also wanted to have my own contract in hand before I started passing million-dollar grants to the corporation.

Dr. Gerald Lowrey, the cardiothoracic surgeon from Houston, proved less patient than me. He resigned two months after he arrived in Glasgow. He left with no warning or prior announcement to the staff. (The hospital administration, however, issued statements questioning his abilities as a surgeon. They were not true. Lowrey's knowledge and talents are outstanding.)

Other doctors were also becoming increasingly restless. The small trickle of patients meant little work for any of us, and none at all for me. None of us held signed contracts. The CEO and the medical director continued to express optimism and constantly reassured us that everything was coming along on budget and on schedule. They told us that marketing agreements from various countries were being finalized, and that the negotiations with Glasgow University and Harvard were progressing well. They even urged us to accept HCI stock in lieu of our promised bonus payments. "It will make you all millionaires." They almost convinced me to go along with the program. Instead, I finally requested that my bonus be paid in dollars. I received only promises.

There were few patients in the hospital and even fewer families in the £100-per-day-hotel. (An increasingly critical local newspaper pointed out that comfortable beds could be had at a nearby rooming house for £12.50 per night.) I told Wiczai that I could no longer accept the accuracy of HCI projections for patients and income. He responded by admitting that he had not recognized the flaws in their assumptions. He explained that the original projections had been based on "misinterpreted signals" rather than solid facts. When I told him that I was considering resignation, he replied that he still believed in the ultimate success of the enterprise and strongly urged my continued loyalty.

Four months after the official opening of the hospital, HCI had made only minimal progress. Assurances that negotiations with other countries were about to be finalized continued to circulate with increased intensity. The medical director called a special meeting to inform us that he had found a replacement for our head of cardiology. A famous Italian heart surgeon had agreed to perform most of his surgery at HCI, although he would continue to have his main surgical practice in Italy. They later gave us similar information about a group of Dutch surgeons.

Despite the fact that HCI had designed our institution only to provide tertiary care, a sheik from Abu Dhabi arrived for his annual
physical examination. (A physical is typically provided by a primary
care physician.) He also brought his harem, and asked that HCI provide them all with complete physicals. As a tertiary-care facility, we
had neither internists nor gynecologists on staff. Worse yet, we discovered that our prized five-star hotel, designed in consultation with
leading international architects, had no private dining room for the
sheik's wives. None of the designers had adequately researched the
most basic requirements of the key target market.

A delegation from the government of Morocco arrived to visit
HCI, supposedly in preparation for the referral of a large number of
patients on a daily basis. The large number of patients never materialized. Groups of physicians and businesspeople arrived with
increasing frequency to tour our facilities. We saw delegates from
Arab countries virtually every week. Others visitors came from
Czechoslovakia, Turkey, Portugal, Spain, Italy, and other countries.
We heard from friends in the local community that HCI executives
wined and dined these visitors most lavishly. We could see for ourselves that the hospital beds remained empty. Our operating rooms
remained idle.

On one occasion, I received notice that our "agent" in Abu Dhabi
had requested a consultation concerning a man suffering from chronic
osteomyelitis on one of his tibias. The infection had been allegedly
present for many years but had failed to respond to various treatments. I immediately wrote a letter, requesting a more detailed history, X rays, and laboratory reports. While I was still awaiting a
response, the patient himself arrived, unannounced, accompanied by
his son.

I observed an indolent ulcer over the middle of his leg with minimal drainage. The X rays concerned me a great deal, and although
the radiologist called it osteomyelitis, I indicated in my records that I
suspected a malignant degeneration of a chronic infectious process. I
performed a biopsy but had to leave for Egypt the next day. (Two
months earlier, I had accepted an invitation from the Cairo Medical
School to serve as a visiting professor.)

Prior to my departure for Cairo, I called our consulting plastic
surgeon and discussed the possibility of having the patient undergo
plastic surgery after we surgically excised his osteomyelitic lesion.

That night, I called him again to inform him that I suspected malignant degeneration. I told him that we would have to wait for a report from the pathologist.

Before I left, Professor David Hamblen came to HCI to consult on the case. I had asked him to give me a second opinion. David did not agree with my tentative diagnosis of malignancy. Two days after my departure for Egypt, the plastic surgeon excised the infected area and covered the surgical defect with a flap of skin from the adjacent area.

As soon as I returned to Glasgow, I obtained the pathologist's report. It identified the biopsy sample as malignant. That meant that the plastic surgeon had performed the wrong surgery. Worse yet, the extensive surgery could well have spread the malignant cells to other parts of the body. I immediately amputated the leg. Because the previous operation had already compromised the healthy skin just below the knee, I had no choice but to amputate above the knee. In practical terms, that meant that the patient, because of his age, would have little likelihood of successfully learning to wear a prosthesis.

The whole unpleasant episode resulted from the inexcusable hurry to accommodate a plastic surgeon who wished to confine his HCI practice to weekends. If he had waited only two more days, he could have benefited from the pathologist's report. He would then have known that he was dealing with a malignant tumor. We could have produced a much-improved outcome. But HCI did not have a plastic surgeon on staff, and had to accommodate the unusual scheduling request.

There would be only two other patients requiring orthopaedic surgery. During my trip to Egypt for guest lectures in Cairo and Alexandria, Peter Grigoris performed a total hip replacement. I later treated a former patient of mine who flew from California to Glasgow so that I could revise a failed prosthetic hip component. Other than those two, and the patient from Abu Dhabi, no orthopaedic patients were admitted to the hospital during the months that I lived and worked in Glasgow.

The hospital administration warned all of us that we were not to discuss anything concerning the number of patients at HCI with anyone not on staff at the hospital. In an attempt to jump-start the facility, the CEO scheduled a second grand opening. This time, many luminaries such as the secretary general of Scotland and members of the local medical community were finally given tours of the hospital.

The HCI administration seemed to believe that the British press would happily pay attention to the ceremonial ribbon cutting and ignore the absence of patients. Instead, the press began to pay closer attention to the luxurious medical facility and reported that we seemed to be having many problems, most notably, an absence of patients. In response, Jim Wiczai issued a statement attacking the local community and their negative attitude.

In a further attempt to assuage the medical staff's concerns, the administration declared that contrary to previous estimates, continued viability did not require the hospital to admit five thousand patients during the first year. Only three thousand admissions would suffice. A later announcement changed the revised figure to two thousand.

The physicians/chiefs of the various medical services were then asked to meet with bankers involved in the financing of HCI. One of them came to my office, accompanied by a senior hospital executive. The HCI executive was the first one to sit down. The banker politely asked him to leave the room. He wanted to talk to me in private.

During the course of the meeting, he asked me if in my opinion the hospital could become a success. I responded by saying that before I could answer his question, it would be necessary for him to respond to a question of mine:

I asked, "How long can the hospital survive in the red?"

He answered without hesitation, "No more than one year."

I looked at him for a few seconds before I answered his first question: "The hospital will not make it."

The following day I prepared a letter to the medical director, with an official copy to the CEO, Jim Wiczai. I told them that I intended to resign and requested a meeting to discuss the terms of separation and the date of final termination of my duties. They met with me but were unable to answer my questions. Instead, they urged me to remain at my post. "Do not jump ship so early. . . . Think about your plans more carefully. . . . All we need is a little more time. . . . Your departure would be a major blow to the hospital in such critical days. . . . We need your support."

I then wrote another letter in which I explained in some detail the reasons for my resignation and departure. I ended the letter saying that although I did not have a written contract, I expected that the verbal agreement would be acknowledged. I also set out the terms of an acceptable financial settlement, including full salary for the year, prorated bonuses, and reimbursement for moving expenses back to the United States.

The next day, I left to attend the meeting of the Hip Society in San Francisco. Just prior to my departure, HCI received two referrals for total hip replacement surgery. One was an elderly gentleman from a nearby town. The National Health Service had a one-year waiting list for the operation. This gentleman did not want to wait, and was willing to pay for the operation himself. I had already examined him in my office and had scheduled his surgery for the day after my return to Glasgow. The other patient was a lady from the Bahamas who wanted to have her hip surgery in Glasgow because her relatives lived nearby. I had not examined her in person, but had corresponded with her. I had also reviewed her X rays and medical history.

I returned to Scotland after a few days in the United States. It was Sunday at noon when the plane landed. I went home and then drove to the hospital to see the two patients who had been scheduled for surgery the following day. Neither appeared on the surgical schedule. Both surgeries had been canceled by the administration.

The next day, Jim Wiczai told me that during my absence, the hospital had accepted my resignation. I no longer had surgical privileges. He said that he had been forced to act abruptly because I had sent a letter to the professor in Cairo discrediting HCI, and because my letter had caused the Egyptian government to terminate important and promising negotiations. He had heard about the letter informally, and had then ordered his staff to locate the letter on my computer.

The letter that I had written to the Egyptian professor was a short one. I had written it to tell him that I would not be able to serve as his visiting professor the following November, because I anticipated returning to the United States. I had written that I would be leaving Glasgow because I had concluded that HCI could not provide me with the academic opportunities I needed. Nothing in that letter discredited the hospital.

I then wrote a formal request for a financial settlement, in which I laid out my claims. I reminded HCI that I had been given an assurance of a five-year work opportunity although it was never put into an official, legal document; that HCI had not honored its commitments to me and had misrepresented the number of patients I would be treating. I had been promised a professorship at the University of Glasgow and the opportunity to develop educational and research programs. They had broken commitments to recruit other physicians. I told them that their commitments had caused me to resign from my professorship at USC, that moving of my books and other possessions back to the United States would cost me in excess of $34,000, and that I would be returning to the States without a professional position.

Wiczai promised to prepare a generous separation package, providing that I would agree not to discuss with anyone my views about the HCI operation or criticize the organization in any way, for a period of six months after my departure. I found his suggestion insulting and demeaning. I informed him that I would be vacating my office within one week, as I had a number of matters to attend to, and expected a full severance package.

That afternoon, the chief surgeon called for an emergency meeting of the medical staff. I did not plan to attend. When his secretary asked if I planned to be at the meeting, I told her that I did not intend to go to it. Then I changed my mind. I suspected that Dr. Hollier had called the meeting to announce my departure. I wanted to be sure that the staff understood my reasons for leaving.

Judging from his expression when he entered the room and saw me, Dr. Hollier had not expected me to be there. He indicated to the packed room that he had called the meeting to let the medical staff know that I was leaving HCI. He handed me a typewritten announcement and asked if its contents met with my approval. I responded by saying that I would be appreciative if the wording of the memorandum was changed to more appropriately reflect the facts. His memorandum had read, "Doctor Sarmiento is leaving HCI immediately." I remarked that such wording suggested that I had been involuntarily terminated, which was definitely not the case. I asked if I could briefly address the group, and he reluctantly agreed.

I summarized the events that had led to my resignation. I said that I did not believe that an orthopaedic program at the hospital could be developed in the foreseeable future. I told them that I had been successful in the United States as an educator and researcher, as well as a hip replacement surgeon, but circumstances in Glasgow were not permitting me to function in any of those capacities.

"I have performed only one surgical procedure in eight months. I do not see the picture changing sufficiently rapidly to justify my remaining here. Perhaps if I were younger, or older, I would have made a different decision. If I were younger, I could sit and wait for things to improve. If I were older, I would have probably tolerated a job where I would be paid large amounts of money while doing nothing to earn it. I want to be productive for the remaining few years I have as a surgeon. Glasgow precludes that opportunity."

I finished my comments by saying that I was happy to have met so many wonderful people. I told them that I treasured their friendship and wished them well.

I went for a cup of coffee and returned to my office. When I got there, I tried to call Dr. David Hamblen to tell him that I was leaving. The phone was dead. The chief surgeon, according to his messenger, had ordered that it be disconnected. Mr. Yick, his assistant, came into my office and asked me when I was planning to vacate the premises. It was already late on the Thursday afternoon. I told him that I would be gone within the next four days. He replied that the chief surgeon had instructed him to tell me that I should be out of the office by the next day.

I left the office on Friday. I gave Peter Grigoris many of my medical books and my entire collection of hardbound American and British journals of orthopaedics. Austin Moore had given me the volumes covering the first three decades. I hated to leave them behind, but by eliminating them, I knew that I could reduce the cost of transportation back to the United States. I was beginning to suspect that HCI would not pay my moving expenses without a fight.

I also drafted a letter to all of the staff physicians, repeating everything that I had said at the meeting. I wanted to be sure that they understood my position. I also wanted to prevent the administration from "revising" the story behind my resignation.

Then came the task of placing the house for sale and packing the books, X rays, and patient files. I had to place this most depressing task in Barbara's hands. I had been invited to keynote the meeting of the Association for Fracture Repair in Kobe, Japan. It was a great honor. I could not cancel the trip, in spite of the enormous inconveniences my travel would bring to my wife.

While I was in Kobe, I received a telephone call from a reporter for Glasgow's major newspaper. He had a copy of a letter, purportedly written by me to Jim Wiczai. He read the first paragraph, and I confirmed that I was the author. It was the letter I had written to the medical staff. The reporter refused to tell me how he had obtained a copy. He only told me that he intended to discuss the issue on the pages of his newspaper the following day.

When I returned to Glasgow from Japan, the newspaper had already printed portions of my letter and discussed many of the issues concerning the viability of the hospital and the reasons for my resignation. The article was accompanied with a recent photograph of me. The picture had been taken by the hospital photographer, but I had never even seen it. For several years following my departure from Glasgow, I thought that someone within the hospital administration must have provided the reporter with the letter and photograph. I was mistaken. I later learned Ann Karg had handed the information and the photograph to the reporter the night before she returned to the United States.

For the next two weeks, I was bombarded with requests for interviews from television stations and newspapers from various parts of the United Kingdom. I declined to meet with anyone. I told them only that we were dealing with a personal matter that I did not wish to discuss in public. One television station called my home and tried to persuade my wife to provide them with information. She also declined to get involved.

Newspapers in the States also published information about the events in Glasgow. One article reminisced about the fact that only a few months earlier, they had written about the exodus of medical talent to the fabulous new hospital, inspired and partially funded by Harvard, and financed by other powerful and prestigious investment groups. Curiously, the U.S. press never explored many of the most fascinating issues surrounding HCI, including the reputed "disappearance" of almost £100 million of the initial underwriting. The British press continued to tear at the story for many months after my departure. Opposition politicians repeatedly demanded full-scale investigations of the affair, and the resignations of everyone who had anything to do with it. I have no idea what, if anything, ever came of those demands.

chapter 38.
greed and hubris

"I am not what I am; I am what I am not."
—Georg Wilhelm Friedrich Hegel

HCI never honored its unwritten contract with me. I did finally receive my prorated salary but none of the promised bonuses. They also never paid any moving costs for my return the United States. I investigated the possibility of filing suit, but my Scottish lawyer convinced me that I would have no chance for recovery. He told me that a Scottish jury would be totally unsympathetic to my viewpoint. From their perspective, they would find that HCI's payment of my salary had been more than adequate, and that since I had been paid so much, I should be willing to pick up my own moving expenses. Reluctantly, I decided not to litigate. HCI's bankruptcy, of course, ended even remote possibilities of recovery.

I never tried to keep in touch with anyone at HCI after I left Glasgow. I know that Dr. Peter Grigoris left HCI a few months after my departure. He went to work with Dr. David Hamblen at the university. To the best of my knowledge, the rest of the original staff returned to the United States. I received a letter from the chief of medicine, who had relocated in the States, commenting that he had judged me incorrectly when I left HCI. He had not been able to accept my gloomy predictions. He acknowledged that I had been correct. He felt sorry for the people who so innocently had embarked upon such a disastrous "nightmare." I share his feelings.

Jim Wicsai was diagnosed with advanced cancer of the prostate during my last days in Scotland. He had ignored ominous signs of his own poor health, just as he had ignored the signs of the collapse of his hospital. By the time he sought medical care, it was too late. He died in Boston, two years later. I was furious with him at the time of my departure from Glasgow. Now, I believe that he was trying to do his best under difficult circumstances. He did things under the specter of disaster that he would never have done under more normal circumstances.

I am still grateful that I had an opportunity to spend eight months in Scotland. We in the United States and the people of Scotland supposedly share a language and a heritage, but the Scots clearly differ from us in many ways. They are genuinely sincere and unassuming people. They live simple, uncomplicated lives. They have not been overwhelmed by the apparently insatiable thirst for money that has become so rampant in our part of the world.

I first encountered this phenomenon when I tried to recruit local orthopaedists who might want to admit their private patients to HCI Hospital. We would have made such transfers financially rewarding to the doctors. I expected them to welcome the opportunity. Instead, they told me that they had no desire to earn more money. They were satisfied with their payment from the National Health Services, even though it is only a small portion of what physicians earn in the United States.

The Scottish doctors I met all exhibited a much broader scope of knowledge about government, philosophy, history, literature, and international affairs than the average American physician. They enjoy cultured conversation with learned friends. They read widely and think clearly about broad and meaningful issues. They are more interesting people than their American counterparts. They also seem to be substantially happier and more content.

On one occasion, many years ago, my daughter asked me about my lifetime of travel. She wanted to know which of the many countries I had visited did I like the most. I responded that every country I had seen had unique beauty. From the physical point of view, I told her, it was impossible for me to answer her question. However, if I were to look for other reasons to judge countries, I had to say that New Zealand was the one that had left the deepest impression on me. The people of New Zealand, I thought, are totally without arrogance but rich in sincerity and warmth.

I told her of an experience I had in Hamilton, New Zealand, at the home of a local orthopaedist. He had seven children, most of them girls. At dinnertime, all of the children sat at the table and joined in an animated conversation with their parents and me. That was something I had rarely witnessed in the United States, where I had learned, when guests come to dinner, the children usually eat separately.

A few years after my trip to New Zealand, I learned that many of the inhabitants of New Zealand are of Scottish descent. Perhaps that explains why I noticed so many similarities between the Scots and the New Zealanders.

I also left Scotland with a new appreciation of the National Health Service (NHS). I now believe that many observers grossly exaggerate reports of widespread problems, especially extended waiting times by those in need of medical care. While some medical conditions require patients to wait months and even years for surgical treatment, those conditions are exceptions to the usual situation. Furthermore, in most instances, the extended waiting can be justified.

In 1970, when I spent several months at Dr. John Charnley's Hip Center, I often heard him tell people with arthritic hips to return in another year. He told them that in the meantime, they should use a cane and take symptomatic medications for their pain or discomfort. At first, I did not understand the logic of his decisions. Only later did I learn to appreciate his wisdom. He knew that artificial replacements of major joints are not always successful. It is best to perform the surgery on people whose disability is significant and who no longer respond to nonsurgical treatments. When I worked in Miami, my patients often had to wait a year for me to operate on them.

In the United States, people with moderately or even minimally painful arthritic conditions often demand replacement surgery as soon as possible, and the sooner the better. Since a total joint replacement usually provides immediate improvement, many find the thought of even the briefest postponement to be totally abhorrent. As one observer recently commented, "Americans invented instant gratification. However, they don't like it anymore because it takes too long."

Emergency care is rendered without any delay in the United Kingdom. When necessary, NHS doctors cancel elective surgeries in order to accommodate urgent conditions. At Los Angeles County Hospital, I often saw patients waiting days before their open fractures received surgical attention. I never saw or heard of any such treatment in the United Kingdom. Neither did I see the "epidemic of surgery and technology" that is sweeping our country. The British seem to be more realistic than we are. They understand that no country, no matter how wealthy it might be, can indefinitely sustain the abuse of high-cost, sophisticated, expensive technology.

I enjoyed the slow pace of Scotland. I found it exhilarating to be far away from the big cities where I had always lived. I prize my memories of the solitude brought on by winter weather in Scotland. I loved the beautiful countryside, and found myself fascinated by the constant change brought on by the changing seasons. I have lived all the rest of my life in tropical climates. I had never before seen winter, or appreciated the coming of spring.

With no medical work to do, I used my evenings and weekends to delve into two of the things I have enjoyed the most since my early adolescence: reading and listening to classical music. Scotland gave me my first opportunity to fully indulge in those pleasures. The isolation of my home from traffic, neighbors, and visitors provided me with my first exposure to true quietude, and time to occupy myself with those activities. I must admit that rarely do I sit down to listen to music without having a book in my hands. I suppose that one really should concentrate on the music. I have always read at the same time, however, and do not seem to be able to break that habit.

The day I entered medical school, I promised myself that I would never go to bed at night reading a medical text. I would never allow medicine to intrude so deeply on my most private time. I have kept that promise diligently. Only books dealing with nonmedical subjects have a place on my night table. I confine my medical books and journals to my library and living room.

During my younger years, I read the philosophers of antiquity as well as the giants of classic literature. In Scotland, I took advantage of my solitude and free time to read anew many of the books I had read in my youth. I found the new experience greatly rewarding. I discovered that maturity brings a remarkably different perspective. With it comes a new appreciation of universal brilliance and a new, deeper, and richer pleasure that comes only with a fuller understanding of great minds.

As I reread Plato's *Dialogues*, I was amazed to rediscover the enduring integrity and relevance of his analysis. Homer's masterpieces and Sophocles' *Antigone* helped keep my intellect from hibernating; I discovered that my lifetime of experiences created a whole new context for understanding the accomplishments of Greek and Roman civilization. As a youth, I had thought Plutarch's *Lives* overlong and somewhat boring. In the brilliance of the brief midday sun reflecting off the Scottish snows, I found it incredibly exciting and filled with intriguing insight. The works of Giovanni Vico, Oswald Spengler, Arnold Toynbee, Bernard Braudel, and Edward Gibbon brought new understanding not only to the rise and fall of the Romans but also to the enduring nature and failings of man. The writings of the great men of the Scottish and French Enlightenment, for which I had always held enormous fascination, continued to bring new appreciation for their enduring lessons.

I found remarkable pleasure in reciting passages from Dante's *Inferno* and *Purgatorio* out loud. Curiously, as I had done in my youth, I stopped reading *Divine Comedy* after the end of the second volume. I have never arrived at Paradise. You are welcome to draw your own conclusions from this peculiar behavior.

I also took full advantage of the solitude and this timely intermission in my life to reread *Don Quixote*, *Les Misérables*, *Crime and Punishment*, and *The Brothers Karamazov*. I also took a fresh look at James Joyce's *Ulysses*, perhaps the greatest twentieth-century novel written in English, which reinforced my realization that we read differently when we are young and must revisit the great books when we have experienced more of life. I had found *Ulysses* extremely difficult to read as a youth. In those younger days I lacked the understanding I now have of the history of Ireland, its turbulent relationship with England, and the profound influence of the Roman Catholic Church in its everyday life. But more importantly I did not have the maturity to truly appreciate the relationship of the book with the Homeric epic that inspired Joyce. T. S. Elliot, upon recognizing the greatness of Joyce's masterpiece remarked that it would be a landmark because "it destroys our civilization."

The Scottish weather even brought new pleasure to the reading of poetry. Even the works of Spanish poets, a literature that had given me much enjoyment in my youth, again became a source of strength and pleasure. Barbara and I also visited the extraordinary museums of Glasgow and Edinburgh, and took surprising pleasure in the rich atmosphere of Scottish culture. The museums of many cities are more widely publicized and more popular with tourists. The collections of Glasgow and Edinburgh have a unique depth and intensity that make them well worth the journey. We also found great pleasure in the castles scattered throughout the Scottish countryside.

Since my return to the United States, I have used far too much of my solitude and leisure reviewing my experience in Scotland and trying to understand the failure of HCI. I have decided the true answer has little to do with market research, international relations, the globalization of the economy, or the international status of U.S. medicine. HCI failed because it was conceived solely as a business venture rather than as a health care facility. Its planners never saw its patients as people in need of medical attention. They saw only customers. Plans for any hospital should evolve from a perceived medical need. HCI emerged only from greed and hubris. The Harvard Medical School physicians who originally conceived HCI were overpowered by both. So, too, were the Harvard Foundation financiers and Harvard Management business experts who never investigated the health care practices ethos and facilities in their target countries. Hubris was everywhere. We are Americans. We are Harvard. If we build it, they will come.

Government authorities in Ireland learned from the DeLorean fiasco and refused to make the same mistakes. The Scottish Development Authority failed to learn from the Irish experience. I, too, failed to learn from history. I should never have moved to Scotland without a contract in hand. I should have learned that from my experience when I first sought to leave Bucaramanga to study with Dr. William Green in Boston. I should have learned it from my disappointments when I first moved to Miami and later to California. I guess that I am a slow learner. I am easily misled by promises. I am still far too trusting.

Barbara and I received more lessons in the errors of excessive trust when the time came to sell our house and our car. We had paid a large sum of money for the house, and had invested even more in repair of sagging floors, termite damage, and termite removal. Only eight months had passed since we had purchased the house. We ended up losing money on our investment.

We waited to sell our British car until we were ready to leave Scotland. Then we placed an ad in the local community newspaper. When a potential buyer arrived, we discovered that we did not have the appropriate documents. Soon afterwards, I discovered that our automobile had been illegally brought into Scotland from Ireland. We soon learned that it had probably been stolen in Ireland, and that the man who sold it to us was a notorious and presumably dangerous underworld figure. Our taxicab driver advised us to forget about reporting the incident to the police.

We had paid cash for the car. Now we were unable to sell it. As our departure date neared, we chose to give the car to our taxicab driver, who promised to send us whatever he could as monthly payments. A few weeks after we left the country, we heard that the driver had been in a serious traffic accident with his taxicab. He was not seriously injured but was out of work. We have not heard from him since.

chapter 39.
back where it all began

"Now that my ladder is gone,
I must lie where all ladders start,
In the foul rag-and-bone shop of the heart."

—W. B. Yeats

"Health Care reform is not needed; what is needed is greed reform"
—Anonymous

We returned to Florida and settled in the small house in Long Boat Key, a town next to Sarasota, that we had purchased several years earlier as a retirement home. It is a lovely little place on the water with a magnificent, relaxing view of the bay.

Although I had passed my sixty-fifth birthday, I did not yet want to retire. I also did not want to return to California, even though I received several offers from friends with practices in the Los Angeles area. I knew that I would only be interested in doing surgery for a few more years. Since I had always planned to retire in Florida, another move to California made little sense to me or to Barbara.

Several old friends in Florida also offered me employment, but none of the offers included educational or research opportunities. I looked most closely at Doctors Hospital in Miami, an old institution that had always enjoyed an outstanding reputation. Doctors Hospital was affiliated with the department of orthopaedics at the University of Miami Medical School. It was home to three university programs. The atmosphere appeared to be conducive to productivity.

The hospital was owned and operated by HealthSouth, a private organization. The hospital officials impressed me with their alleged commitment to excellence. I suggested that they establish a Center of Musculoskeletal Disorders and pointed out that no such facility existed in the state of Florida. As a first step leading to the development of the center, I proposed to organize an Arthritis and Joint Replacement Institute. They displayed great enthusiasm for the idea and offered to support such an effort if I chose to join their team at Doctors Hospital.

I had originally assumed that the university presence provided an environment that would be conducive to my plans to develop parallel orthopaedic programs. I failed, however, to recognize that Health-South required overnight economic success. They would not entertain my idea of establishing an Arthritis and Joint Replacement Institute as a first step in the creation of a major Musculoskeletal Center. Although some of the major ingredients for the center were already in place, they were not willing to make the necessary short-term investment. I knew that I had to improve the financial prospects of my plans if I wanted to attract corporate support.

Accordingly, I gathered all the necessary information needed for an official presentation, along with blueprints for existing space within the hospital where I could locate the program. The hospital CEO approved my request to use the space and authorized me to continue planning. I then convinced all related hospital departments to join the endeavor. They all realized that such a center would be in their best interest. It would bring cohesiveness to a disparate and autonomous collection of programs with no identifiable philosophy or goals.

When all the ducks were lined up, I finally made my presentation to a representative of HealthSouth. When a representative from its headquarters came to Miami to meet with me, I made the presentation. For all practical purposes, existing physical structures were to be used without the need for new construction. The personnel needed to get the program moving were already onboard. The only substantial expenses involved new educational activities and the introduction of clinical research. The HealthSouth representative assured me that my proposal was in line with the corporate philosophy. He promised that HealthSouth would provide the necessary support.

I then established weekly conferences for orthopaedists and rheumatologists. Since the hospital did not have facilities for the conduct of those courses, and because we needed some marketing and basic audiovisual equipment, we planned to hold these conferences at a nearby hotel. I also initiated negotiations to organize the first of an anticipated long series of educational seminars. I organized the course myself and recruited distinguished faculty from across the country.

My office prepared announcements and brochures. We sent them to the hospital's business office for production and distribution.

The course was to take place in December of 1995. About forty-five days before the scheduled start of the conference, we discovered that the fliers announcing it had not been mailed. When my secretary called the hotel to go over last-minutes details, the hotel informed her that the hospital had not as yet honored its financial commitments. While the course eventually took place, the hospital paid its bills from the hotel only several months later. One year after running an advertisement for the course, I finally personally issued a check to the *Journal of Bone and Joint Surgery*. Eventually, the hospital reimbursed me.

I cancelled all future continuing education activities and moved our weekly conferences to a monthly schedule. I finally discontinued these conferences altogether. Not only had the hospital withdrawn most of its logistical support for the activities but attendance at the meetings had also declined dramatically. It seemed that these academic programs held little attraction for either the local medical community or hospital staff. The era in which I had grown up was the era when doctors sought to participate in frequent informal debates and conferences of the nature I had proposed. Now they seek information mainly from industry-sponsored meetings and publications and from the vendors of surgical products. The new era, the age of applied medical technology and medicine as a business has begun, and who knows where it will take us.

chapter 40.
medicine as a business

"Modern civilization which beguiled itself in its youth with dreams of eternal progress . . . is facing a more premature senility than any previous culture."

—Reinhold Neibuhr

The U.S. medical profession is deeply concerned over its increasing loss of social status and professional autonomy. It never occurred to us that one day, authorities outside of medicine would dictate professional practices to physicians. We still find it hard to accept that such a change is taking place. Government agencies and private insurers now monitor and in various degrees control treatment, hospital stays, medication, and other aspects of care for many medical conditions.

Many of my colleagues find themselves stunned by the decline in professional income. A surgeon from San Diego recently told me that one local HMO reimbursed only $250 for a particular procedure for which we once routinely charged $2,500. I asked him if there were any orthopaedic surgeons in the community willing to perform the procedure for such a small amount. "Of course," he replied. "It beats driving a cab."

Stripped of its autonomy and adequate financial compensation, the practice of medicine becomes unpleasant and underpaid. Intelligent, ambitious, self-assured individuals will be more attracted to other careers. Do we really want to divert more of our most talented, creative, imaginative young people away from medicine and toward advertising, public relations, marketing, and the "virtual" universe?

We can no longer leave issues of health care delivery to be resolved by the private business sector of our society. With a great deal of philosophical reluctance, I now think that we will soon reach the conclusion that we need more government intervention, not less.

I have reached the point where I believe that the United Sates soon will move in the direction of a National Health Insurance. The private sector has clearly demonstrated that it cannot be trusted to do the job. We must not allow entrepreneurs to dominate health care any longer. They wish only to maximize their own personal revenues. They do not hesitate to compromise and damage quality of care. We have already allowed too many HMOs and for-profit hospitals to do too much damage. I still believe that medicine is a calling, and therefore it cannot and should not be treated as a business.

Many factors have influenced the developments that concern us today. In retrospect, we could have prevented many of them. We lacked the wisdom and the unselfishness to address them while they were still in their infancy, when our actions could still have prevented these problems from reaching today's monstrous proportions.

Neither our social critics, nor the media, nor the medical profession itself realized how rapidly and explosively the scientific and technical revolutions that began in the sixties and seventies would change our culture. We assumed that change would be gradual, that the new knowledge and technology would be assimilated into the daily practice of medicine. Instead, the benefits and costs of the new technology overwhelmed the system.

In orthopaedics, the technological revolution fostered a fragmentation of our discipline. The availability of new techniques and devices seduced us into a spiral of overspecialization. We stopped treating patients with disorders of the musculoskeletal system and became subspecialists in regions of the body. Soon we started to treat hips, hands, feet, knees, and backs as isolated components. Then came the most fashionable and medically irrelevant of them all—sports medicine. Surely, we do not really wish to ignore both the patient and the condition, and base treatment only on the environment in which the condition occurred.

Such overspecialization increased profits but trivialized medicine. Academia and the profession in general quickly followed the trail that led to unlimited riches. So, with the full support of our teachers and our leaders, we learned to pay more attention to business and less attention to our patients. That is how we have reached the point where we are no longer educating physicians but are training highly specialized body part repair technicians. I think of many contemporary orthopaedists as sophisticated cosmetic surgeons of the skeleton.

An orgy of surgery and technology is sweeping the world of orthopaedics. I suspect this to be true for all other branches of surgery. While visiting a prestigious trauma center in Europe, a junior faculty member proudly told me that the staff treated all fractures surgically. I expressed skepticism about this sweeping statement. He showed me the evidence. Even simple fractures of the wrist had surgery, regardless of the patient's age or the degree of severity. The staff even treated fractures of the long bones of the hand in the same manner. I expected to hear that fractures of the collarbone were an exception. Not so. My guide happily showed me how these fractures were stabilized by closed nailing. He easily rationalized this excessive use of surgical intervention by pointing out that patients no longer want to accept the small lump that nonsurgical treatment might produce.

Unexpectedly, I found myself in a situation that appeared to give me the opportunity to do something meaningful to effect change in the pervasive pattern sweeping the Western world. I could do something in a major way. Unexpectedly, I was approached by a group of orthopaedists from Europe who had also become concerned about the increasing cost of orthopaedic care and had concluded that the exaggerated emphasis on the surgical approach was a major cause. They had organized and planned the creation of a society devoted to the dissemination of information about the benefits of conservative treatment of fractures.

I was invited to attend one of their meetings in Amsterdam, where their philosophy and plans were enthusiastically explained to me. Though I thoroughly agreed with their concerns, I disagreed with their proposed methodology. I felt that their worldwide educational efforts aimed at bringing back interest in the nonsurgical treatment of fractures was condemned to failure. The world of trauma care had changed radically during the past three decades, and to anticipate a reversal of the trend was not only unrealistic but counterproductive. The society would be identified with an attitude that ignored the reality of change, and the great benefits that surgery had brought to victims of fractures. In addition, the awesome power of industry was strongly in support of treatment modalities that require the use of their highly profitable products. To pursue that route would have been suicidal. I suggested that if the venture were to become successful, it had to clearly and openly recognize that the surgical approach to fractures was the best one in many instances; that no orthopaedist in the modern world could effectively provide good care, unless he was well trained and competent in the performance of surgery. However, there was also a definite place, and a major one, for the conservative approach in many instances. That promulgating a rational balance between the approaches was the most effective philosophy for the nascent organization.

Though there was some opposition and concern expressed by several members of the group, eventually my views prevailed. I was offered the presidency of the society, which we called The Association for the Rational Treatment of Fracture; ARTOF for short.

With enthusiasm and commitment I jumped into the arena. I was going to be successful, I told myself, and that the ideas of the group would eventually change the thinking and practices of orthopaedists all over the world. I was convinced that we would be presenting—not only to orthopaedic surgeons but also to politicians and economists— a sound and logical approach to an important segment of medicine.

I proceeded to plan and organize a series of educational ventures in various countries. Members of the new society shared my enthusiasm and dreams. Within the next two years we held meetings in approximately ten different countries, most in conjunction with already-scheduled meetings of national and international orthopaedic societies. The first of such meetings took place in Barcelona, working in concert with the European Association of Orthopaedics and Traumatology.

The meeting was a success. We had a large audience and the speakers performed extremely well while discussing their various nonsurgical and surgical approaches to a group of fractures. At the end of their presentations we tried to draw conclusions regarding the most appropriate indications for the various treatment modalities.

After Spain we held similar courses in a number of countries. We went to Peru, where the meeting of the Latin American Orthopaedic Association was held. Afterward, we met in the Czech Republic, New Zealand, Finland, Japan, Italy, Hungary, Austria, Germany, Holland, and other countries.

In June 1998, I found my most supportive audience for the ideas behind the formation of ARTOF. Ironically, the occasion was my keynote speech before the meeting of the AO in Switzerland. The AO, more than any other organization, has led the movement toward excessive surgical treatment. Judging by their reception of my keynote speech, however, the AO may well become a powerful instrument of reform. My address was published in the bulletin, which reaches all corners of the world.

The president of the Orthopaedic Trauma Association, a U.S.-based international organization, was in the audience, and he promptly invited me to be his presidential guest speaker at the annual meeting of his organization a few months later. At the meeting in Switzerland I had an opportunity to observe for three days the trustees of the AO in action. I recall that the orthopaedist in charge of the meeting gave the attending trustees the assignment of discussing and making recommendations to the assembled body at the end of the meeting regarding an important issue. The assignment was presented in this manner: picture in your mind a twenty-five-year-old man who sustained an open fracture of his leg after being hit by an automobile in a small village a hundred miles from either Calcutta or Bogota. The young man was taken to the local hospital where a surgeon, who had attended a basic AO course, practiced his profession. The operating room, however, had only six different plates that could be used to stabilize the fracture. Apparently they were either too long or too short to fit his leg. After giving instructions to the group, and dividing it into smaller groups, the participants went to their respective rooms to discuss the issue and prepare their recommendations.

It had become obvious to me from the very outset that the expected recommendations would be proposals for the AO to provide more complete sets of instruments, so the surgeons taking care of injured patients would effectively be able to choose the plates of appropriate length.

On the last day of the meeting the trustees reassembled and presented their recommendations. I was sitting in the back of the room, carefully listening to the reports given by the appointed leaders of the teams. Unexpectedly, the chairman said, "Doctor Sarmiento, we would like to hear from you. Please, give us your opinion." I was not prepared to articulate my feelings. I said that I was there only as an observer and preferred not to say anything. He insisted, however, that I should say a few words.

I stood up and said,

In my view, the alleged problem of the hospital not having enough plates, was not a problem. The real problem was that the hospital had too many plates. If enough plates had been available the chances were that following surgery the fracture would have gotten infected and eventually the leg would be amputated. Under the precarious circumstances surrounding the accident, the best possible treatment for the fracture was an appropriate cleansing of the wound, the application of a cast, and the administration of antibiotics. In that manner, it was very likely that the fracture would have healed without an infection, though with shortening of the extremity and perhaps with some deformity. But that slightly deformed limb was better than an amputation."

I then added, "Rather than spending money supplying the operating rooms of underdeveloped regions of the world, use it to educate their physicians on the basic principles of fracture care, not those of internal fixation, which are practical only in areas of the world, which have the financial resources and the infrastructure required for the implementation of sophisticated technology." Noticing that my words were being listened to carefully I concluded, "The issue you are discussing is analogous to another one, which frequently attracts commentary. The alleged highly civilized Western countries passionately preach peace and urge other people in poor countries to avoid violence and war. However, the 'civilized' countries are the ones who supply the uncivilized ones with the weapons of war and destruction. They should not be so hypocritical."

I completed my tour of duty as president of ARTOF satisfied with the accomplishment we had made in such a short time, and with the apparent favorable reaction the orthopaedic community had given to our philosophy. Unfortunately, two years later, at the time of this writing, it appears that soon ARTOF might disappear from the radar screen. Perhaps due to a lack of true interest and commitment to the cause, the enthusiasm that is required to maintain momentum has dwindled. I suspect ARTOF will be nothing but a memory in the minds of those who, like myself, dreamt of a better world.

This bad experience proved once more that without passion nothing can be accomplished. To expect others, who lack true dedication and devotion to an idea, to succeed in bringing skeptical people to accept change is futile to say the least.

One other subject that has occupied my mind in recent years is the exaggerated interest that my profession has placed on subspecialization. The inability or unwillingness of organized orthopaedics to recognize the potential damage that excessive subspecialization has gen-

erated speaks poorly of the vision of its leaders. One gets the feeling
that they have not yet recognized the threat that spiraling medical
costs represent to our society and the role that subspecialization has
played in the creation of that phenomenon. They have not yet taken
any steps or initiated any programs to assume responsibility for controlling the costs of medical care. The welfare of their own personal
lives and that of their organizations seems to have been their highest
priority.

Today, we are paying the price of such blindness. The powerful
third-party payers are punishing us unmercifully by decreasing payment for services and by encouraging other medical disciplines to
usurp territory that for a long time was ours.

In the meantime patient care suffers. Hospitals curtail basic services and expand borderline and medically questionable programs.
Through brilliant marketing, rehabilitation has become a darling of
the media and a medical sacred cow. With the smiling, beatific
approval of the media, for-profit hospitals continue to milk rehabilitation for far more than it is worth.

I recently treated a woman who had been suffering pain in one of
her hips for several years. A rheumatologist had treated her, but her
symptoms persisted. Whenever she visited her physician in her office
she was given the ubiquitous injection of intraarticular cortisone to
temporarily reduce inflammation and alleviate pain. She had been
twice admitted to the Arthritis Unit for the Medicare-approved seven
days. After several years, she became impatient with the lack of
improvement and sought a referral to an orthopaedic surgeon. Her
primary care "provider" referred her to me.

I replaced the hip joint and she recovered quickly. She was soon
able to walk without support and without pain. I reported her
progress to the referring physician. The patient herself informed the
rheumatologist's office about the good results she had from the
surgery. Remarkably, her rheumatologist insisted that she should
again be admitted for one week to the Arthritis Unit of a local hospital. The medically unnecessary treatment generated substantial fees
for the rheumatologist and income to the hospital. Because the treatment fell within Medicare guidelines, everyone (except the patient)
benefited.

When I told this story at a dinner party, an orthopaedist on the
same hospital's staff topped it. He told me about a patient of his with

Alzheimer's disease. The patient's senility had advanced to the point that he was unable to recognize even his wife. He was an elderly gentleman who spent most of his time staring into space. Nonetheless, a staff physician suggested to his wife that the man should be admitted to the arthritis unit for one week of rehabilitation. When she informed the physician that her husband needed her around the clock for supervision, he told her that he would arrange for her to be admitted as well! Her history of chronic back pain was all that she needed to qualify for treatment. Husband and wife became in-patients together for the Medicare-approved one-week farce that enriched the hospital but helped neither of them.

Just a few weeks earlier, I had submitted an article for publication in one of our major journals. It dealt with my twenty-five years of experience using aspirin as the prophylactic of thromboembolic disease in total hip surgery. It reported a detailed review of nearly two thousand patients treated in that manner. Our study confirmed the work of others who have in the past reported on similar good results using the inexpensive drug. The paper indicated a mortality rate of 0.13 percent. This low complication rate compares well with the best rates achieved with other, much more expensive methods of prophylaxis.

The editor rejected our paper upon recommendations from two "independent reviewers." The reviewers objected to the fact that the study was not a randomized, double-blind, perspective- and placebo-controlled study. Those requirements are indeed the rigorous standards by which newly released medications are now typically judged. However, they are not necessary requirements for appropriate retrospective recording of review of actual patients and experience-based outcomes. It made no sense to deny publication on such a basis.

I wrote to the chief editor, stated my objections, and pointed out that no manufacturer has sufficient vested interest to underwrite the massive expense of a randomized, double-blind, perspective- and placebo-controlled study of aspirin. I also sent the paper to another journal, one that is published in England. The second journal rejected my article because they had already published several papers documenting the good results achieved with aspirin.

I was caught in a trans-Atlantic ideological tug-of-war. The U.S. journal would not publish the article because the reviewers felt that my presentation did not document the good results achieved with aspirin in ways that met the journal's standards of proof. The British, meanwhile, claimed that the effectiveness of aspirin had been so well documented that another article on the subject was not needed.

A few months later, I received a telephone call from the chief editor of the U.S. journal telling me that he and his associate editor had given further thought to the rejection of the paper. They wanted to take a fresh look at it. Accordingly, we responded to several earlier editorial criticisms and sent the paper back to them. Several weeks later, they wrote that they were seriously considering publication and asked for some clarifications. We again responded to their requests and again mailed the manuscript. Two weeks later, I received another letter requesting answers to thirty-five additional questions. We responded accordingly.

Throughout my career, I have published more than 170 papers in peer-reviewed journals but never had such a detailed review of any of them. The whole thing gave me frequent headaches. I probably should just have taken two aspirin tablets and called the editor again in the morning. The article was eventually published. It read well, thanks to the hard work of the editors.

Prophylactic medications of thromboembolic disease have become in recent years a big business. Journals advertise in big letters accompanied by attractive drawings the expensive drugs that generate the greatest profit to the manufacturers. The advertisement for one such drug depicts a bomb about to explode, clearly suggesting that in the absence of its administration to surgical patients, death will be inevitable. The cost of the usage of this drug is, according to hospital charges, $100 a day. The cost of aspirin as a prophylactic drug is only a few pennies. Almost without exception, every paper dealing with thromboembolic disease praises the virtues of the expensive drugs and ignores the even better results obtained from the use of cheaper and safer drugs.

The success of marketing these expensive medications has been extraordinary. The manufacturing companies have skillfully recruited a handful of orthopaedists to market the product. They are sent around the world, obviously accompanied by a host of vendors, to lecture at every conceivable medical meeting, society, or medical school. Industry has helped these vendors' departments, and I suspect that they have also received handsome personal financial perks.

For as long as nearly two years, our five-physician office has received free samples of two of the most commonly used nonsteroidal anti-inflammatory analgesics in quantities that in over-the-counter prices could easily represent over $100,000 a year. This bothers me greatly. In our offices we are allowed to see only "paying patients" who are well covered with medical insurance. I do not question that among them there are some who still find it difficult to pay out-of-pocket for the prescribed drugs. Nonetheless, free samples of expensive medications should go to the truly needy.

A physician in the office must acknowledge receipt of the drugs by signing a document prepared by the delivering rep. I refuse to sign such documents, and several times I have said to the industrial representative to donate the free samples to the indigent clinics at the local public hospitals where the poor are cared for. Or if that is not possible, they should suggest to their superiors to ship the samples to countries where poverty and disease are endemic.

What aggravates this situation is the fact that neither of the manufacturers of these medications is letting the lay community know that those drugs may have very undesirable side effects. The medications are marketed to alleviate pain associated with bone, muscle, and joint conditions. Among those conditions are muscle tears and fractures. Though it is true that the medications provide some temporary relief, the fact remains that they interfere with tissue healing. It has been well documented in animal studies that fracture healing is delayed. Why is it that this important information is not passed on to physicians and patients as well? Because making profit is more important than being ethical and professional. By the time the drugs become fully discredited, new ones will be released, which allegedly no longer have any undesirable side effects. And the game goes on.

At our local hospital, a friend and colleague of mine was asked to conduct a research study by the manufacturers of a nonsteroidal analgesic, aimed at finding out if their drug was very effective when administered to "Spanish" patients. "Spanish patient" means anyone who happens to have a Spanish sounding name, be it the first or the last name. My children, who obviously have a Spanish last name, fall in that category. It does not matter that their mother is Anglo-Saxon and they do not speak Spanish.

The research project was brought for possible approval to the appropriate committee of the hospital. I called the project "Mickey Mouse research" and indicated that this type of investigation was not scientific at all, and was structured simply for political reasons. There are many people in Miami who have a Spanish name, and many of them indeed have Spanish or Latin American roots. No one I know has ever suggested that any medication has a different effect on "Spanish" patients.

I felt that we could anticipate the local newspapers, published in Spanish in the local area, reporting a few months later that a "distinguished physician/scientist in Miami had documented that a certain medication was very effective among 'Spanish patients.' I added that I suspected that a similar study was being conducted in neighborhoods heavily populated with African Americans. The local paper will later announce that the drug is very effective when taken by "black people."

In the summer of 1996, a family practitioner asked me to consult about a patient of mine who had spontaneously dislocated a hip prosthesis. I had inserted the prosthesis twenty-five years earlier. I had kept in touch with him since the original operation, and had personally communicated with him every year while I lived in Miami. The man was now ninety years old.

When I visited him in the hospital, I discovered that he was in bad medical condition and appeared to be seriously ill. He was bowel- and bladder-incontinent. During the last two years, he had been treated with laminectomies on his neck and low back to relieve his advanced arthritic pains. Those surgeries had not helped him at all. His balance was extremely poor and he was barely able to take only a couple steps with the aid of a walker while his wife stood by and further supported him. His mind, however, was in good condition.

It appeared that he had dislocated his hip while in bed or trying to get out of it. The hip had been dislocated for quite some time without his being aware of it. It was discovered accidentally, during a radiological examination of his abdomen. The dislocation was causing only mild, decreasing discomfort. His main pain was coming from his low back and neck.

I told his family doctor that I could not recommend aggressive treatment of the dislocated hip because I did not feel that it would be in the best interest of the patient. If left alone, the dislocated joint would become completely free of pain within a short time. The patient could continue to transfer from his bed to a wheelchair, much as he had done during the previous years. I emphasized that in my opinion, heroic measures on an individual his age and in such poor medical condition were difficult to justify.

His physician argued vehemently that it would be inappropriate to leave the hip unreduced. I found myself becoming quite annoyed by his reaction and suggested that he consult with another orthopaedist. I assured him that he could easily find somebody who would agree with him.

As I was in the process of putting my recommendations in writing on the patient's hospital chart, I looked at the treatment he had received since his admission to the unit. I was appalled to find out that he had had a shunt procedure to improve his balance. It had not, of course, done him any good. A gastroenterologist had evaluated his bowel incontinence; an urologist had evaluated his bladder dysfunction; a cardiologist had requested electrocardiograms and echocardiograms. His physician had also consulted a neurologist regarding the condition of his muscles and peripheral nerves. Following electromyography studies, the neurosurgeon who had previously performed surgery on the patient's neck and lower back reevaluated his condition. Finally, a physiatrist had evaluated the patient in anticipation of a transfer to a rehabilitation unit for further care.

Before I gave my report to the requesting physician, I spoke to the patient and his wife. They both knew that his walking days were over and that the most logical and practical solution was for him to accept the need for confinement to a wheelchair. The couple knew that hope for further recovery was unrealistic. They were extremely complimentary about the efforts of their family physician. They said that he was devoted to his patients and anxious to find any possible way to assist in their recovery. He had been their doctor for nearly thirty years.

A local orthopaedic surgeon then saw the man. A few hours later, the orthopaedist performed an open reduction of the dislocated joint and replaced the hip socket with a new one. They told me that the surgery went well. Two days later, the patient returned to surgery. This time, he was suffering with an acute abdominal obstruction. He eventually recovered from the abdominal surgery, but his new hip dislocated again, as I had predicted. The surgeons then applied a heavy and cumbersome brace that made it impossible for the patient to even get out of bed. He remained bedridden for the remainder of his hospitalization. When he used the allotted in-patient Medicare days, he transferred to a rehabilitation center. Mercifully, he died a few months later.

I am disturbed by the cynicism that infects me as I look at my profession in a more mature and objective way. I know that the actions and behavior of the family physician caring for this patient were not appropriate. I also disagree with the way my fellow orthopaedic surgeon subjected him to an unnecessary and useless surgical procedure. No hospital review board would support my view, however. Organized medicine would never criticize the treatment I have described. Instead, it closes its eyes and looks the other way. We can expect nothing more from the new generation of future physicians who are now training at medical schools around the world.

It is painful to admit that similar episodes are repeated throughout the country with increasing frequency. They are no longer occasional. I witness them with regularity even though I am not involved in medical/political issue in an official capacity. Last year I listened to a young orthopaedist lecture at the medical school in Miami. He had volunteered to address the orthopaedic staff. I had never met him before but had heard about his great success performing an operation about the hip, which had not as yet proven to be effective, and which obviously required further study.

The procedure is performed for painful symptoms in the groin, which are not associated with radiological evidence of osteoarthritis. Within the last two years, the young surgeon informed us, he had performed more than one hundred such procedures. I immediately sensed that he was abusing surgery and was performing the procedure in some instances unnecessarily. I said, "Many of your patients will experience within a short time the need to have their hips replaced. Why not then limit the operations only for the appropriate indications?" I had already anticipated his reply. "On the contrary, I am keeping those patients from having a major replacement procedure."

Less than year later, a thirty-three-year-old man came to my office seeking a second opinion regarding a proposed surgery that had already been scheduled for the following week. He informed me that the surgeon, who had given the lecture at the medical school a few months earlier, was going to replace his hip with an artificial one. The surgeon had moved out of the Miami area, but the patient was willing to travel the long distance because he had "great confidence" in the surgeon.

The young man told me he was an avid soccer player, and enjoyed the game a great deal. He played it every chance he had. However, lately the hip had become painful at the end of the game, keeping him from enjoying the game the way he used to. He had visited the surgeon, who, after informing him that he had arthritis in the hip, proceeded to recommend an arthroscopic procedure and repair of the "labrum" normally found in the hip socket.

He had the procedure performed without any improvement. Three months later the surgeon took new X rays and said that the arthritis had increased a great deal to the point that the joint needed to be replaced with an artificial one. He was scheduled for surgery.

Upon examining the patient and questioning him about his perception of his incapacitation and expectations from surgery, it became obvious to me that his pain was minimal. "After a long day of major activity, my hip aches at the end of the day. Some time I take some pills, which get rid of the discomfort." He insisted, however, that he wanted to get rid of all problems and be able to live a "totally" normal life. He was convinced that the surgery would make that possible.

His X rays showed moderately advanced osteoarthritis of a degree that can often be associated with marked pain and disability. Such X rays in an older person would be in all likelihood sufficient to justify the replacement procedure. We know that the elderly do not use and abuse the hip the way younger people do. Their remaining life span is also shorter.

I realized then that my comments during the surgeon's lecture a year earlier had been accurate. The arthroscopic procedure was not indicated, because the disease process at that time contraindicated it. The surgeon was misleading when he told the patient that the arthritis had "gotten a lot worse" since the arthroscopy was performed. The fact is that his type of arthritis never progresses radiologically in a rapid manner. Years must elapse before marked changes can be detected. No one benefited from this episode, only the surgeon, who performed two surgical procedures within a very short time.

On the day that I examined the elderly hip replacement patient with the dislocated hip, I came home early. Barbara was busy discussing a cover for the Jacuzzi we had in the backyard of the house. I spoke to the young man who was doing the work. I don't remember much about our conversation but at some point he said that the only thing that was certain in this life was death. Then he added, "That may not even be the case any longer. Nowadays, they keep you alive forever so they can make money."

He did not know that I was a physician and I did not want to pursue the issue. His statement, nonetheless, made an indelible impression. I have continued thinking about it. Has cynicism spread so far? Do his views represent the views of his generation? Have we already totally lost everyone's respect? Was he right? Has our profession become so corrupt?

I fear that the number of people who see doctors as opportunists is growing rapidly. When I first began my practice, my patients' faces were usually filled with trust in me and confidence in my profession. Today, I see suspicion and distrust. We have sown those seeds ourselves. Now we must reap the whirlwind.

The medical profession at this time feels very strongly that malpractice litigation has reached a crisis level. The problem is without a doubt a major one begging for a solution. Hope for tort reform that will alleviate the malpractice crisis sweeping the country dwindles as our legislative representatives watch the crisis escalate but seem incapable or unwilling to act upon it. The medical profession and the lay community as a whole seem to have concluded that the current situation favors the legal profession, and therefore no change can be anticipated.

The media broadcast in alarming terms the errors committed by physicians and argue for government intervention. Ads from legal firms encourage people to seek their advice following any accident or a less than perfect result from any medical treatment. Suing somebody for any possible reason has become an automatic reaction to many people in contemporary U.S. society. This has resulted in a spectacular growth in the number of litigation attorneys, larger settlements, and an exponential increase in the cost of medical malpractice insurance.

Although the genesis of this festering problem is complicated, I will venture to add my perceptions to the discussion.

Medicine cannot and should not claim to be an innocent bystander in the issue of malpractice litigation or, in fact, the entire health care crisis. Some commit medical malpractice; therefore a control system is necessary. Organized medicine has failed to effectively monitor and prosecute physicians guilty of wrongdoing. This is public knowledge, which has fueled support for the legal profession's intervention.

The technical revolution that our profession experienced in the last few decades has contributed to the problem. Our greater dependency on technology for the diagnosis and treatment of an increasing number of medical conditions has fostered undesirable changes in the relationship between physicians and patients. Oftentimes laypeople outside the doctor's office conduct many tests, and subsequent visits and conversations with the treating professional may not take place again. Some surgeons complete the surgical intervention and do not see their patients again until a few weeks later in his office. Patients are followed in the hospital by an ever-decreasing number of nurses, who in turn are instructed to transfer them to a Skilled Nursing Unit or a Rehabilitation Center. These scenarios compromise a healthy relationship between patient and doctor. Therefore a less than perfect result, or even a result that does not meet the patient's expectations, serves as an excuse to seek legal advice. Subsequent litigation becomes a matter totally in the hands of the attorney, who by then is perceived as the "true friend" of the unhappy patient.

epilogue

My professional life spanned one of the richest periods in the history of medicine. I witnessed a technological and scientific revolution of unprecedented dimensions. I entered my residency training the same year that Jonas Salk discovered a vaccine against poliomyelitis and sophisticated internal fixation of fractures became a practical procedure. Within a few years, we had learned to replace arthritic joints and correct spinal deformities. The invention of the arthroscope, the sophisticated imaging technology of the CAT scan and the MRI followed in short order.

My patients and I profited from all of those developments. I was also fortunate enough to make my own small contributions in the advancement of knowledge and technology in the areas of total hip surgery, fracture healing, and fracture care.

I had the opportunity to practice medicine at the height of its glory. The profession might never again be the same. I doubt that the world will ever again see a profession where so many practitioners subordinate their interests to the interests of those they serve. Never again will we see an entire profession exhibit genuine altruism; lofty ideals; and powerful, positive values.

Tragically, my generation chose to ignore the warnings of a collapsing system. Organized medicine and academic medicine have chosen to abandon their cultural responsibilities and ceased to maintain their leadership roles. Since no one in medicine stepped forward to accept that vacated responsibility, industry and insurance companies have filled the void. The staff of Aesculapius has fallen. The false values of business and commerce have taken its place.

Regardless of my level of success in each of my ventures, I have a clear conscience. I did my best to be an honest physician and to lead by example. I focused on the big issues. I knew that others could concentrate on the details.

I am by nature a lonely person who relishes solitude. For much of my life, I had but few opportunities to indulge that need. My eight months in Scotland brought a wonderful opportunity to assuage my hunger for lonely isolation. Now I have learned to create the necessary time and space. On weekends, I take long walks through the quiet streets of our neighborhood. I take a tape player with me, and listen to the recorded works of great philosophers and the other builders of civilizations When I read at home, I now find that I need to have music playing in the background. Usually I listen to classical music, but I am also finding pleasure in the popular music of my younger years, especially the music of my native Colombia.

Through my entire career my family has always been the needle in the compass of my life, though it is only recently that I have recognized its true value. Without my family, my life would have been empty. My triumphs and the accolades I received would have been meaningless. As I have grown older, I have gained increasing awareness of the importance of family. I now understand and appreciate the importance of family in European and Latin American cultures. The triumphs and problems of my children assume proportions greater than I ever dreamed in my younger days. I long for their companionship. I look forward to their presence with the anticipation of a young lover. Even the sound of their voices over the telephone brings great pleasure.

I often have wondered what would have happened if I had been less selfish with my time and devoted more of it to my family. I remain ambivalent; I don't really have an answer. Nietzsche once said that parents learn more from their children than children learn from their parents. If this is true, maybe I simply deprived myself of their teachings.

On one occasion, during one of those days when I was feeling guilty on account of my long absences from home, I took my children to the backyard of the house and tried to teach Gregory, our youngest son, how to hit a baseball. My daughter, who at that time was probably no more than eleven years old and was watching the scene, said to me, "Dad, let me teach Greg how to do it right. This is not what you like to do. It looks phony when you pretend to enjoy throwing balls."

In retrospect, there was a hidden message in her remarks: My contribution to their welfare and education rested in a different arena. Whatever love and attention I was giving them was enough as far as they were concerned. There was no need for me to change my ways. Nonetheless, I still wonder: What if?

I have stubbornly questioned many traditions in medicine and successfully challenged some of them. Several times, my criticism proved to be wrong. That does not bother me. I sought the truth, and in doing so I played the role of the gadfly and irritated many. If I pursued projects and ideals with more passion than tact, I have no apologies. I remain more certain than ever that professional medicine must rediscover its core values, its mission, and its ideals. It must restore its focus on patient welfare. It must find a way to throw down the symbol of Hermes and once again raise the staff of Aesculapius. Medicine is a gravely ill profession. It must cure itself. I will continue to fight the excesses of the Medical Industrial Complex as long as I am able to write and speak.

My thoughts never stray far from the trials and tribulations of orthopaedics and health care. Over the years, I have devoted many words and hours to issues related to the future of medicine, particularly to my own specialty, orthopaedic surgery. I have viewed my profession from many different perspectives. Regrettably, I see mainly serious problems ahead for years, possibly decades to come.

At times, I am confused, however, about the true meaning of my perceptions. Are these really problems that I see, or are they merely changes? Are they the products of our mistakes or just the latest manifestations of professional evolution? Should I attend the pronouncement of the French social philosopher Jean-Jacques Rousseau, that "material progress has always lead to decadence" or that of Reinhold Neibuhr's remark "In every civilization, its most impressive period seems to precede death by only a moment. Like the woods of autumn, life defies death in a glorious pageantry of colors"?

Deprived of his illusions and forced to accept reality in all its ugliness, Don Quixote embraces death. In his name and memory, I prefer to remain defiant.